CARCINOMA OF THE CERVIX

DEVELOPMENTS IN OBSTETRICS AND GYNECOLOGY

VOLUME 6

1. J.E. Jirásek, Human fetal endocrines, 1980. ISBN 90-247-2325-6.
2. P.M. Motta, E.S.E. Hafez, eds., Biology of the ovary, 1980. ISBN 90-247-2316-7.
3. J. Horský, J. Presl, eds., Ovarian function and its disorders, 1980. ISBN 90-247-2326-4.
4. D.W. Richardson, D. Joyce, E.M. Symonds, eds., Frozen Human Semen, 1980. ISBN 90-247-2370-1.
5. E.S.E. Hafez, W.A. van Os, eds., Medicated Intrauterine Devices. 1980. ISBN 90-247-2371-X.

Series ISBN 90-247-2334-5

CARCINOMA OF THE CERVIX

BIOLOGY AND DIAGNOSIS

edited by

E.S.E. HAFEZ *and* J.P. SMITH

School of Medicine, Wayne State University, Detroit, Michigan, U.S.A.

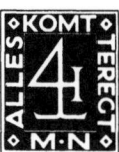

1982

MARTINUS NIJHOFF PUBLISHERS

THE HAGUE/BOSTON/LONDON

Distributors:

for the United States and Canada

Kluwer Boston, Inc.
190 Old Derby Street
Hingham, MA 02043
USA

For all other countries

Kluwer Academic Publishers Group
Distribution Center
P.O. Box 322
3300 AH Dordrecht
The Netherlands

Library of Congress Cataloging in Publication Data   CIP

Main entry under title:

Carcinoma of the cervix.

    (Developments in obstetrics and gynecology,
ISBN-13: 978-94-009-7487-6
    Includes index.
    1. Cervix uteri--Cancer--Congresses. 2. Cervix
uteri--Cancer--Diagnosis--Congresses. I. Hafez,
E. S. E. II. Smith, Julian P. III. Series.
[DNLM: 1. Cervix neoplasms--Congresses. W1
DE998M v. 6 / WP 480 C265 1980]
RC280.U8C374   616.99'4   81-22436
ISBN-13: 978-94-009-7487-6   AACR2

ISBN-13: 978-94-009-7487-6   e-ISBN-13: 978-94-009-7485-2
DOI: 10.1007/978-94-009-7485-2

TABLE OF CONTENTS

III. ETIOLOGY

IV. DIAGNOSIS AND PROGNOSIS

PREFACE

Various scientific evaluations taken from these chapters were presented during the international symposium, 'Carcinoma of the Cervix,' which was held from September 4–7, 1980 in Kiawah Island, Charleston, South Carolina, U.S.A. An international selection of research investigators have contributed reviews designed to be informative to medical, graduate and post-graduate students, as well as clinicians, oncologists and investigators working in the area of female carcinoma.

An attempt has been made to provide a total coverage of current progress in carcinoma of the cervix. In particular, the following major areas are included: Epidemiology, Histology & Histochemistry, Ultra-structure, Physiology & Biochemistry, Genetics & Cytogenetics, Immunology, Diagnosis, and Patho-physiology & Complications. Major changes have occurred in incidence and mortality rates for carcinoma of the cervix in the past decade. Mass screening programs and their ability to detect earlier stage diseases have attributed to a reduction in invasive diseases. Most cervical cancers could be prevented by an extension of cytologic screening programs in high risk areas. Greater resources must be provided to reach high risk areas in order to prevent the occurrence of cervical cancer.

Outreach clinics, for example, have been established to screen hard-to-reach women. These clinics are mobile units which specifically screen high risk neighborhoods. Epidemiologic studies have shown an association between cervical cancer and low income, limited education, and Black and Hispanic populations. In developed countries, with an affluent, better educated, white population, Papanicolaou (Pap) smears are better accepted and used as a screening procedure. A further reduction of morbidity and mortality from invasive carcinoma of the cervix is most likely to be achieved by developing strategies to screen women of 50 years and older and by incorporating routine screening for women under 50 years into examinations that are less dependent upon mode of contraception.

It is hoped that this volume will serve as a stimulus to research scientists, clinicians and oncologists concerned with female carcinoma in order to intensify their research in conquering the existence of carcinoma of the cervix.

April 1982

E.S.E. HAFEZ
Detroit, Michigan
U.S.A.

CONTRIBUTORS

ALLEN, J.M.: Birmingham Maternity Hospital, Queen Elizabeth Medical Centre, Edgbaston, Birmingham, B15 2TG United Kingdom.

AMIRIKIA, H.: Department of Gynecology and Obstetrics, Wayne State University School of Medicine, Detroit, MI 48201, U.S.A.

BALTZER, J.: I. Frauenklinik der Universität München, Maistrasse 11, D-8000 München 2, F.R. Germany.

BARBER, H.R.K.: Department of Obstetrics and Gynecology, Lenox Hill Hospital and New York Medical College, 100 East 77 Street, New York, NY 10021, U.S.A.

BELLE, S.H.: Medical Division, Department of Social Oncology, Michigan Cancer Foundation, Detroit, MI 48201, U.S.A.

BRENES, M.M.: Gorgas Memorial Laboratory, Apartado 6991, Panamá 5, República de Panamá.

BRENNAN, M.J.: Medical Division, Department of Social Oncology, Michigan Cancer Foundation, 110 E. Warren Avenue, Detroit, MI 48201, U.S.A.

DE BRITTON, R.C.: Instituto Oncológico Nacional, Apartado 6-108, El Dorado-Panamá, República de Panamá.

CABRAL, G.A.: Department of Microbiology, Medical College of Virginia/VCU, MCV Station, Richmond, VA 23298, U.S.A.

CASTELLANO, C.J.: Departments of Gynecology and Pathology, Instituto Nacional Enfermedades Neoplásicas, Av. Alfonso Ugarte 825, Lima 1, Peru.

CAVANAGH, D.: Division of Gynecologic Oncology, Department of Obstetrics and Gynecology, University of South Florida, 12901 North 30th Street, Tampa, FL 33612, U.S.A.

CHRISTOPHERSON, W.M.: Department of Pathology, University of Louisville, Health Sciences Center, Louisville, KY 40292, U.S.A.

CLARK, BARBARA A.: Department of Obstetrics and Gynecology, University of Minnesota Medical School, 420 Delaware Street S.E., Box 395 Mayo Memorial Building, Minneapolis, MN 55455, U.S.A.

CONROY, L.: Departments of Gynecology and Pathology, Instituto Nacional Enfermedades Neoplásicas, Av. Alfonso Ugarte 825, Lima 1, Peru.

COPPLESON, M.: King George V Memorial Hospital, Sydney, Australia.

DABANCENS, A.: Service of Cytopathology and Control of Cancer, University of Chile, Casilla 6606, Correo 4 – Santiago, Chile.

DAVINA, J.H.M.: Department of Submicroscopic Morphology, Catholic University of Nijmegen, Geert Grooteplein Zuid 24, 6500 NB Nijmegen, The Netherlands.

DÍAZ-BAZÁN, N.: Department of Surgery 'Hospital Rosales', National Medical Center, Oncology School of Medicine, University of El Salvador, San Salvador, El Salvador, C.A.

DINGES, H.P.: Pathologisches Institut, A.ö. Landeskrankenhaus, A-7400 Oberwart, Austria.

DINI, M.M.: Division of Gynecologic Oncology, Department of Obstetrics/Gynecology, Cook County Hospital, 1835 W. Harrison Street, Chicago, IL 60612, U.S.A.

FAIFERMAN, I.: Department of Pathology, University of Illinois, Chicago, IL 60612, U.S.A.

FRENCH, P.W.: Queen Elizabeth II Research Institute, The University of Sydney, Sydney, 2006 Australia.

FRY, D.: Department of Microbiology, Medical College of Virginia/VCU, MCV Station, Richmond, VA 23298, U.S.A.

GOPLERUD, D.: Department of Obstetrics/Gynecology, Medical College of Virginia/VCU, MCV Station, Richmond, VA 23298, U.S.A.

GORE, HAZEL: Division of Gynecologic Oncology, Department of Obstetrics/Gynecology, The University of Alabama in Birmingham, University Station, Birmingham, AL 35294, U.S.A.

GROSSBART, ANN: Medical Division, Department of Social Oncology, Michigan Cancer Foundation, 110 E. Warren Avenue, Detroit, MI 48201, U.S.A.

HAAN, R.W. DE: Division of Gynecological Oncology, Department of Obstetrics and Gynecology, Catholic University of Nijmegen, Geert Grooteplein Zuid 14, 6500 HB Nijmegen, The Netherlands.

HAFEZ, E.S.E.: Department of Gynecology and Obstetrics, Wayne State University School of Medicine, Detroit, MI 48201, U.S.A.

HALL, D.: Department of Obstetrics/Gynecology, Medical College of Virginia/VCU, MCV Station, Richmond, VA 23298, U.S.A.

HALL, J. ST. E.: Department of Obstetrics and Gynecology, University of the West Indies, Mona, Kingston 7, Jamaica.

HASSAN, S.: Department of Pathology, Al-Sabah Hospital, P.O. Box 4078, Kuwait, Arabia.

HATCH, K.D.: Division of Gynecologic Oncology, Department of Obstetrics/Gynecology, The University of Alabama in Birmingham, University Station, Birmingham, AL 35294, U.S.A.

HATHOUT, H.: Department of Obstetrics and Gynecology, Faculty of Medicine, Kuwait University, P.O. Box 24923, Kuwait, Arabia.

HAYASHI, S.: Department of Obstetrics and Gynecology, School of Medicine, Keio University, Tokyo, Japan.

HERMANNS, U.: Städtische Frauenklinik, Osnabrück, West Germany.

ISHIWATA, I.: Department of Obstetrics and Gynecology, School of Medicine, Keio University, Tokyo, Japan.

IZUMI, S.: Department of Obstetrics and Gynecology, School of Medicine, Keio University, Tokyo, Japan.

JOPLIN, C.F.B.: Gorgas Memorial Laboratory, Apartado 6991, Panamá 5, República de Panamá.

JORDAN, J.A.: Birmingham Maternity Hospital, Queen Elizabeth Medical Centre, Edgbaston, Birmingham, B15 2TG United Kingdom.

KENEMANS, P.: Division of Gynecological Oncology, Department of Obstetrics and Gynecology, Catholic University of Nijmegen, Geert Grooteplein Zuid 14, 6500 HB Nijmegen, The Netherlands.

KOMOROWSKI, R.A.: Department of Pathology, The Medical College of Wisconsin, Milwaukee County Medical Complex, 8700 West Wisconsin Avenue, Milwaukee, WI 53226, U.S.A.

KORHONEN, M.: Department of Obstetrics and Gynecology, University of Helsinki, Helsinki, Finland (currently at Departments of Obstetrics and Gynecology, and Pathology, Baylor College of Medicine, Houston, TX 77030, U.S.A.).

KURIHARA, S.: Department of Obstetrics and Gynecology, School of Medicine, Keio University, Tokyo, Japan.

LABI, L.: Department of Gynecology/Obstetrics, Padua University School of Medicine, Via Giustiniani 3, 35100 Padua, Italy.

LINDGREN, J.: Department of Bacteriology and Immunology, University of Helsinki, Helsinki, Finland.

LOHE, K.J.: I. Frauenklinik der Universität München, Maistrasse 11, D-8000 München 2, West Germany.

MARCIANO-CABRAL, F.: Department of Microbiology, Medical College of Virginia/VCU, MCV Station, Richmond, VA 23298, U.S.A.

MOTAWY, S.: Department of Radiotherapy, Al-Sabah Hospital, P.O. Box 4078, Kuwait, Arabia.

NOZAWA, S.: Department of Obstetrics and Gynecology, School of Medicine, Keio University, Tokyo, Japan.

OKAGAKI, T.: Department of Obstetrics and Gynecology and of Laboratory Medicine and Pathology, University of Minnesota, Medical School, 420 Delaware Street S.E., Box 395 Mayo Memorial Building, Minneapolis, MN 55455, U.S.A.

OKUMURA, H.: Laboratory of Cell Biology, National Institute of Health, Tokyo, Japan.

ONNIS, A.: Department of Gynecology/Obstetrics, Padua University School of Medicine, Via Giustiniani 3, 35100 Padua, Italy.

OOTA, H.: Department of Obstetrics and Gynecology, School of Medicine, Keio University, Tokyo, Japan.

PRAPHAT, H.: Division of Gynecologic Oncology, Department of Obstetrics and Gynecology, University of South Florida, 1290 North 30th Street, Tampa, FL 33612, U.S.A.

RAMIREZ, G.: Departments of Gynecology and Pathology, Instituto Nacional Enfermedades Neoplásicas, Av. Alfonso Ugarte 825 Lima 1, Peru.

REEVES, W.C.: Gorgas Memorial Laboratory, Apartado 6991, Panamá 5, República de Panamá,

REID, B.L.: Queen Elizabeth II Research Institute for Mothers and Infants, The University of Sydney, Sydney, 2006 Australia.

ROMOFF, A.: Lenox Hill Hospital, 100 East 77 Street, NY 10021, U.S.A.

RUFFOLO, E.: Division of Gynecologic Oncology, Department of Obstetrics and Gynecology, University of South Florida, 12901 North 30th Street, Tampa, FL 33612, U.S.A.

SCHMIDT, W.A.: Department of Pathology and Laboratory Medicine and Obstetrics and Gynecology, University of Texas Health Science Center, Houston, TX 77030, U.S.A.

SCHRODT, G.R.: Department of Pathology, University of Louisville, Health Sciences Center, Louisville, KY 40292, U.S.A.

SEPPALA, M.: Department of Obstetrics and Gynecology, University of Helsinki, Helsinki, Finland.

SESKI, J.C.: Department of Gynecology, M.D. Anderson Hospital and Tumor Institute, Houston, TX 77030, U.S.A.

SHEPHERD, J.H.: Division of Gynecologic Oncology, Department of Obstetrics and Gynecology, University of South Florida, 12901 North 30th Street, Tampa, FL 33612, U.S.A.

SHINGLETON, H.M.: Division of Gynecologic Oncology, Department of Obstetrics/Gynecology, The University of Alabama in Birmingham, University Station, Birmingham, AL 35294, U.S.A.

SINGER, A.: Department of Obstetrics/Gynecology, University of Sheffield, Sheffield, S37RE United Kingdom.

SOMMERS S.: Lenox Hill Hospital, 100 East 77 Street, New York, NY 10021, U.S.A.

SPORNITZ, U.M.: Anatomisches Institut der Universität Basel, CH-4056 Basel, Switzerland.

STADHOUDERS, A.M.: Department of Submicroscopic Morphology, Catholic University of Nijmegen, Geert Grooteplein Zuid 24, 6500 HB Nijmegen, The Netherlands.

SWANSON, G. MARIE: Medical Division, Department of Social Oncology, Michigan Cancer Foundation, 110 E. Warren Avenue, Detroit, MI 48201, U.S.A.

TOMLIN, H.: Department of Obstetrics/Gynecology, Medical College of Virginia/VCU, MCV Station, Richmond, VA 23298, U.S.A.

TSUKAZAKI, K.: Department of Obstetrics and Gynecology, School of Medicine, Keio University, Tokyo, Japan.

TSUTSUI, F.: Department of Obstetrics and Gynecology, School of Medicine, Keio University, Tokyo, Japan.

TWIGGS, L.B.: Department of Obstetrics and Gynecology, University of Minnesota Medical School, 420 Delaware Street S.E., Box 395 Mayo Memorial Building, Minneapolis, MN 55455, U.S.A.

UDAGAWA, Y.: Department of Obstetrics and Gynecology, School of Medicine, Keio University, Tokyo, Japan.

VALDÉS, P.F.: Instituto Oncológico Nacional; Apartado 6–108; El Dorado-Panamá, República de Panamá.

VALENTE, S.: Department of Gynecology/Obstetrics, Padua University School of Medicine, Via Giustiniani 3, 35100 Padua, Italy.

VOOYS, G.P.: Department of Pathology, Catholic University of Nijmegen, Geert Grooteplein Zuid 24, 6500 HB Nijmegen, The Netherlands.

WAHLSTROM, T.: Department of Pathology, University of Helsinki, Helsinki, Finland.

WILKINSON, E.J.: Department of Pathology, The Medical College of Wisconsin, Milwaukee County Medical Complex, 8700 West Wisconsin Avenue, Milwaukee, WI 53226, U.S.A.

WILTERS, J.H.: Division of Gynecologic Oncology, Department of Obstetrics/Gynecology, The University of Alabama in Birmingham, University Station, Birmingham, AL 35294, U.S.A.

YOUNG, J.L., JR.: Biometry Branch, National Cancer Institute, Landow Building, 7910 Woodmont Avenue, Bethesda, MD 20205, U.S.A.

ZANDEN, P.H.T. VAN DER: Division of Gynecological Oncology, Department of Obstetrics and Gynecology, Catholic University of Nijmegen, Geert Grooteplein Zuid 14, 6500 HB Nijmegen, The Netherlands.

ZANDER, J.: I. Frauenklinik der Universität München, Maistrasse 11, D-8000 München 2, West Germany.

ZEITLHOFER, J.: Department of Pathology, Kaiser-Franz-Jozef-Spital, Kundratstrasse 3, A-1100 Vienna, Austria.

ACKNOWLEDGEMENTS

Basic research, clinical trials, preparations of manuscripts, editorial assistance and presentation of results related to this volume have been generously supported by the following institutions and organizations:

Department of Gynecology/Obstetrics, Wayne State University, Detroit, Michigan, U.S.A.

Hutzel Hospital, Detroit Medical Center, Detroit, Michigan, U.S.A.

Department of Obstetrics/Gynecology, Medical University of South Carolina, Charleston, South Carolina, U.S.A.

Pan American Health Organization, New York, New York, U.S.A.

Wayne State University School of Medicine, Detroit, Michigan, U.S.A.

Thanks and appreciation are due to the contributors who meticulously prepared their chapters; to Ms. Jane Wittersheim for editorial skills and assistance; to Ms. Jackie Mucci for editorial help; and to Ms. Jackie Smieska for her excellent secretarial assistance. Thanks are also due to Mr. Jeffrey K. Smith of Martinus Nijhoff Publishers for his fine cooperation during the publication of this volume.

April 1982

E.S.E. HAFEZ
Detroit, U.S.A.

I. EPIDEMIOLOGY

1. U.S. TRENDS IN CARCINOMA OF THE CERVIX: INCIDENCE, MORTALITY AND SURVIVAL

G. Marie Swanson, S.H. Belle and J.L. Young, Jr.

I. USES OF INCIDENCE AND MORTALITY DATA

Trends in cervical cancer in the United States are best expressed by incidence rates. Cancer incidence rates are defined as the annual rate of newly diagnosed cases within a specific population and are usually expressed as the number of cases per 100,000 persons in the population. In general, incidence data are considered the most useful type of descriptive measure because they reflect the probability of the development of a disease within a population and its sub-groups (Lillienfeld 1967). For carcinoma of the cervix in the United States, one can understand trends only through incidence data, since more than 75% of all cases are diagnosed as *in situ* disease.

Mortality data are frequently utilized to describe disease trends, but they are useful only when they accurately reflect the true frequency of a disease within a population (Lillienfeld 1980). Use of mortality rates to attempt to understand the frequency of cervical cancer in the United States female population today would result in an underestimate by more than 75%.

Until 1970, the most widely utilized descriptions of U.S. trends in carcinoma of the cervix were based on mortality data. In addition to the problem inherent in using mortality rates to describe cervical cancer, death certificates did not specify cervical cancers as distinct from uterine cancer until 1940. Analysis of 1966 death certificates revealed that 30% of all deaths from cancer of the uterus were described as cancer of other and unspecified parts of the uterus (Kessler and Aurelian 1975).

II. HISTORICAL DATA FOR THE UNITED STATES

Incidence data for the United States were available for the first time in 1937, but did not distinguish between cancers of the cervix uteri and corpus uteri (Dorn 1944). They did, however, recognize for the first time higher occurrence among black females than among white females, with incidence rates (based on the 1950 U.S. standard population[1]) for uterine cancer of 109 for black females and 60 for white females. At that time it was thought that excess frequency among black females was partially explained by lack of proper medical care during childbirth, since a smaller proportion of black women than white had deliveries in hospitals (Dorn 1944).

Cervical cancer incidence rates for the United States were presented for the first time in 1947 and were for invasive cervical cancer only. Again, based upon the 1950 U.S. standard population, the incidence rate for white females was 35 and for non-white females was 61. These rates must be utilized with caution, since, in 1947, the importance of distinguishing between cervical and endometrial cancer was not adequately recognized when recording diagnoses, with the primary site frequently specified merely as uterus (Dorn and Cutler 1959).

In 1969–1971, incidence rates for invasive cervical cancer based on the 1950 standard population were 15 for white females and 34 for black females. At the same time, endometrial cancer rates were higher among whites (20) than among blacks (11). The proportion of *in situ* cervical cancer was 69%, with 31% invasive cases for 1969–1971 (Cutler and Young 1975). One must compare these rates with the 1947 rates with caution because of the likelihood of inadequate specification of cervix as the primary site in the 1947 data and because the survey

Hafez, E.S.E., Smith, J.P. (eds.), Carcinoma of the Cervix: Biology and Diagnosis. ISBN-13: 978-94-009-7487-6
© 1982, Martinus Nijhoff Publishers, The Hague/Boston/London.

2

populations are not totally comparable due to the inclusion of three different cities in the 1969–1971 survey.

The relative frequency of invasive cervical cancer compared with other cancers among the U.S. female population has declined over the thirty years from 1947 to 1977. For white females, invasive cervical cancer was the second most frequently occurring tumor in 1927, fourth in 1969–1971 and sixth in 1973–1977. Among black females, there was a smaller decline, with invasive cervical cancer progressing from the most common malignant tumor in 1947 to second in 1969–1971 and third in 1973–1977. For both black and white women cancers of the lung and bronchus and colon are now beginning to occur at rates similar to those of the female genital system.

Incidence, mortality and survival data for the United States since 1973 are provided through the National Cancer Institute Surveillance, Epidemiology, and End Results program, known as SEER. SEER includes eleven population-based cancer registries located throughout the United States and representing a 10% sample of the U.S. population. In addition to the registry for metropolitan Detroit, SEER includes the San Francisco-Oakland metropolitan area; the states of Connecticut, Hawaii, Iowa, New Mexico, and Utah; Metropolitan New Orleans, the Seattle-Puget Sound area, Metropolitan Atlanta, and Puerto Rico (Young et al. 1978). The SEER program is designed to supersede the national incidence surveys as well as the End Results Program, which described survival trends, in order to achieve the objective of producing comparable time trends for malignant neoplasia in the United States (Young et al. 1978).

III. INCIDENCE TRENDS

Incidence of *in situ* cervical cancer, in all SEER areas combined, declined for black females in 1977 compared with 1973, and increased slightly among white females. Black women experienced a 16% decrease in *in situ* carcinoma of the cervix over the five year period, while white women experienced a 7% increase (Figure 1a). With rates (1973–1977) of 32 for white females and 60 for black females,

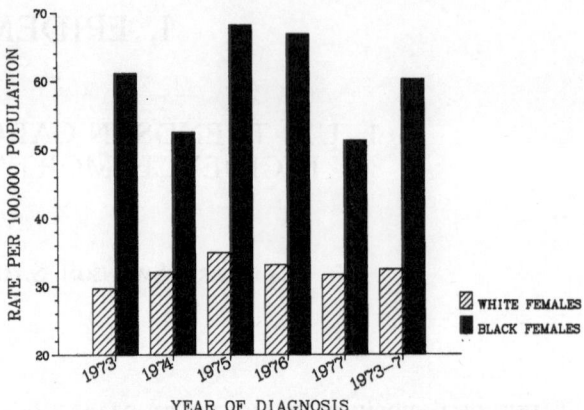

Figure 1a. Age adjusted incidence rates, 1973–1977; *in situ* cervical cancer – all SEER areas.

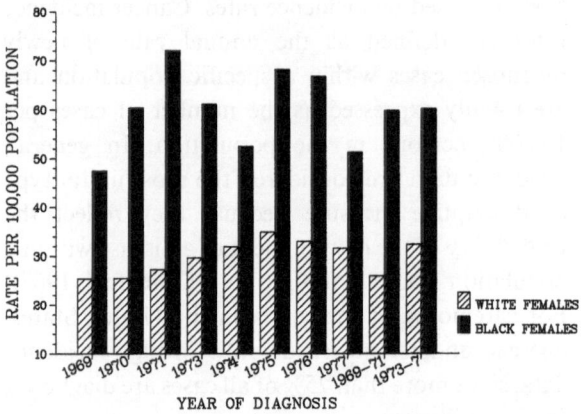

Figure 1b. Age adjusted incidence rates, 1969–1977; *in situ* cervical cancer – Detroit.

blacks have nearly twice the incidence of *in situ* carcinoma of the cervix. For the combined years 1973–1977, *in situ* carcinoma of the cervix was the second most frequent cancer occurring among women of both races, surpassed only by breast cancer.

From Detroit data, annual comparisons for the 1969 through 1977 period reveal an increase in *in situ* carcinoma of the cervix for the nine year period (Figure 1b). The rates increased by 12% among white females (25 in 1969 to 28 in 1977) and 21% among black females (47 in 1969 to 57 in 1977).

Invasive cervical cancer for all SEER areas combined occurred among black women at greater than twice the incidence rates for white women, with age-adjusted rates of 26 for blacks and 11 for whites for 1973–1977. During the five year time period of 1973 through 1977, rates of invasive carcinoma of the cervix declined 25% among whites and 27% among blacks (Figure 2a). As presented in Figure 2a, white women experienced annual decreases, ranging from 10% between 1976 and 1977 to 1% between 1975 and 1976. Black women had their largest decrease between 1973 and 1974 – 22% – and did not drop below 1974 rates again until 1977. Invasive cervical cancer had the eighth highest incidence rate among white females in all SEER areas combined for 1973–1977, surpassed by breast (86), *in situ* cervical (32), colon (31), uterine corpus (30), lung (22), ovary (14), and rectal (11) cancers. Among all SEER area black females, invasive carcinoma of the cervix had the fourth highest incidence rates, surpassed by breast (72), *in situ* cervical (60) and colon (31) cancers.

Detroit data for 1969 through 1977 reveal a slow, but continuous annual decrease in invasive disease among white women and an increase among black

women from 1969 to 1971, followed by a decrease through 1974, an increase in 1975, with further decreases occurring in both 1976 and 1977 (Figure 2b). The total decline among white females was 44% in 1977 (9) compared with 1969 (16), with 70% of this decrease accounted for by the more rapid decline from 1973 (13) through 1977 (9). Among black females, the decrease in incidence of invasive cervical cancer from 1969 (33) to 1977 (22) was 33%.

Age-specific incidence rates for *in situ* cervical cancer for all SEER areas combined, 1973–1977, indicate that it is a disease of younger women (Figure 3a). For both black and white women, the highest incidence rates occur among those in the age groups between 25 and 34, with sharp declines occurring in most age groups over 35. Substantial incidence rates for *in situ* carcinoma of the cervix begin with the 20–24 age group (46 for white females and 116 for black females, 1973–1977). In the 25–29 group, these rates increase to 116 and 203 for whites and blacks, respectively. *In situ* rates drop rapidly after 45, declining to 35 among white women and 55 among black women aged 45–49 (Figure 3a).

The age distribution for women diagnosed with invasive carcinoma of the cervix is quite different from that for *in situ* disease. There are continuing increases in incidence rates among women from all SEER areas combined for 1973–1977 as age at diagnosis increases, with rates at age 50 rising to over 20 per 100,000 for white females and to over 50 per 100,000 among black females (Figures 3b). Specifically, white females have rates of 21 among

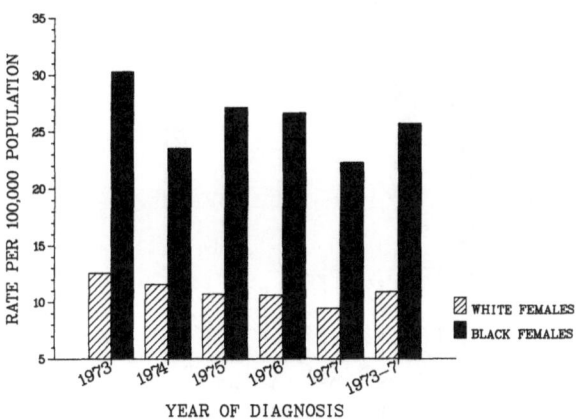

Figure 2a. Age adjusted incidence rates, 1973–1977; invasive cervical cancer – all SEER areas.

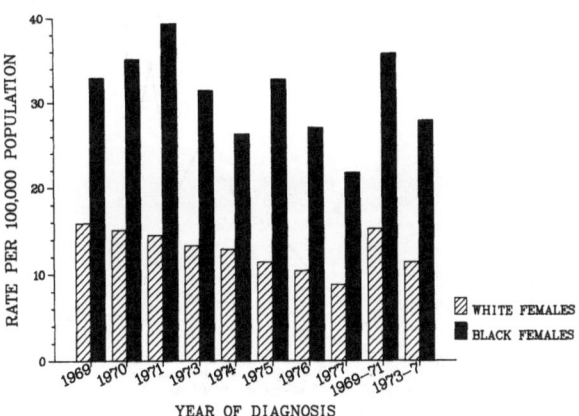

Figure 2b. Age adjusted incidence rates, 1969–1977; invasive cervical cancer – Detroit.

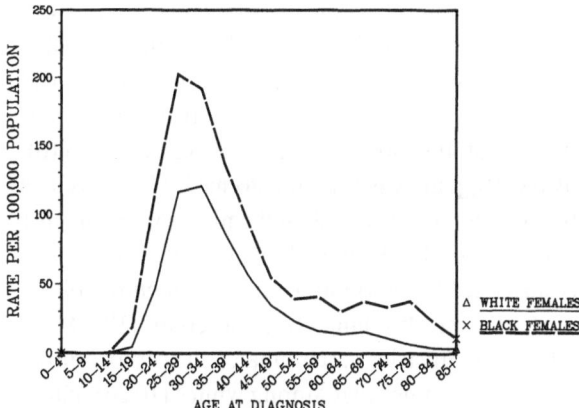

Figure 3a. Age-specific incidence rates, 1973–1977; *in situ* cervical cancer – all SEER areas.

4

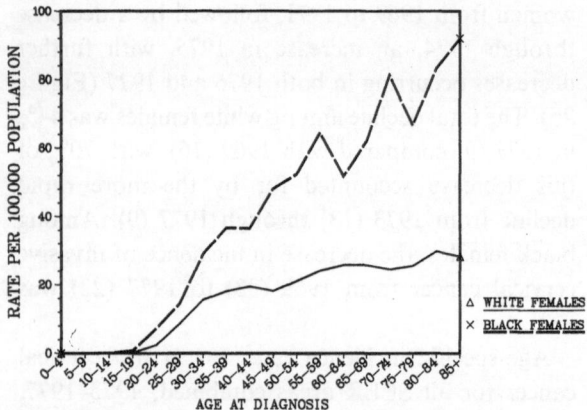

Figure 3b. Age-specific incidence rates, 1973–1977; invasive cervical cancer – all SEER areas.

women 50–54, 26 among those 65–69 and 28 in women over 80. Black females experience rates of 52 among those 50–54, 62 among women 65–69, and 92 in women over 80 (Figure 3b).

IV. MORTALITY TRENDS

The decline in incidence of invasive carcinoma of the cervix has been accompanied by a decline in mortality from this disease. Reductions in mortality from malignant neoplasia of the cervix have occurred in both black and white females in all SEER areas combined between 1973 and 1977 – 23% and 25% respectively (dropping to 10 in 1977 from 13 in 1973 for blacks and to 3 in 1977 from 4 in 1973 for whites, Figure 4a). Mortality from this disease is low, with all SEER areas having had mortality rates for 1973–1977 of 3 for white females and 10 for black females. Compared with mortality from cancer of other sites among women, these rates are ninth highest for white females and fourth for black females. For whites, deaths from invasive cervical cancer are surpassed by deaths from malignant tumors of the breast (28), colon (17), lung (16), ovary (9), pancreas (7), and stomach (4), as well as by lymphomas (5) and leukemias (5); while for blacks, mortality from malignant cervical neoplasia is surpassed by mortality from malignant neoplasia of the breast (28), lung (18), and colon (17). Mortality from invasive carcinoma of the cervix among blacks is 3.0 times that among whites (10 compared with 3).

Age-specific mortality from invasive cervical can-

cer displays a pattern quite similar to incidence of invasive carcinoma of the cervix. The highest mortality rates occur about ten years later than was observed for incidence, beginning at age 60 (Figure 4b). For white females, mortality rates are 12 among women 60–64, 12 among those 70–74, and 20 in women 80 and older. For black women, mortality rates are 31 in women 60–64, 34 among women 75–79, and 37 among those 80 and older (Figure 4b).

V. SURVIVAL TRENDS

In Detroit, five-year relative survival for women diagnosed with invasive carcinoma of the cervix between 1973 and 1977 ranges from 54% among black women to 59% among white women (Figure 5a). For localized disease (Figure 5b), white females

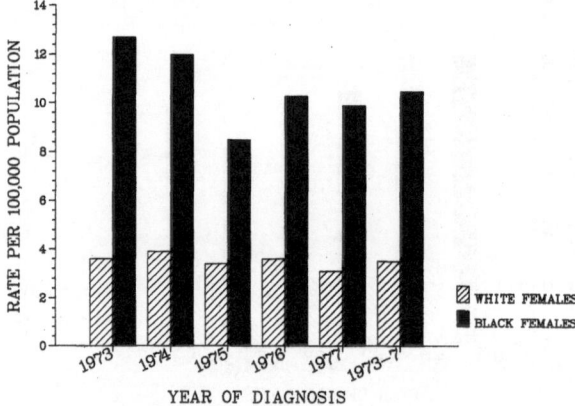

Figure 4a. Age adjusted mortality rates, 1973–1977; invasive cervical cancer – all SEER areas.

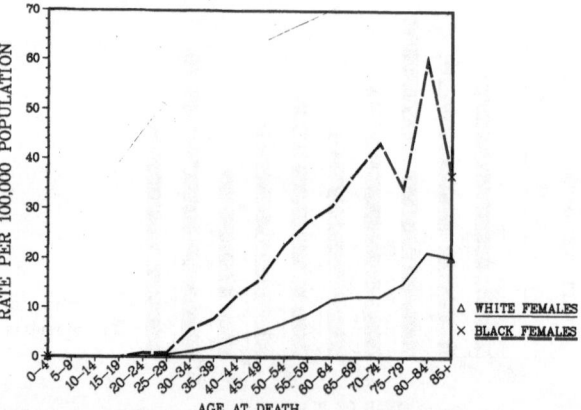

Figure 4b. Age-specific mortality rates, 1973–1977; invasive cervical cancer – all SEER areas.

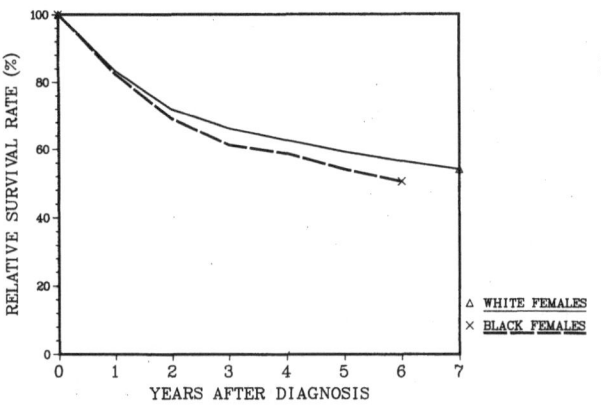

Figure 5a. Relative survival rates for patients diagnosed 1973–1977; invasive cervical cancer – Detroit.

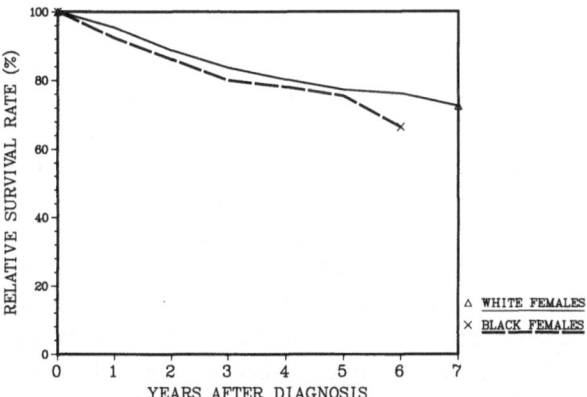

Figure 5b. Relative survival rates for patients diagnosed 1973–1977; localized cervical cancer – Detroit.

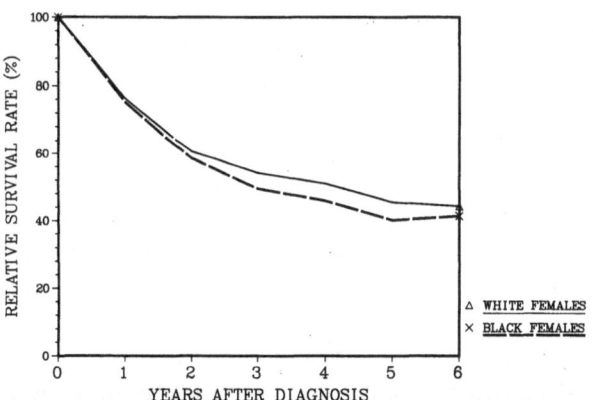

Figure 5c. Relative survival rates for patients diagnosed 1973–1977; regional cervical cancer – Detroit.

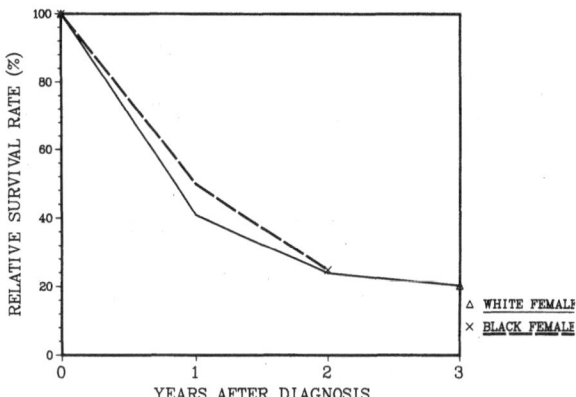

Figure 5d. Relative survival rates for patients diagnosed 1973–1977; remote cervical cancer – Detroit.

Among women diagnosed with remote disease, blacks have higher one-year relative survival than is experienced by whites (50% compared to 41%), while two-year relative survival is nearly identical (25% for blacks and 24% for whites, Figure 5d).

Median survival time for invasive carcinoma of the cervix decreases with increasing age at diagnosis (Figure 6; Axtell et al. 1976). Both black and white females have longest median survival (ten years or more) when invasive cervical cancer is diagnosed among women 34 or younger. White females diagnosed with invasive disease at age 35 to 44 retain better than ten year median survival, while for black females in this age range median survival drops to 7 years. As age at diagnosis advances, white females continue to experience longer median survival than black females, ranging from three times higher in the 45–54 age group (9 years compared with 3) to 50% higher in the 65 and older group (3 years compared with 2 years).

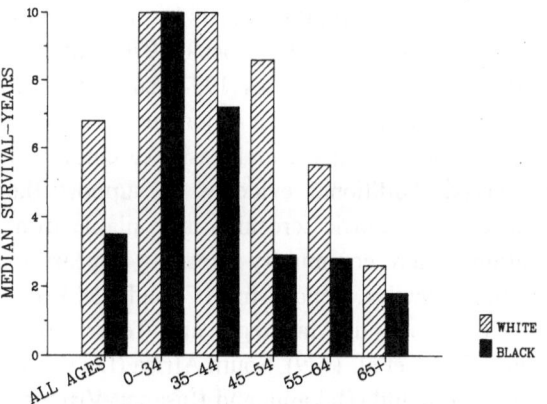

Figure 6. Invasive cervical cancer diagnosed 1960–1973; observed median survival time – U.S. *Source:* Cancer Patient Survival, Report No. 5, NCI, 1976.

have slightly higher five-year relative survival than black females (77% compared to 75%). Five-year relative survival from regional disease shows a higher rate for white females compared with black females (45% and 40%, respectively, Figure 5c).

VI. INFLUENCES UPON DECLINING MORBIDITY AND MORTALITY

The decline during the 1970s in both incidence and mortality from invasive carcinoma of the cervix may be partially attributed to four factors: (1) prevalence of screening by Papanicolaou smears within the U.S. female population, (2) prevalence of hysterectomy among U.S. women, (3) changing patterns of contraception, and (4) shift in incidence from invasive to *in situ* disease.

The 1970 National Fertility Study conducted by the Office of Population Research at Princeton University and data from the 1973 National Health Survey reveal variation in prevalence of Pap smears among selected groups of women. There is higher frequency of Pap smears among white compared to black women, women between the ages of 25 and 44 contrasted to women 65 and older, urban compared with rural females, for women with a college education compared with women with less than a high school education, for women with a family income of more than $15,000 in comparison with women with a family income of less than $5,000, and for women from western states compared with those from southern states (Rochat 1976; National Center for Health Statistics 1977).

An additional factor that has influenced the frequency with which women obtain Papanicolaou smears is method of contraception. Women who utilize oral contraceptives (84%) and intrauterine devices (83%) are more likely than women using other methods of contraception to have an annual Pap smear (Rochat 1976). Overall prevalence of Papanicolaou smears among U.S. females at approximately 80%, with Pap smears beginning widespread use in the late 1950s (Rochat 1976; National Center for Health Statistics 1977) suggests that cytologic screening has had a major role in reducing incidence and mortality from invasive carcinoma of the cervix. Additional evidence to support the influence of cytologic screening is available from programs where community screening appears to have been effective. Reports from Canada (Miller et al. 1976), Scotland (Macgregor and Teper 1978), France (Berlie et al. 1979), South Africa (DuToit et al. 1978), Finland (Hakama and Rasanen-Virtanen 1976), Denmark (Berget 1979), British Columbia (Boyes et al. 1977), Iceland (Johannesson et al.

1978), Hawaii (Dickinson 1975), Louisville, Kentucky (Christopherson 1976), and Toledo, Ohio (Kim et al. 1978) provide world-wide evidence that declining morbidity and mortality from cervical cancer has occurred in areas of active mass screening programs. There is, however, some contradictory evidence from other communities with mass screening programs for cervical cancer that have not achieved reductions in morbidity and mortality from this disease (Yule 1978; McLaren 1979; Green 1978; Green 1979).

Reasons for these negative results are not clear, but both supportive and non-supportive data regarding the extent to which Papanicolaou smears have influenced world-wide reductions in mortality and morbidity from invasive cervical carcinoma must be considered in the context of proper targeting for high risk population groups and adequacy of follow-up to ensure timely therapy. In estimating the magnitude of effect of Papanicolaou smear screening on these rates, one must attempt to account for the influence of prevalence of hysterectomy among U.S. females. A statistical procedure for adjusting rates of cervical cancer incidence and mortality for the time period 1960 to 1973 was developed to correct for effects of rates of hysterectomy (Lyon and Gardner 1977). Hysterectomy is the second most common operation among females, with 690,000 performed in 1973. The rate of hysterectomy in 1973 ranged from 2,011 per 100,000 women between the ages of 35 and 44 to 93 per 100,000 among women 15 through 24 (Lyon and Gardner 1977). Recalculating mortality rates from cervical cancer by incorporating the hysterectomy correction factor increased mortality rates by about 27%, but did not eradicate the decline in mortality from carcinoma of the cervix between 1960 and 1973. Change in type of procedure over time may also have influenced rates of cervical cancer by reducing the number of cervixes at risk. Comparing subtotal to total hysterectomy over time, in the 1940s, all hysterectomies were subtotal; by 1950–1959, 29% were subtotal; and by 1975, only 5% were subtotal (Stern et al. 1977). Increasing prevalence of hysterectomy combined with increased prevalence of examination by Papanicolaou smears are likely to have had the predominant role in reducing incidence and mortality from invasive carcinoma of the cervix in the United States.

Reductions in invasive cervical carcinoma are not simply a reduction in total disease, but rather express a major shift from invasive to *in situ* disease. This shift first became apparent in data from the Third National Cancer Survey (Cutler and Young 1975). During the 1969–1971 period, 69% of newly diagnosed cervical cancers were *in situ* disease, with the proportion of cases diagnosed at that stage rising to 76% for the 1973–1977 period. This shift may partially explain the fact that the reduction in U.S. mortality from invasive cervical carcinoma began to appear in the 1950s for white females and in the 1960s for black females (Kessler and Aurelian 1975), the years during which improved ability to diagnose cases at the *in situ* stage was more readily available.

VII. EXPLANATION OF RACIAL VARIATION

Although definitive studies of the relative influence of socioeconomic status and race upon the incidence of various types of cancer remain to be made, there is evidence which suggests that cervical cancer incidence rates would be comparable for black and white females in the United States, if one could control for socioeconomic factors.

Where socioeconomic data have been available, there is a higher incidence of cervical cancer in lower socioeconomic groups (Graham et al. 1963; Petrakis 1979). A study of geographic patterns of cancer mortality found that highest mortality from cervical cancer among white females occurred among those with median family income of $4,402 and that, overall, there was 25% greater mortality from invasive cervical carcinoma among women in lower socioeconomic categories compared to those in higher categories (Hoover et al. 1975). Definitive data regarding the interaction between race and socioeconomic status are required to more thoroughly understand characteristics of highest risk groups of women.

VIII. AGE VARIATION AND NATURAL HISTORY OF CERVICAL CANCER

Variations in high-risk age groups for *in situ* carcinoma of the cervix compared with invasive cervical cancer are assumed to be related to the natural history of the disease (Walton Report 1976). The occurrence of high risk for *in situ* disease at ages 25–34, for invasive disease at 50 and older, and for mortality at 60 and older suggests a latent period of 25 to 30 years. This age trend suggests that *in situ* disease would progress to invasive cervical cancer over time if permitted to follow its natural course. At least two studies provide evidence of epidemiologic similarity between *in situ* and invasive carcinoma of the cervix. The earlier study suggested that some women with severe dysplasia may also have epidemiologic characteristics similar to women with *in situ* and invasive disease (Thomas 1973). The current study supports the concept that *in situ* and invasive cervical cancer are different aspects of a single process, but found no similarity in epidemiologic characteristics among women with dysplasia to those with *in situ* and invasive disease (Terris 1980). Further elucidation of the natural history of cervical cancer seems critical to achieving an understanding of reasons for variation in age-specific incidence patterns among women with invasive disease when contrasted to those with *in situ* disease.

IX. PRACTICAL IMPLICATIONS

In order to continue the decline in incidence and mortality from invasive carcinoma of the cervix, and perhaps even to maintain current low rates in the United States, it may be necessary to incorporate cytologic screening into routine, preventive health care examinations for women that are less dependent upon mode of contraception. Such action will require changes in the behavior of women as well as in medical practice.

Age and socioeconomic factors appear to be the best indicators for selecting women at highest risk. Routine screening examinations among women 20 to 40 are critical to maintaining the large proportion of cases now diagnosed at the *in situ* stage. Women in the lowest socioeconomic categories are the least likely to obtain Pap smears at their own initiative (Rochat 1976; National Center for Health Statistics 1977), thus constituting a high risk group that requires innovative approaches if reductions in cervical cancer are to be achieved within this group. Finally, stronger emphasis must be placed upon establishing appropriate intervals for routine screening among women over 50. These women are at highest risk for incidence of invasive disease and for mortality from invasive carcinoma of the cervix. The National Health Survey indicates that 40% of women over 65 never had a Pap smear, while only 41% had a Pap smear within the prior 12 months (National Center for Health Statistics 1977). This is the largest, single category of never-screened women identified by the survey. Women 65 and over account for 25% of total incidence and mortality of invasive carcinoma of the cervix, while women 50 and older constitute 56% of all women diagnosed with and dying from this disease. Improvements in survival from malignant neoplasia of the uterine cervix can be achieved only through reductions in invasive disease among women 50 and older.

X. CONCLUDING REMARKS

Black females in the United States are clearly at greater risk for carcinoma of the cervix than are white females. They experience higher incidence rates for both *in situ* and invasive disease, greater mortality, and lower survival. Women between the ages of 25 and 29 have the greatest frequency of *in situ* carcinoma of the cervix, while women 50 and older are at highest risk for invasive cervical cancer. The best median survival results when invasive

carcinoma of the cervix is diagnosed among women under 35. Incidence rates for invasive cervical cancer declined by more than 22% between 1973 and 1977. A concomitant decrease in mortality from malignant cervical neoplasia of approximately 12% occurred between 1973 and 1977.

Although the relative importance of invasive cervical cancer as a health problem among women in the United States has been reduced over the past 30 years, it remains a significant form of illness requiring continued attention if further gains are to be realized. Based upon SEER data, it is estimated that in 1979 in the United States there were 16,000 new cases of invasive cervical carcinoma and 7,400 deaths from this disease (Eddy 1980). Further reduction of morbidity and mortality from invasive carcinoma of the cervix is most likely to be achieved by developing strategies to screen women of 50 and older and by incorporating routine screening for women under 50 into examinations that are less dependent upon mode of contraception.

ACKNOWLEDGEMENT

This research was supported by the National Cancer Institute Contract NO-CP-61028 and by the United Foundation. Data were provided by the National Cancer Institute Surveillance, Epidemiology, and End Results (SEER) program and by the Michigan Cancer Foundation SEER registry for Metropolitan Detroit.

REFERENCES

Berget A: Screening for Cervical Neoplasia. Dan Med Bull 26: 313, 1979.

Berlie J, Janin ML, Hucer M, Gest J, Brunet M: Mortalité par Cancer du Col d'Utérus en France, de 1950 à 1976. Bull Cancer 66: 395, 1979.

Boyes DA, Nichol TM, Millner AM, Worth AJ: Recent results from the British Columbia Screening program for Cervical Cancer. Am J Obst Gyn 128: 692, 1977.

Christopherson WM: Mass Population Screening for Cervix Cancer. Tumori 62: 297, 1976.

Cutler SJ, Young JL Jr (eds): Third National Cancer Survey; Incidence Data. NCI Monograph 41. Bethesda, MD: US-DHEW, 1975.

Cutler SJ, Young JL Jr: Demographic Patterns of Cancer Incidence. *In* JF Fraumeni (ed): Persons at High Risk for Cancer. NY: Academic Press Inc., 1975.

Dickinson LE: Control of Cancer of the Uterine Cervix by Cytologic Screening. Gyn Onc 3: 1, 1975.

Dorn HF: Illness from Cancer in the United States. Reprint No. 2537 from the Public Health Reports. Washington, D.C.: U.S. Gov't. Printing Office, 1944.

Dorn HF, Cutler SJ: Morbidity from Cancer in the U.S. Public Health Monograph No. 56. Washington, D.C.: U.S. Gov't. Printing Office, 1959.

Eddy D: ACS Report on the Cancer-Related Health Check-up. CA 30: 215, 1980.

Graham S, Levin ML L, Lillienfeld AM, Sheehe P: Ethnic Derivation as Related to Cancer at Various Sites. Cancer 16: 13, 1963.

Green GH: Cervical Cancer and Cytology Screening in New Zealand. Br J Obst Gyn 85: 881, 1978.

Green GH: Screening and cervical Cancer. Lancet, January 6: 40, 1979.

Hakama M, Rasanen-Virtanen U: Effect of a Mass Screening Program on the Risk of Cervical Cancer. Am J Epi 103: 512, 1976.

Hoover R, Mason TJ, McKay FW, Fraumeni JF Jr: Geographic Patterns of Cancer Mortality in the United States. *In* JF

Fraumeni, Jr (ed): Persons at High Risk of Cancer.NY: Academic Press, Inc., 1975.

Johannesson G, Geirsson G, Day N: The Effect of Mass Screening in Iceland, 1965–74, on the Incidence and Motality of Cervical Carcinoma. Int J Cancer 21: 418, 1978.

Kessler I, Aurelian L: Uterine Cervix. In D Schottenfeld (ed): Cancer Epidemiology and Prevention. Springfield, Ill.: C. Thomas, 1975.

Kim K, Rigal RD, Patrick JR, Waltes JK, Bennett A, Nordin, W, Claybrook JR Parekh RR: The Changing Trends of Uterine Cancer and Cytology. Cancer 42: 2439, 1978.

Lillienfeld AM, Pedersen E, Dowd JE: Cancer Epidemiology: Methods of Study. Baltimore: The Johns Hopkins Press, 1967.

Lillienfeld AM, Lillienfeld DE: Foundations of Epidemiology. NY: Oxford U Press, 1980.

Lyon JL, Gardner JW: The Rising Frequency of Hysterectomy; Its Effect on Uterine Cancer Rates. Am J Epi 105: 439, 1977.

MacGregor JE, Teper S: Mortality from Carcinoma of the Cervix Uteri in Britain. Lancet, October 7: 774, 1978.

McLaren HC: Leaves from the Arbor Vitae. Acta Cyt 23: 522, 1979.

Miller AB, Lindsay J, Hill GB: Mortality from Cancer of the Uterus in Canada and Its Relationship to Screening for Cancer of the Cervix. Int J Cancer 17: 602, 1976.

National Center for Health Statistics: Use of Selected Medical Procedures Associated with Preventive Care, U.S. – 1973.

DHEW Publication No. (HRA) 77–1538. Rockville, MD.: USDHEW, 1977.

Petrakis NL: Historic Milestones in Cancer Epidemiology. Sem Onc 6: 433, 1979.

Rochat RW: The Prevalence of Cervical Cancer Screening in the United States in 1970. Am J Obstet Gyn 125: 478, 1976.

Stern E, Miscyzynski M, Greenland S, Damus K, Coulson A: 'Pap' Testing and Hysterectomy Prevalence: A Survey of Communities with High and Low Cervical Cancer Rates. Am J Epi 106: 296, 1977.

Terris M, Wilson F, Nelson JH Jr: Comparative Epidemiology of Invasive Carcinoma of the Cervix, Carcinoma In Situ, and Cervical Dysplasia. Am J Epi 112: 253, 1980.

Thomas DB: An Epidemiologic Study of Carcinoma In Situ and Squamous Dysplasia of the Uterine Cervix. Am J Epi 98: 10, 1973.

Toit JP du, Van Niekerk WA: Cervical Cytologic Screening Among Females with Nongynecologic Hospital Admission. Obst Gyn 51: 342, 1978.

Walton Report: Cervical Cancer Screening Programs. CMAJ 114: 1003, 1976.

Young JL Jr, Asire AJ, Pollack ES (eds): SEER Program: Cancer Incidence and Mortality in the U.S., 1973–1976. DHEW Publication No. (NIH) 78–1837. Bethesda, MD: USDHEW, 1978.

NOTE

1. Rates are adjusted for age distribution of persons within a population and are based upon a standard population for the U.S. for specific time periods. Rates can be compared over time only when they are based upon the same standard population. Cancer rates presented in this chapter are the number of cases per 100,000 females. Incidence data for 1937, 1947 and 1969–1971 for the U.S. were obtained by the National Cancer Institute's First, Second and Third National Cancer Surveys, respectively.

2. MASS SCREENING FOR CERVICAL CANCER: STRATEGIES FOR REACHING HIGH RISK WOMEN IN AN URBAN-INDUSTRIAL SETTING

M.J. Brennan, Ann Grossbart and G. Marie Swanson

I. OBJECTIVES OF MASS SCREENING

Mass screening programs for the detection of carcinoma of the cervix have been conducted in Canada (Bryans et al. 1964) and the United States (Calabresi et al. 1958; Burns et al. 1968) since the late 1940s. Such programs gained an increasing popularity worldwide in the 1960s which continued throughout the 1970s. Mass screening for cervical cancer has been an especially emphasized element of public health programs in Scandinavia (Pederson et al. 1971; Hakama and Rasanen-Virtanen 1976; Berget 1975), the United Kingdom (Samson et al. 1971; deBono et al. 1978), Canada (Walton Report 1976), and the United States (Christopherson 1976; Kessler and Aurelian 1975).

The purpose of mass screening programs for cancer is to detect malignancies at the earliest possible stage by identifying precursor lesions and early cancerous lesions in asymptomatic persons. Entire population groups or selected high-risk subgroups may be screened. Not unexpectedly, the most cost-effective programs have proven to be those which concentrate on high risk segments of a population (Schottenfeld 1975).

For cervical cancer, the objective of mass screening is to detect cases at the *in situ* stage and provide treatment which prevents progression to invasive disease. High-grade dysplasias, which many believe to be precursors of carcinoma *in situ*, are also sought. Women at higher risk for cervical cancer have been shown to include those of lower socioeconomic status; those of younger age at first coitus, pregnancy, and marriage; those living in urban areas; and those who have had multiple sexual partners (Walton Report 1976). The use of known risk factors to identify population groups among whom screening programs are most likely to find a high proportion of early cases is the most effective approach to improving disease control through screening (Breslow 1978).

II. CRITERIA FOR MASS SCREENING

Criteria that are basic to any screening program were proposed by the World Health Organization. Among these are: (1) the disease for which screening is carried out should be viewed as an important public health problem, (2) there should be a valid screening technique which is acceptable to the target population, (3) an accepted mode of treatment should be widely available, (4) there should be an understanding of the natural history of the disease, and (5) the cost of screening and treatment should be reasonable when compared to the total health expenditures (Wilson and Jungner 1968).

The practical application of these criteria must be viewed in terms of the social context in which screening programs are to be implemented. The extent to which selective screening programs can be effective is directly related to their acceptability to the population at risk. For cervical cancer screening, the relative importance of risk for cervical cancer to women in the target group must be compared with other health, family, economic, and personal concerns. Since women of lower socioeconomic status are at highest risk for cervical cancer (Walton Report 1975), there are likely to be other health concerns – either of the woman herself or her family – and economic concerns that take priority over the need for having a Pap test. Therefore, if the program is to be effective, a plan which educates women about the benefits of screening and motivates them to participate in the program must be combined with a screening strategy

Hafez, E.S.E., Smith, J.P. (eds.), Carcinoma of the Cervix: Biology and Diagnosis. ISBN-13: 978-94-009-7487-6

that is unobtrusive – one which facilitates participation with minimal intrusion upon the woman's primary concerns.

III. STRATEGIES FOR CERVICAL CANCER SCREENING

Detroit mass screening for cervical cancer in higher risk populations was carried out in a two-phase program. The first phase, known as Project 'CODAC' (Community Outreach, Detection, and Care), was organized in June, 1974 and continued through June of 1977. The second phase was a cervical cancer screening intervention of the Metropolitan Detroit Cancer Control Program (MDCCP). It began in July, 1977 and continued through June, 1981.

During Project CODAC, the specific goal was to promote utilization of and provide access to cytological screening services for women living in medically-underserved areas where a high incidence of invasive carcinoma of the cervix had been recorded. Three screening strategies were employed.

The first method, standing clinics, were permanent neighborhood health facilities in which CODAC nurse examiners offered cervical cancer screening during the day, five days a week. These facilities included hospital outpatient clinics, health department clinics, and other private and neighborhood health clinics. The clinics generally offered a variety of health services such as family planning, maternal and child health services, and general medical services, but had not previously offered free cytological screening. Specialized clinics, such as that of the Michigan Cancer Foundation, which had ongoing programs of free screening for cervical cancer were also utilized.

Outreach clinics utilized a combined strategy of community outreach health workers and movable equipment to provide cervical cancer screening in non-medical facilities located in high-risk communities. The outreach health workers were women recruited from high risk neighborhoods who were trained to provide health education regarding risk for cervical cancer, and the need for regular cytological examination.

Outreach health workers placed leaflets and posters in grocery stores, churches, and neighborhood clubs; then recruited women in the community for mobile clinics by contacting them in their homes and providing them with direct, personal information. Mobile clinics were held two or three days after such community outreach and were usually conducted in churches, schools, or community social clubs. The third strategy was to conduct cervical cancer screening clinics at the work place for employees of a variety of companies in Metropolitan Detroit. Arrangements for these clinics were made with management of the companies or with unions. The clinics were advertised in advance, then held at the workplace on scheduled dates. Follow-up examinations for both employee and outreach clinics were conducted by CODAC nurses at the Michigan Cancer Foundation clinic.

All cytological samples were taken by specially trained nurses. Training was provided by physicians and experienced nurse examiners of the Michigan Cancer Foundation. All slides were interpreted centrally by a single cytology laboratory and results of tests were communicated to screenees and their physicians by central staff or Project CODAC until 1977 and by MDCCP staff thereafter. This ensured consistency in the quality of examinations, and in re-examination, referral, follow-up, and analytical procedures.

During the second phase, information gained during Project CODAC about the relative effectiveness of these three strategies was utilized to develop a system for a smaller scale, high-risk population screening involving the Detroit City Health Department, Oakland County Health Department, and the Michigan Cancer Foundation.

IV. PROFILES OF CLIENTS AND DETECTION RATES OF ALTERNATE STRATEGIES FOR CERVICAL CANCER SCREENING

For the total screening program from June of 1974 through December of 1979, there were 78,431 women screened and 189 cancers (*in situ* and invasive) found, for a case-finding rate of 2.4 per 1,000 women screened (only histologically confirmed cancers are included in these analyses). During the Project CODAC phase, 103 cancers were found among 45,797 women screened, resulting in a case-finding rate of 2.3 per 1,000. The case-finding rate for the MDCCP phase of the screening program was 2.6 per 1,000 (86 cancers found among 32,634 women screened). Thus, even with differences in the objectives of the two phases – field-testing the strategies in Project CODAC and transferring them to ongoing organizations in MDCCP – the results were stable over time.

In order to evaluate the productivity and effectiveness of the three approaches to cervical cancer screening, four variables were selected as most important to the assessment: (1) race of participants, (2) age of participants at first screening, (3) socioeconomic status of participants and (4) type of clinic.

The age distribution of black and white women at first screening differs considerably. There were 57% of the black participants in the cervical cancer screening program who were under 35 years of age, while 54% of the cancers detected among blacks were found in this age group. Only 25% of white screenees were under 35 and 23% of the cancers found among whites were in this group. The largest proportion of cancers found among white screenees was concentrated in the 50–59 year age group. There were 22% of the white participants in this age group, but 48% of the cancers found among whites were in this group. No cancers were detected in either black or white screenees under the age of 20, while 13% of cancers found among both black and white participants were in women 60 or older.

There were differences between black and white screenees in terms of family income level. The 1970 poverty level income for a family of four was $5,500 (U.S. Bureau of Census 1971). For this study, the lower income group is constituted by those with an annual family income of $8,000 or less; the middle income group includes those in the $8,001–15,000 family income range; and the upper

income group consists of women with a family income of $15,001 or more.

Using these income figures as crude indicators of socioeconomic status (SES), 79% of black screenees were in the lower SES group and 78% of the cancers in black women were in this group. In the middle SES group of black screenees there were 10% of cervical cancers among black participants, while 4% were in the upper SES group. The results among white screenees were less concentrated in the lower SES group, which included 44% of the screenees and 32% of the cancers in white participants. In the middle SES group of white screenees, 32% of the cancers were found, while 32% were detected in women in the upper SES category.

Data describing insurance status of the screening clinic participants lends support to data on income for purposes of SES distribution. Persons covered by Medicaid have a poverty-level or lower income. Thirty-nine percent of the cancers found in black screenees were among women with Medicaid insurance. None of the white cancer cases had Medicaid coverage. In contrast, 68% of the cancers found among white screenees were women with private insurance, while only 23% of black screenees found to have cancer had private coverage.

Analysis of results by clinic type shows a large variation in productivity. For screening clinic clients who were white, equal proportions of cancers were found in standing clinics (32%) and outreach clinics (32%). For black participants, outreach clinics were clearly the most effective, producing 83% of all cancers found in this group. The high proportion of black screenees entering the outreach clinics reflects the fact that most of the outreach clinics sessions were organized in predominantly black lower income neighborhoods with known high incidence of invasive cervical cancer. Employee clinics were not effective for either black or white women, with less than 3% of screenees and cancers in this group.

Analyzing clinic type by age and race, the only strategy effective in finding cervical cancers among women of both races in all age categories was the outreach strategy. The outreach strategy was also the only successful method for detecting cervical cancer among black women 50 and older. There were differences in the type of cancer found among black and white screenees. *In situ* cervical cancer

Table 1. Cancer cases by type and race[a]; July 1976 – December 1979.

Type of cancer	White	Black
	%	%
cervical cancer, *in situ*	68	86
cervical cancer, invasive	23	11
endometrial cancer	10	3

[a] 41,596 women screened, 109 cancers detected.

was detected in 86% of the cases found among black females, while only 68% of the cancer cases among white screenees were *in situ* (Table 1). A few endometrial cancers were found in both the black and white screened populations. Improvement in stage at diagnosis for screenees compared to that for the general population in Detroit occurred only for black females. There was essentially no difference in the proportion of cervical cancers found among white screenees at the *in situ* stage compared with Metropolitan Detroit (75% for both). For black screenees, however, there was a 9% improvement in the proportion of cases detected as *in situ* disease (88% – screenees; 79% – Metropolitan Detroit).

V. THE NEED FOR VARIABLE SCREENING INTERVALS

The appropriateness of annual Pap tests for all sexually active women has been questioned (Foltz and Kelsey 1978; Marx 1979). A recent panel organized by the National Institutes of Health was unable to reach a consensus for recommending appropriate screening intervals for women in different risk groups (Henderson 1980).

The critical factor from all these discussions for mass screening and for routine cytological examination is the need to properly target high risk groups of women for mass programs, rather than attempting to screen entire populations and to establish appropriate intervals for Pap smears for women at high, average, and low risk for cervical cancer. Targetting for previously unscreened women is particularly important, since studies conducted by Princeton University and the National Center for Health Statistics indicate that approximately 80% of all women in the United States have had at least one Pap smear, while nearly 62% have routine examinations for cervical cancer (Rochat 1976; National Center for Health Statistics 1977).

VI. GUIDELINES FOR URBAN MASS SCREENING PROGRAMS

Results from the Detroit cervical cancer screening program provide practical guidelines for the development of similar programs in other metropolitan areas of the U.S. which have substantial black populations. First, since the highest case-finding rates (4.3 per 1,000 for blacks compared to 1.3 for whites) and the only improvement in stage at diagnosis were obtained among black screenees, selective screening in urban areas is likely to be most effective among black women. Further support is provided by a survey describing prevalence of previous Pap smears among U.S. females, which indicates that a higher percentage of black women living in cities have never been screened (12%) compared to white women living in cities (7%, Rochat 1976).

Second, the only age group in which no cancers were detected among black screening clinic clients was among women under 20. Therefore, it seems practical to target for women 20 and older. Also, women 60 and older should be included in these programs, since case-finding remains high.

Third, the target population for urban programs of mass cervical cancer screening can be further refined by orientation towards black women of low socioeconomic status. In the Detroit program, for black women for whom family income was known, 78% of the cancers were detected among women in the low income group. Only 32% of the cancers detected among white screenees were in the same low SES category. The Princeton survey again lends support, indicating that 30% of black women in the lowest income category had never been screened for cervical cancer, compared to 13% of white females in the same income group (Rochat 1976).

Finally, the community outreach strategy was found, in Detroit, to be the most effective method for reaching high risk black women and detecting cancers among black women of all age groups, from 20 through 80. This strategy is likely to be effective among other low SES women who are not involved in routine health care programs.

VII. CONCLUDING REMARKS

Mass screening for cervical cancer in urban areas similar to Detroit will be most effective when targeted for low income black women. These women are less likely to have private insurance which would enable them to obtain Pap smears from private physicians or clinics and are most likely,

14

therefore, to benefit from a community screening program. Community outreach is an effective strategy for reaching these women at all ages from 20 to 80 and for achieving high case-finding rates.

ACKNOWLEDGEMENT

This research was supported by the National Cancer Institute, Contracts NIH-NCI-CN-74-15, NO1-CN65252 and NO1-CP-61028 and by the United Foundation. Data were provided by Project CO-DAC, the Metropolitan Detroit Cancer Foundation SEER registry for Metropolitan Detroit. The authors wish to thank Ms. Kathleen Lynch-Brown and Ms. E. Jean Christian for their efforts in organizing and maintaining the data base for the 80,000 patients screened for cervical cancer.

REFERENCES

Berget A: Epidemiologic Characteristics in Patients with Epithelial Dysplasia, Carcinoma *In Situ*, and Invasive Carcinoma of the Uterine Cervix: The Population Screening for Cervical Carcinoma in Maribo County, 1967-69. Dan Med Bull 22: 252, 1975.

deBono AM, Kingley-Pillers EM, Kirk NM: The Pattern of Presentation of Carcinoma of the Uterine Cervix in East Anglia, 1960 to 1975. Br J Obst Gyn 85: 887, 1978.

Breslow L: Risk Factor Intervention for Health Maintenance. *In* Abelsom PH (ed): Health Care: Regulation, Economics, Ethics, Practice. Washington: AAAS, 1978.

Burns EL, Hammond EC, Percy C, Seidman H, Gorski TW: Detection of Uterine Cancer: Results of a Community Program of 17 Years. Cancer 22: 1108, 1968.

Bryans FE, Boyes DA, Fidler HK: The Influence of a Cytological Screening Program Upon the Incidence of Invasive Squamous Cell Carcinoma of the Cervix in British Columbia. Am J Obst Gyn 88: 898, 1964.

Calabresi P, Arbold NV, Stovall WD: Cytological Screening for Uterine Cancer Through Physicians' Offices: Report of 65,153 Women Examined Over a Period of Ten Years (1947–1956). JAMA 168–243, 1958.

Foltz AM, Kelsey JL: The Annual Pap Test: A Dubious Policy Success. Mil Mem Fund Quar 56–426, 1978.

Hakama M, Rasanen-Virtanen U: Effects of A Mass Screening Program on the Risk of Cervical Cancer. Am J Epi 103: 152, 1976.

Henderson M: National Institutes of Health, Consensus Development Conference Statement. Unpublished Report. Washington: NIH, 1980.

Kessler I, Aurelian L: Uterine Cervix. *In* Schottenfeld D (ed): Cancer Epidemiology and Prevention. Springfield, Ill.: C. Thomas, 1975.

Marx JL: The Annual Pap Test: An Idea Whose Time Has Gone? Science 205: 177, 1979.

National Center for Health Statistics: Use of Selected Medical Procedures Associated with Prevention Care, U.S. – 1973. DHEW Publication No. (HRA) 77–1538. Rockville, Md.: USDHEW, 1977.

Pedersen E, Hueg K, Kostad P: Mass Screening for Cancer of the Uterine Cervix. In Ostfold County Norway: An Experiment. Acta Obst Gyn Scand 50: 1, 1971.

Rochat RW: The Prevalence of Cervical Cancer Screening in the United States in 1979. Am J Obst Gyn 125: 478, 1976.

Sansom DC, Wakefield J, Ule R: Trends in Cytological Screening in the Manchester Area, 1965 to 1971. Comm Med 26: 253, 1971.

Schottenfeld D: Cancer Detection Programs. *In* Fraumeni JF Jr (ed): Persons at High Risk of Cancer. NY: Academic Press, Inc., 1975.

U.S. Bureau of the Census: Characteristics if the Low-Income Population, 1970. Washington, D.C. 1971. Curr Pop Rep m Series P-60, No. 81.

Walton Report: Cervical Cancer Screening Programs. CMAJ 114: 1003, 1976.

Wilson JMG, Jungner G: Principles and Practice of Screening for Disease. Public Health Paper No. 34, World Health Organization. Geneva: WHO, 1968.

3. INVASIVE CARCINOMA OF THE UTERINE CERVIX IN WOMEN YOUNGER THAN 25 YEARS

C.J. CASTELLANO, L. CONROY and G. RAMIREZ

Invasive carcinoma of the uterine cervix is rare in young women, particularly of women less than 20 years old. Only one case was reported in a large series (Truelsen 1949), and only 30 cases from one report were found in women younger than 20 years of age (Pollack and Taylor 1947). Several studies have been reported on young women with cancer of the uterine cervix under 35 years of age (Berkowitz et al. 1979), under 34 years of age (Kjörstad 1977) and under 30 years of age (Kyriakoset al. 1971). The results of these studies have been contradictory in many instances, and their common denominator is that the reported rarity of cervical cancer in younger women is of limited validity due to the small number of patients studied.

The only Peruvian Cancer Registry is located in Lima, and it covers approximately one-quarter of the country's population. The majority of cancer cases are diagnosed or referred for treatment to the Instituto Nacional de Enfermedades Neoplásicas, devoted exclusively to the management of malignant tumors. The incidence of cancer of the uterine cervix in Metropolitan Lima from 1968 to 1970 was 28.61/100,000 women of all ages, and 44.54/100,000 women older than 15 years. Cervical cancer is the malignancy most frequently encountered. A large sector of this population is of low socio-cultural-economic status, thus giving rise to a large population at high risk of developing cervical cancer. Although methods for screening and detection have increased, it has not yet had a great impact on the incidence and distribution of invasive carcinoma.

The frequency of cervical cancer in patients under 35 years of age is less than 10%, and is only 2.6% for patients under 30 years (Lindell 1962). The cervical cancer series from this study has a distribution of: 11% in the under-35 age group; 4% in the under-30 age group; and 0.7% in the under-25 age

group, with 123 registered cases of invasive cancer of the cervix. This younger group (under 25 years) was selected for an analytic study of the parameters that affect this age group and that may differ from those of the older age groups.

I. CLINICAL STUDY

There were 17,326 cases of invasive carcinoma of the uterine cervix registered over a period of 27 years, from 1952 to 1978, of which 123 patients were age 25 or less. To serve as a total statistical control, all invasive cervical cancer cases of all age groups from this period studied were tabulated for: age, gravidity, association with pregnancy, age at first coitus, latent period, histology, clinical stage distribution, influences of gravidity.

Data from the National Office of Statistics was also used as a partial statistical control for age at first coitus in the general female population, in relation to the age group. A histochemical study was conducted of cervical carcinoma associated with pregnancy in the so-called apparent mucoepidermoid carcinoma to determine the real nature of the intracytoplasmatic component responsible for the clear aspect which those cells possess. Stains were made with P.A.S. and Best Carmine using previously digested cases as controls. The results of this investigation will be reported in the chapter on histopathology.

II. STUDY PARAMETERS

II.A. Age

The youngest patient in the series of 123 cases was

Hafez, E.S.E., Smith, J.P. (eds.), Carcinoma of the Cervix: Biology and Diagnosis. ISBN-13: 978-94-009-7487-6

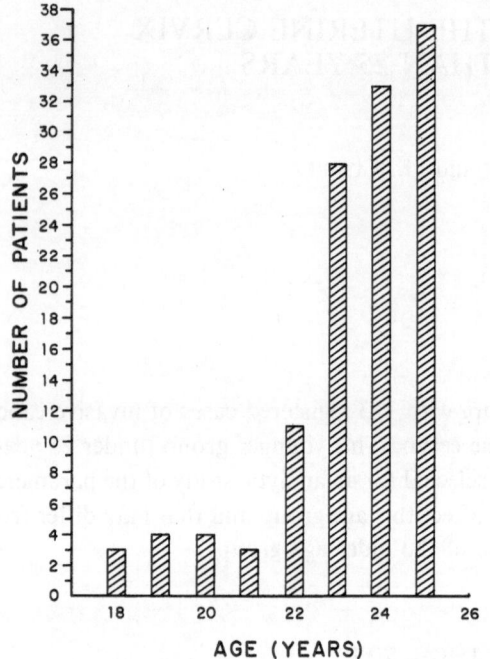

Figure 1. Age distribution in 123 women with invasive cervical cancer younger than 25 years.

18 years old (Figure 1). Three patients were 18 years of age; and of these, two had adenocarcinoma, and the third had epidermoid carcinoma. The average age was 23.3 years, with a median of 23.5. The average age for all patients with invasive cervical carcinoma registered from this 27 year period was 51.2 years. This report studies women younger than 25 years, being almost entirely a product of the prevalence of this disease in a population definitively at high risk. There is only one institution in the country exclusively devoted to the management of malignant tumors.

Although cancer detection and screening in Peru was initiated in 1953, it was only in the private sector and covered a limited population. In 1972, a Public Health Program for control of cervical cancer was initiated. This program has not yet had a recognizable impact, due to the short period of time since its inception.

Several large clinical series (Cavenagh et al. 1966; Diddle and Watts 1962; Lindell 1962; Handy et al. 1965) have reported that the proportion of patients in their 30s has varied from 1.5% to 14%. Many of these papers deal with time periods before the adoption of routine cytologic screening. A large series of 2,918 patients (Truelsen 1949) reported on only 83 patients from age 20–29 (3%) and only one

patient under 20. Another series (Kurohara et al. 1970) reported on 77 patients younger than 30 years old. A review of the world literature (Boyes et al. 1956) found only 19 patients less than 15 years of age had adenocarcinoma.

II.B. *Gravidity*

There were a total of 405 pregnancies of 113 patients, for an average of 3.5 per patient. Ten patients (8.1%) had never been pregnant (Figure 2). The group of 113 patients with previous pregnancies was distributed as follows: 105 patients with from one to five pregnancies (85%), and 8 patients with six or more pregnancies (6%). When the gravidity of this group was compared to that of older women in the 26 to 90 years of age group (Table 1), statistically significant differences were found. The group of older women was composed of: 1% nulligravid; 30%, gravida one to five; and 69%, gravida six or more.

This gravidity data has been compared to a control group of the female population of reproductive age, of apparent good health and who have had sexual intercourse. The control group had 2.6% nulligravids under 25 years of age (Oficina Nacional de Estadística 199). The percentage of nulligravids under 25 years of age was three times more

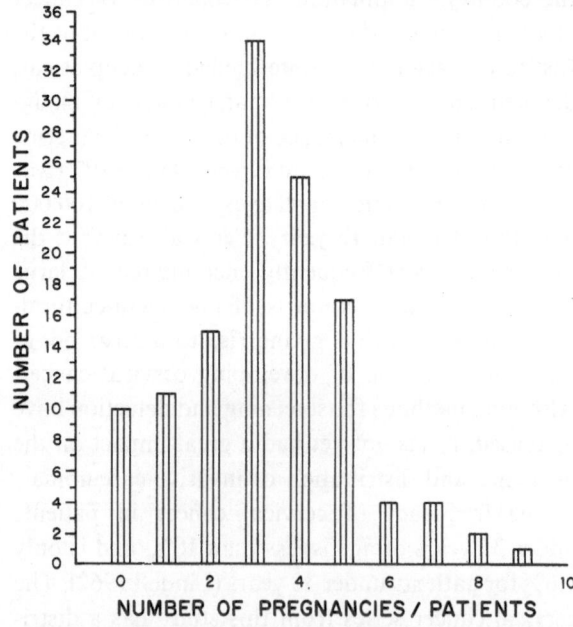

Figure 2. Gravidity distribution in 123 women with invasive cervical cancer younger than 25 years.

Table 1. Gravidity in women with invasive cervical cancer older and younger than 25 years.

Gravidity	≤25 years		26–90	
	Number of cases	%	Number of cases	%
0	10	8	191	1
1–5	105	85	5,128	30
≥6	8	7	11,884	69
	123	100	17.203	100

$P < 0.001$

frequent (8%) in women with cervical cancer, a statistically significant difference.

Approximately 10% of patients with cervical cancer have never been pregnant (Christopherson et al. 1965; Boyd and Doll 1964; Rotkin 1967). The number of women with cervical cancer that were gravida six or more times, was six times larger than in the normal control group, 6% and 1% respectively. 69% of the women age 26 to 90 were gravida six or more times. This was more than three times the rate of the normal control group (18%). Several studies (Christopherson and Parker 1965; Rotkin 1967; Terris and Oalmann 1960) have shown an increased prevalence of the disease with an increasing number of pregnancies, but others have shown no such correlation. In this series, only the groups gravida six times or more, regardless of age, have shown a direct correlation with increased prevalence of cervical cancer.

II.C. Association with pregnancy

There were 39 cases out of the 123 associated with pregnancy (32%), including patients diagnosed within the period of pregnancy or during the 12 months following delivery. Of the 39 cases, 24 were diagnosed in the postpartum period; 10 were diagnosed following abortion; and only five cases were diagnosed during the first two trimesters of pregnancy. Of the cervical carcinomas associated with pregnancy, histology was distributed as follows: 32 of the epidermoid type; 4 mucoepidemoid; and 3 adenocarcinoma.

The frequency of cervical cancer associated with pregnancy is evidently very high in the series of women younger than 25 years. A significant statistical difference is revealed when this series is compared to an isolated series of patients of all ages

from 1952 to 1970, in which 242 cases of cervical cancer associated with pregnancy were found in a total of 11,644 cases (2%) (Castellano 1973). An excellent opportunity is presented for cervical cancer screening during the prenatal care of those young women at high risk of developing cervical cancer. Screening of the young high risk population should also be encouraged.

II.D. Age at first coitus and latent period

Data on age at first coitus was obtained for 100 out of the 123 patients (Figure 3). Nineteen patients (19%) were age 14 or less at the time of first coitus; 60 were age 16 or less (60%); and 88 were younger than 20 years of age (88%). The mean and median ages at first coitus were 16.4 years with a range of 12–23 years.

Extensive epidemiological data (Barron and Richart 1971; Beral 1974; Rotkin 1973; VillaSanta 1971) suggests that early cervical carcinoma might be considered a mildly contagious sexually transmitted disease. Women with cervical cancer started intercourse at an earlier age than women without cervical cancer. Data from 17 investigators, concludes that only early sexual intercourse before the age of 17, as well as multiple sexual partners were

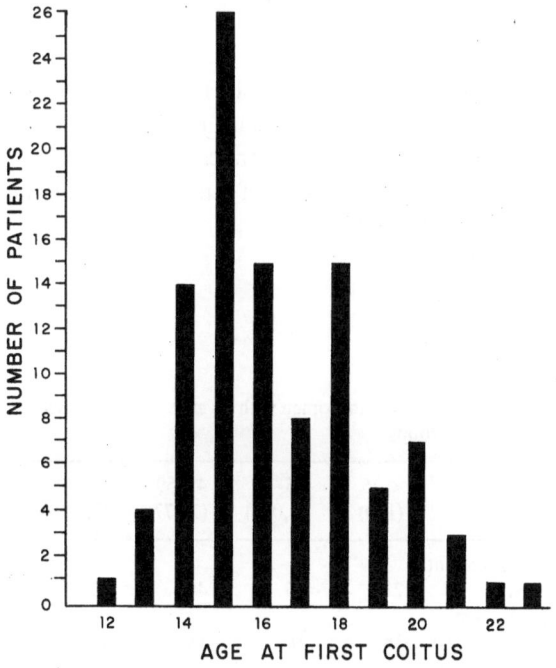

Figure 3. Distribution of age at first coitus in 123 women with invasive cervical cancer younger than 25 years.

18

two main reasons influencing the risk of cervical cancer (Rotkin 1973; Briggs 1979). Out of the 123 patients studied, 88% had intercourse before the age of 20, as compared to only 60% in the control group (Oficina Nacional de Estadística 1979). In the group with cervical cancer, the onset of coitus before the age of 17 was 60% out of 100 cases, as compared to only 20% in the control group. The relation of cervical cancer in young women to onset of first coitus before 20 years and 17 years has a ratio of 1.4 and 3.0 respectively, as compared to a ratio of 1.5 and 2.2 respectively (Rotkin 1973). The latter ratio is highly significant when compared to that found in the cancer group with earlier onset of first coitus.

The latency period between the age at first intercourse and the diagnosis of cervical cancer is approximately 30 years, with a range from 8 to 61 years (Rotkin 1962), and 9.3 years (Kyriakos et al. 1971) for women younger than 30 years. The average latent period, or the time interval between first intercourse and the diagnosis of carcinoma, was 6.9 years for the entire group, with a range from 0 to 12 years (Table 2). Comparison with the latent period for other age groups revealed that it was 17 years for the 26 to 40 years of age group; 29 years for the 41 to 59 years of age group; and 48 years for the oldest group, from 60 to 90 years of age.

The latent period was 6.9 years for the epidermoid type (range one to twelve), being lower, 4.4 years, for the adenocarcinoma type. One patient with mesonephric type adenocarcinoma was 18 years old when the onset of first coitus and the diagnosis was made.

Table 2. Latent period in women with invasive cervical cancer at different age groups.

	≤25 (100)	26–40 (3,070)	41–59 (7,677)	60–90 (3,338)
Average patient's age (yrs)	23	35	48	67
Average first coitus age (yrs)	16	18	18	19
Average latent period (yrs)	7	17	29	48

Table 3. Hisologic type in women with invasive cervical cancer younger than 25 years (123 cases).

Histologic type	%
Epidermoid	84.6
Adenocarcinoma	6.5
Mucoepidermoid	6.5
Undifferentiated	2.4
	100.0
Mucoepidermoid →	Glucoepidermoid

II.E. Histopathology

There were 104 tumors classified as epidermoid carcinoma (85%); 8 as adenocarcinoma (6.5%); 8 as mucoepidermoid (6.5%); and 3 were undifferentiated.

The grade of histologic differentiation of the epidermoid type was well-differentiated in 20%, moderately differentiated in 58%; and poorly differentiated in 22%. Among the eight cases of adenocarcinoma, there was one well-differentiated; two moderately differentiated; one poorly differentiated; two clear cell adenocarcinoma; one of the mesonephric type; and one adenoacanthoma.

Of the total series of 17,326 patients with carcinoma of the uterine cervix, 351 cases of adenocarcinoma were found (2%). This frequency was three times less than that found in the series of women younger than 25 years of age (6.5%). This greater frequency of adenocarcinoma in young women is statistically significant. A rate of 9.6% adenocarcinoma of the cervix has been reported in women over 35 years of age (Berkowitz et al. 1979), in contrast with a rate of 26% for those women 35 years of age or younger. Another study (Kjörstad 1977) reported the histologic distribution in a series of 2,002 cases of women of all ages, finding 92,5% squamous cell carcinoma and 5% adenocarcinoma, with this histologic distribution being the same for all age groups. If these data are comparatively evaluated, the findings have no uniformity.

The term mucoepidermoid has been reported as a growth composed of squamous cells with variable amounts of mucin content in tumors of the salivary glands (Stewart et al. 1945). A later report (Helweg 1957) applied this histologic type to carcinoma of the uterine cervix. When the mucoepidermoid cases in this series of carcinoma of the cervix associated

Table 4. Clinical stage distribution in women with invasive cervical cancer all ages and younger than 25 years.

Clinical stage	All ages		≤25 years	
	Number of cases	%	Number of cases	%
I	1,448	8	14	11
II	5,488	32	60	49
III	8,875	51	43	35
IV	1,515	9	6	5
Total	17,326	100	123	100

≤25 Years: 123 / 17,326, 0.7%.

with pregnancy were reviewed (Castellano 1973), the apparent mucoepidermoid was really glucoepidermoid.

II.F. Clinical stage

The patients were staged according to the classification of the International Federation of Gynecology and Obstetrics. Table 4 shows the number of patients in each stage comparatively in women at all ages and under 25 years. Out of the total 17,326 cases, 123 were younger than 25 years (0.7%). An analysis of this table reveals a clear predominance of lesions in the advanced stages with a differing distribution in both groups. The proportion of patients in Stage II is greater in the group of patients 25 years of age or less, and the number of Stage III patients is lower than expected. Due to the small number of cases in Stage I and IV, it cannot be determined that the proportion differs between the patients under 25 years of age and those of all ages.

Of the 14 cases in Stage I, four corresponded to Stage I-A and 10 were Stage I-B. The 60 cases in Stage II were all II-B. The 43 cases in Stage III were

all III-B; and of the six patients in Stage IV, two were IV-A and four were IV-B. Within the 27 year period, 1,247 cases of carcinoma *in situ* were registered, representing 7% of the total cases of cervical cancer, both *in situ* and invasive. Of the 1,247 *in situ* cancer cases, 21 (1.7%) corresponded to women aged 25 years or less.

One study (Kyriakos et al. 1971) reports on a series showing a preponderance of Stage I lesions (64%) and concludes on this basis that cervical cancer does not run a more rapid and fulminating course in younger women. This is in contrast to the findings of this series and to those of other published reports (Kottmeir 1964; Arneson and Williams 1960; Fidler et al. 1968), indicating a higher percentage of Stage II lesions in patients with cervical cancer. This difference may partially depend on the grade of usage of the cervical cytology and on the different grades of prevalence in the female population.

The distribution of cervical carcinoma by clinical stage has been compared between women younger than 25 years and women older than 76 years, having greatest frequency in the older group with 455 cases (3%) compared to the youngest group of 123 patients in this study (0.7%). The staging distribution of cervical cancer in women older than 76 years for stages I–IV were respectively 5%, 22%, 55% and 18%, which shows a highly significant difference when compared to the youngest age group with a distribution of 11%, 49%, 35% and 5%, respectively.

II.G. Influence of gravidity on clinical stage

Gravidity has some influence on clinical stage (Table 5). The frequency of clinical stages III and IV is higher in the nulligravids group and in the

Table 5. Influence of gravidity on clinical stage in women older and younger than 25 years.

Age	Gravidity 0			1–5			≥6		
	Number of cases III–IV	Number of cases grav. 0	%	Number of cases III–IV	Number of cases grav. 1–5	%	Number of cases III–IV	Number of cases grav. ≥6	%
26–90	111	191	58	3,269	5,128	64	6,714	11,884	56
≤25	8	10	80	34	105	33	7	8	87
P	>0.05			<0.05			<0.05?		

group gravida six or more, than in the group gravida one to five, for women younger than 25 years. Women aged 26 to 90 years, there was little difference in the frequency of stages III and IV in relation to gravidity. Comparing such influence between the two age groups, there is a statistically significant difference between the groups with gravida one to five, and gravida six or more, with stages III and IV being more frequent in the age groups of 26 to 90 years and younger than 25 years respectively. In the nulligravid group, although there is an apparent difference, there is no statistical significance due to the low number of cases.

Moderate gravidity is favorable among patients in the age group 30 to 59 years (Kurohara et al. 1970), and is associated with relatively earlier lesions. More advanced diseases were observed in those patients with either no pregnancy or many previous pregnancies, as in the group gravida six or more. Those relationships were not observable in those patients in whom cancer was diagnosed after the fifth decade of age. These clinical alterations may be explained by certain pathophysiologic changes occurring in the cervix with successive pregnancies and increasing age.

II.H. Age at first coitus and its influence on the clinical stage distribution at different age groups

The age at first coitus has been distributed in two different groups: from age 17 or less and from age 17 or greater (Table 6). In the group 25 years of age or less, the frequency observed in women having intercourse between age 11 and 16 is greater than expected, and is less than expected in the group of women who had intercourse at age 17 or older.

In the group of women with cervical cancer, aged

26 to 90, the findings are reversed. The frequency of intercourse begun at ages 11 to 16 progressively decreases as the patient's age increases. This is contrary to that group of women who had intercourse after age 17. The frequency of the advanced clinical stages III and IV increases for both groups that had intercourse before or after age 17 (Table 6). A statistically significant difference has been found in the group of women aged 60 to 90 years, being that stages III and IV are more frequent in women who had intercourse at an earlier age. In the group of women younger than 25 years, there is no statistical significance due to the small number of cases, although its higher frequency in the group having intercourse at an earlier age could be determined with a large number of cases.

III. SPECIAL CONSIDERATIONS FOR DEVELOPING
COUNTRIES

The fact that cervical carcinoma rarely occurs in women under 20 years of age, and is uncommon under the age of 30, has resulted in low yields when mass cytologic screening is performed; thus making the economic cost of detection in this age group very high. It is sometimes believed that this group should be given low priority in mass screening programs (Christopherson and Parker 1959), whereas others agree with this on philosophic criteria (Kyriakos et al. 1971).

On an individual basis, any woman who is no longer a virgin should have a yearly Papanicolaou smear regardless of age. This point must be emphasized in order to alert not only the gynecologist, but especially those physicians seeing patients for

Table 6. Age at first coitus and its influence on the clinical stage distribution at different age groups.

Age at 1st coitus	≤25 years		26–40		41–59		60–90	
	Number of cases III–IV	All stages	Number of cases III–IV	All stages	Number of cases III–IV	All stages	Number of cases III–IV	All stages
11–16	27 (47%)	58 (58%)	675 (50%)	1,350 (44%)	1,341 (55%)	2,456 (32%)	552 (64%)	868 (26%)
≥17	17 (40%)	42 (42%)	826 (48%)	1,720 (56%)	2,902 (56%)	5,221 (68%)	1,435 (58%)	2,470 (74%)
Total:		100		3,070		7,677		3,338

nongynecologic problems. Attention to the occurrence of cervical cancer in young women should be increased in the developing countries, especially by those physicians and paramedical personnel seeing women at risk.

IV. CONCLUDING REMARKS

The percentage of nulligravids in women younger than 25 years with cervical cancer is more frequent when compared to the normal control group and to the group of women with cervical cancer older than 25 years. There was an increased prevalence of the disease with increasing number of pregnancies for the group gravida six or higher in both age groups. There were 39 patients (32%) out of the total 123

associated with pregnancy. The onset of coitus before the age of 17 years was found to be three times more frequent (60%) in the cervical cancer group than in the control group (20%). The average latency period for the group of women younger than 25 years was 6.9 years. There was a statistically significant greater frequency of adenocarcinoma in this series of young women. The apparent mucoepidermoid cancer associated with pregnancy proved to be glucoepidermoid. The clinical stage II lesions were predominant (48%). Gravidity has an influence on the clinical stage only in the groups of women younger than 25 years $P < 0.001$). Attention to the occurrence of cervical cancer in young women should be increased in the developing countries, especially by those physicians and paramedical personnel seeing women at risk.

REFERENCES

Arneson AN William CF: Long Term follow-up observations in cervical cancer. Amer J Obst Gynecol 80: 775, 1960.

Barron BA, Richart RM: An epidemiological study of cervical neoplastic disease. Based on a self-selected sample of 7,000 women in Barbados, West Indies. Cancer 27: 97, 1971.

Beral V: Cancer of the cervix: A sexually transmitted infection. Lancet: 1037, 1974.

Berkowitz RS, Ehrmann RL, Lavisso-Mourey R, Knapp RC: Invasive Cervical Carcinoma in young women. Gynecol Oncology 8: 311, 1979.

Boyd JT, Doll T: A study of the etiology of carcinoma of the cervix uteri. Brit J Cancer 18: 419, 1964.

Boyes DA, Hardie M, Agnew AM: Carcinoma of the cervix in an infant. Amer J Obst Gynecol 72: 1353, 1956.

Briggs RM: Dysplasia and early neoplasia of the uterine cervix. A review. Obst and Gynecol Survey 34: 70, 1979.

Castellano CJ: Carcinoma de cuello uterino asociado con gestación. Thesis for Doctor in Medicine Degree. Universidad Peruana Cayetano Heredia, Lima, Perú, 1973.

Cavenagh D, McLeod AGW, Ferguson J.H.: Carcinoma of the cervix amoung women in their twenties. JAMA 195: 834, 1966.

Christopherson WM, Parker JE: Relation of cervical cancer to early marriage and childbearing. New Eng J Med 273: 235, 1965.

Christopherson WM, Parker JE: Economic considerations of the control of cervix cancer in high risk patients. CA 19: 107, 1969.

Diddle AW, Watts J: Cervical carcinoma in woman under 30 years of age. Amer J Obst Gynecol 84: 745, 1962.

Fidler HK, Boyes DA, Worth AJ: Cervical Cancer Detection in British Columbia. J Obst Gynecol Brit Comm 75: 393, 1968.

Handy VH, Wieben E: Detection of cancr of the cervix. A public health approach. Obst Gynecol 25: 348, 1965.

Helweg G: Uber Schleimbildung in Plattenepithelkarzinomen, insbesondere an der Portio uteri (Mucoepidermoidcarcinome). A Krebsforch 61: 688, 1957.

Kjörstad K: Carcinoma of the cervix in the young patient. Obstet Gynecol 50: 28, 1977.

Kottmeir HL: Surgical and radiation treatment of carcinoma of the uterine cervix. Acta Radiol (Suppl 92) 1, 1952.

Kurohara SS, Selim MA, Graham JB: Relation of gravidity and age to prognosis and clinical stage in uterine Cervix Cancer. Cancer 26: 39–45, 1970.

Kyriakos M, Kempson RL, Perez CA: Carcinoma of the Cervix in young women. Obstet Gynecol 38: 930, 1971.

Lindell A: Carcinoma of the uterine cervix. Incidence and influence of age. Acta Radiol Suppl. 92, 1962.

Oficina Nacional de Estadistica: Encuesta Nacional de Fecundidad del Perú. Dirección General de Censos, Encuestas y Demografía. Dirección de Demografía, 1979.

Pollack RS, Tayler HC: Carcinoma of the Cervix during the first two decades of life. Amer J Obstet Gynecol 53: 135, 1947.

Rotkin ID: Relation of adolescent coitus to cervical cancer risk. JAMA 179: 486, 1962.

Rotkin ID: Sexual characteristics of a cervical cancer population. Amer J Public Health 57: 815, 1967.

Rotkin ID: A comparison review of key epidemiological studies in cervical cancer related to current searches for transmissible agents. Cancer Res 33: 1353, 1973.

Stewart FW, Foots FW, Becker WF: Mucoepidermoid tumors of the salivary glands. Ann Surg 122: 820, 1945.

Terris M, Oalmann MC: Carcinoma of the cervix: Epidemiologic study. JAMA 174: 1847, 1960.

Truelson F: Cancer of the uterine cervix. Copenhagen: Rosenkilde and Bagger, 1949.

VillaSanta U: Diagnosis and prognosis of cervical displasias. Obstet Gynecol 38: 811, 1971.

4. CERVICAL CARCINOMA IN PANAMA

R.C. DE BRITTON, W.C. REEVES, P.F. VALDÉS, C.F.B. JOPLIN and M.M. BRENES

I. CANCER AS A HEALTH PROBLEM IN PANAMA

I. A. Mortality

Tropical countries have historically devoted most of their health resources to infectious diseases. In countries such as Panama with rapidly improving environmental and health standards, infectious diseases remain the principal cause of morbidity but not mortality. Along with the population's increasing life span, non-infectious chronic diseases have emerged as major public health problems. Panama's published cause-specific mortality rates show this (Table 1); cancer has been among the three principal causes of death since 1968 (Dirección de Estadística y Censo 1979). These crude death rates contradict the fact that more than half of Panama's population is younger than 15 years. A

Table 1. Leading causes of certificated deaths in Panama, 1974–1978.

	Cause of death	% Total deaths	Rate per 100,000
1.	Ischaemic heart disease	12.7	45.1
2.	Accidents – suicide homicide	12.2	43.4
3.	Cancer	12.2	43.1
4.	Cerebro-vascular disease	8.6	30.3
5.	Pneumonia	5.8	20.5
6.	Enteritis diarrhea	3.8	13.9
	Infant mortality per 1,000/ live births	31.5	

similar mortality pattern appears to be evolving in other tropical countries.

I. B. Incidence

The National Oncology Institute of Panama initiated a National Cancer Register in 1974 to document cancer incidence (Valdés et al. 1979). The Panama National Cancer Register actively ascertains all histologically diagnosed cancers by annually reviewing every certified pathologist's histology reports. Registration includes each cancer patient's name, age, sex, hospital/clinic/chart numbers, date of diagnosis, anatomic site, and town where the tissue specimen was obtained (this allows a crude estimation of residence). Registry information is coded (cancer site according to the Ninth Revision of the International Classification of Diseases), and all data is maintained on interactive disc files on the Gorgas Memorial Laboratory computer. Duplicate registration is monitored by checking the patient's name and hospital/clinical/chart number; when necessary specific charts are retrieved to verify information.

The National Cancer Register records only histopathologically diagnosed cancers. No attempt has been made to search hospital or clinic records for clinically diagnosed malignancy nor to include death certificate data. Limiting registration to histopathologically diagnosed malignancy eliminates local variation in clinical criteria and defines cases by objective histologic criteria. Pathologic criteria were constant between 1974–1978 because only three of Panama's nine Provinces (Panama, Colon, Chiriqui) had pathologists. Tissue specimens from all other provinces were sent to Panama City and evaluated by the Pathology Department of either Santo Tomas or Seguro Social Hospital. Both have

Hafez, E.S.E., Smith, J.P. (eds.), Carcinoma of the Cervix: Biology and Diagnosis. ISBN-13: 978-94-009-7487-6

Table 2. Most commonly diagnosed cancers in Panama, 1974–1978.

Male		Female	
Site	Rate[a]	Site	Rate[a]
Skin	16.9	Uterine[b] cervix	37.8
Prostate	14.4	Skin	14.7
Stomach	10.4	Breast	14.4
Trachea, Bronchus, Lung	5.0	Stomach	6.1
Rectum	3.2	Corpus uteri	4.1
Mouth	3.2	Ovary	3.1
Larynx	2.7	Mouth	3.7
Connective tissue	2.3	Rectum	3.1
Bladder	2.4	Colon	2.4
Liver	2.1	Other fem. genital	2.4
Penis	1.9	Connective tissue	1.8

[a]Incidence per 100,000 population adjusted to standard world population.
[b]Includes only invasive cervical cancer.

active Pathology Resident training programs and maintain frequent interchange with pathologists from major U.S., South American, and European Medical Schools.

Although the National Cancer Register underestimates true cancer incidence, it has high specificity. Table 2 summarizes the age standardized rates of the most common registered cancers between 1974–1978. Cancer of the uterine cervix was overwhelmingly the most frequent, accounting for 33% of all female cancers. This age-adjusted cervical cancer incidence was among the highest reported in the world.

II. CERVICAL CANCER IN PANAMA

II. A. Epidemiology

In order to investigate this high cervical cancer incidence, Standardized Cervical Cancer Register was established. Registry personnel visited every hospital and regional health center and enumerated all patients diagnosed as having, or certified as dying with, cervical cancer since 1974. The Standardized Register includes all data recommended by the IARC (World Health Organization 1976). It abstracts each patient's entire medical record and frequently includes data from several clinic and hospital charts. All data is maintained on computer files using the Conversational Statistical System for Medical Records (Kronmal et al. 1970).

The Standardized Cervical Cancer Register includes all patients seen between 1974–1978 at Panama City's three Medical Center teaching hospitals (The National Oncology Institute, Santo Tomas Hospital, and Social Security Medical Center). There have been 1,013 cervical cancers registered, 685 invasive and 328 intraepithelial. There were 708 cases detected by the National Cancer Register, and we discovered 305 previously unknown cases. These registered cases represent approximately 60% of all cervical cancers known to occur between 1974–1978. There were only three hospitals in Panama where invasive cervical cancer could be properly evaluated and treated; residents from anywhere in Panama had unrestricted access to their facilities; and physicians from every province were well-indoctrinated to the importance of rapidly referring cancer patients. Thus, these registered cases comprised a representative country-wide sample of invasive cervical cancer.

This sample revealed an invasive cervical cancer incidence of 28.2 per 100,000 women older than 15 years of age (the population at risk). Age-adjusted to the standard world population (Doll 1976) comprises 23.9 cases per 100,000. Six of seven provinces (including the capital) had a uniform age-adjusted invasive cervical cancer incidence of 20.7, while women from Herrera Province, with an age-adjusted rate of 66.3, had a 3.2 fold greater risk.

In addition to presenting a higher invasive cervical cancer incidence, 39/90 cases (43%) registered from Herrera involved women younger than 40 years. The age specific Herrera invasive cervical cancer incidence was significantly different from that seen in the remainder of Panama or in other countries (Henderson 1977; Waterhouse et al. 1976; Persaud 1977). This geographic clustering of unusually young cases was reported based on previous data from the National Cancer Register (Reeves et al. 1979; Valdés et al. 1979).

Confounding factors did not account for this clustering. Errors in denominator enumeration would cause an excessive rate. However, Panama maintained an extremely accurate census and the rural population was not affected by large-scale immigration. Biased case ascertainment did not occur; most Herrera cervical cancers (93%) were confirmed by biopsy (evaluated at the capital). Lastly, Herrera resembled other rural provinces with respect to physician: population ratio, availability of primary health care facilities and patient utilization of such facilities.

Other factors were similar among all provinces. Essentially all women were sexually active with an average of 2.0 life-time sex partners and multiple pregnancies. Most of them were from lower socioeconomic strata. Overall, 661 of 685 (96%) invasive cervical cancers were confirmed by biopsy; 629/661 (95%) were classified as epidermoid carcinoma, the remainder were adenocarcinoma. The ratio was similar in all provinces.

II. B. Clinical parameters

The National Oncology Institute is the only place in Panama with the capability to administer radiation therapy. Therefore virtually all invasive cervical cancer patients were referred, classified and treated there (592 of 685, 86%). Most women presented with advanced disease. However, between 1974–1978, *in situ* and lower staged cancers showed a relative increase in frequency (Figure 1). This may reflect an increased awareness of cervical cancer

and implementation of cancer detection programs in rural areas.

III. CONCLUDING REMARKS

Chronic non-infectious diseases are the most important contributors to mortality in Panama. Cancer has been among the first three causes of death since 1968, and invasive cervical cancer accounted for 33% of all female malignancies. In addition, Panama's age-adjusted invasive cervical cancer incidence ranked among the highest reported in the world. This is consistent with published data showing that cervical cancer mortality rates have steadily increased in developing countries of Asia, Africa and Latin America (Hill 1975), while concurrently decreasing in industrialized countries (Persaud 1977). The Latin America-Caribbean area supports the highest documented cervical cancer incidence (Caorsi et al. 1976; Hendersen 1977; Madrigal et al. 1976). The three areas reporting cervical cancer incidences comparable to Panama's (Cali, Colombia, Recife, Brazil; Kingston, Jamaica) have many cultural and ethnic similarities.

In addition to an overall high country-wide cervical cancer incidence, Herrera had an incidence three times greater than the rest of the country. Herrera Province also demonstrated a unique age profile with almost half the cases occurring before

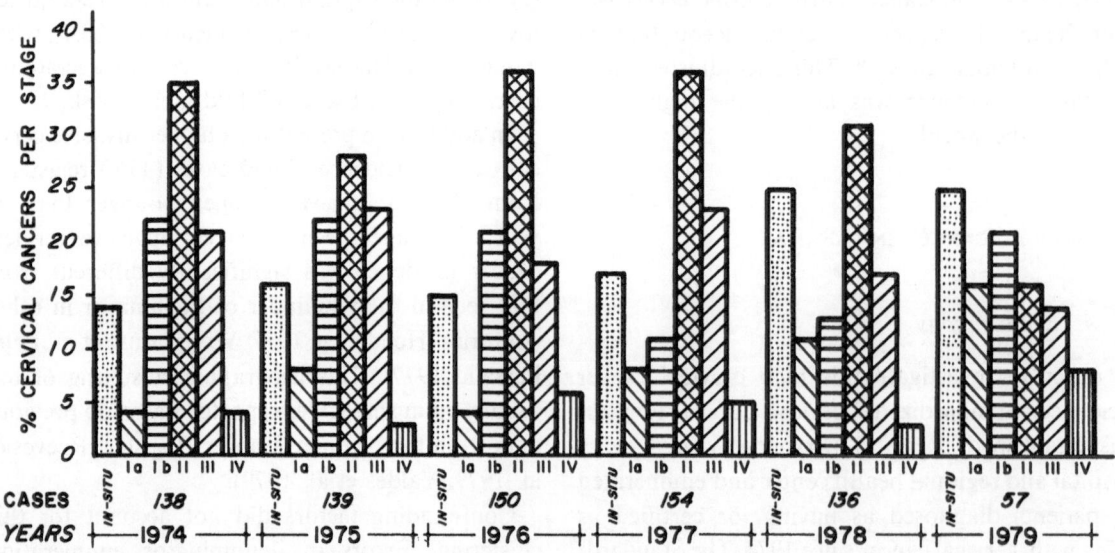

Figure 1. Percent cervical cancers in each clinical stage who were treated at the National Oncology Institute, 1974–1979.

40 years of age. Young women from Herrera were evidently exposed to unique risk factors (Alexander 1973; Kessler and Aurelian 1975). An understanding of these risk factors would not only contribute to the basic epidemiology of cervical cancer but would also allow development of effective local cancer prevention programs.

A cervical cancer situation similar to Panama's also exists in other Central American countries but has not as yet been well documented. It is possible to implement an accurate population-based cancer register in a developing country in spite of limited resources devoted to chronic diseases. Accurate documentation of disease occurrence is necessary to convince and enable individual governments to initiate and support well-planned, effective, cervical cancer detection and treatment programs.

ACKNOWLEDGEMENT

This investigation was partly supported by grant number 1 RO1 CA 25419-01, awarded by the National Cancer Institute, DHEW.

REFERENCES

Alexander ER: Possible etiologies of cancer of the cervix other than herpes virus. Cancer Res 33: 1485–1496, 1973.

Caorsi I, Norambuena ML: El cáncer cervicouterino en el sur de Chile. Bol Ofic Sanit Panamericana 80: 68–77, 1976.

Dirección de Estadística y Censo: Panamá en Chifras, Años 1972 a 1976. Panama. Contraloría General de la República, 1977.

Doll R: Comparison between registries, age standardized rates. *In* Waterhouse J, Muir C, Correa P, Powell J (eds): Cancer incidence in five continents Vol III. Geneva: IARC, 1976: 453–459.

Henderson BE (ed): Epidemiology and cancer registries of Pacific basin. National Cancer Institute Monograph 47, 1977.

Hill GB: Mortality from malignant neoplasm of the uterus since 1950. WHO Statistical Report 28: 323–338, 1975.

Kessler IL, Aurelian L: Uterine-Cervix. *In*: Schottenfeld (ed): Cancer Epidemiology and Prevention, Current Concepts. Springfield, Ill: Thomas, 1975: 262–317.

Kronmal RA, Bender L, Mortenasen J: A conversational Statistical System for Medical Records. J Roy Stat Soc Series C 19: 82–92, 1970.

Madrigal LM, Assal NE, Anderson PS: Cáncer de los organos de la reproducción en Costa Rica. Bol Ofic Sant Panamericana 81: 345–354, 1976.

Persaud V: Geographical pathology of cancer of the uterine cervix. Trop Geogr Med 29: 335–345, 1977.

Reeves WC, Britton R, Valdés PL, Benenson AS: Cervical cancer in Panama. Am J Epidemiol 110: 369, 1979.

Valdés PF, Britton R, Reeves WC, Benenson AS: Cáncer del cuello uterino en Panamá. Rev Med Panama 4: 236–245, 1979.

Waterhouse J, Muir C, Correa P, Powell J (eds): Cancer Incidence in Five Continents Vol III. Geneva: IARC, 1976: 486–535.

World Health Organization: WHO Handbook for Standardized Cancer Registries. Geneva: World Health Organization, 1976.

5. CERVICAL CARCINOMA DETECTION AND MORTALITY IN CHILE

A. DABANCENS

The final objective of a cervical cancer control program is to diminish the rates of mortality from such disease in a determined population.

The survival for a woman with symptomatic cervical cancer of five years does not reach 50%. However, if the disease is diagnosed in its intraepithelial stage, its prognosis is most favorable, since 100% of success can be attained with an adequate treatment while at the same time, the therapeutic methods involved, diminish substantially their complexity and costs.

For these reasons it was decided that the national program for the control of cervical cancer should focus its efforts towards the development in Chile, of an infrastructure capable of detecting, diagnosing and treating of uterine cervical carcinoma in its preclinical stages.

This present report analyzes the characteristics which represent the rates of mortality caused by uterine cervical cancer, with the double object of identifying the groups of major risk and to evaluate the influence of the cytologic detection program on this disease.

The information relating to deaths from cervical cancer was obtained from the yearbook on 'The General Mortality and Causes of Death' published by the Health Ministry. Data regarding population were taken from the records of the National Institute of Statistics whilst information referring to the program was taken from the files of the Cytopathology and Cancer Control Service.

I. RESULTS

I. A. Standardized rates of mortality.

The evolution of the specific rates of mortality from uterine cervical cancer showed a gradual growth from 1961 to 1974 and a sustained diminution in the last three years.

Although the rate of mortality from cancer of the cervix in Chile fluctuates around 22 per 100,000 women as an average, the specific rates for each age group reflect a marked increment in older people duplicating the average value after 55 years of age (Figure 1).

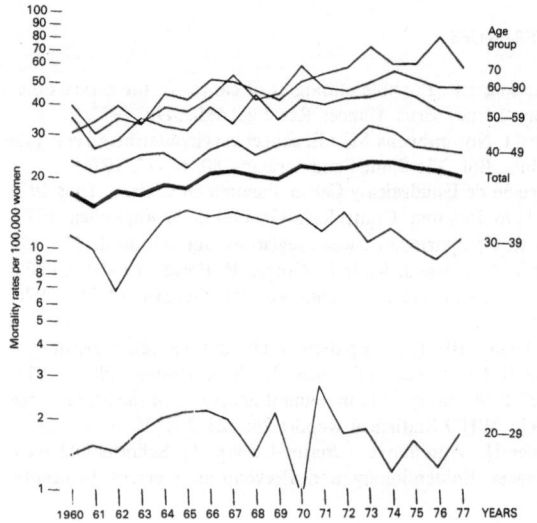

Fig. 1. Mortality rates of uterine cervical cancer, Chile, 1960–197'

I. B. Evolution of the rates of mortality

Between 1960 and 1977, the evolution of specific rates of mortality from cancer of the uterine cervix demonstrates how the distinct age curves have been spread out in the last ten years while the group of 30 to 39 years has been particularly favored by a decreasing tendency which contrasts with the upward tendency in the group of over 60 years of age.

I. C. Influence of the cytologic detection program

In order to analyze the influence of the cytologic detection program on the rates of mortality from cervical cancer, the results achieved by the preventive program in the northern area of Santiago, on which complete data are available, are given here.

On July 1st, 1978, there were 161,443 women of

Hafez, E.S.E., Smith, J.P. (eds.), Carcinoma of the Cervix: Biology and Diagnosis. ISBN-13: 978-94-009-7487-6

over 20 years of age. Between 1966 and 1978 cytologic examination had been made on 86,197 women, or 53,39% of that population. The early detection of uterine cervical cancer has covered preferentially the groups of younger women where the prevalence of intraepithelial lesions is higher. As a result of the cytologic screening in the northern area of Santiago, 546 asymptomatic patients with intraepithelial lesions have been diagnosed and treated. This figure represents an important number of women in whom the appearance of an invading cancer of the uterine cervix has been avoided (Table 2).

The adventageous effect of the program should lead to a precocious diminution in the rates of clinical cancer so that in the future, a reduction in the rates of mortality will occur. From the lists of women who died from cancer of the cervix in the northern area of Santiago, search was made in the Cytopathologic Program and the Control of Cancer registers for the cytologic antecedents attending the deceased persons. In this way, it was possible to determine the rates of mortality both of the women submitted to the program as also of those who did not figure in the registers and who, presumably have had no cytologic controls.

Comparing the rates of mortality found in both groups, it is shown that women forming part of the detection program present diminution superior to 90% with respect to the rate affecting those women who had not practised cytologic examinations and that the said rate only reached 26% of the hoped-for

value.

In consequence, 43.2 deaths per 100,000 adult women, or 53,39% of that population (Table 1). The early detection of uterine cervical cancer has covered

II. COMMENTS

In Chile, rates of mortality from cancer of the cervix have shown an increasing tendency since there are registers which reflect a better diagnosis as well as a real increment of the disease consecutive to the greater ageing of the population.

The value of the cervix cancer control program shown in the Northern Hemisphere and accepted universally by health organisms had not been demonstrated numerically in our country owing to the low coverage level reached after twelve years of operation. We believe, nevertheless, that the slight diminution of the rate of mortality from cervical cancer in the last three years will be maintained and accentuated in the coming years. It may be foreseen, however, that the national rates of mortality will not be able to show material decreases until the coverage of the program reaches the majority of the population at risk.

Although the strong impact produced by the program for the early detection of cancer does not constitute an academic reality, it represents the first demonstration that health organization in Chile is adequate for implementing this type of preventive programs and that, in our environment, the struggle against uterine cervical cancer can be successful.

Table 1. Percentage of the population with one or more Pap smears in different age groups.

Age group	Number of women	Northern area population	% of population studied
20 – 44	66,609	106,268	62.68
45 – 65	16,546	42,400	39.02
65 and more	3,042	12,775	23.81
	86,197	161,443	53.39

Table 2. Expected and observed mortality rates of uterine cervical cancer in the northern area of Santiago (1970–1977) (per 100,000 women above 20 years old).

	Expected rate	Observed rate
Without previous Pap	27.90	47.84
With previous Pap	17.40	4.64

III. CONCLUSIONS

It is necessary to emphasize the conclusions of this analysis which have major operational importance in the field of Public health:

1. After an increase noted up to 1974, the rate of mortality from cervical cancer with standardized population tends to diminish.
2. The rate of mortality shows a declining tendency in the group of 30–39 years (cytologically examined).
3. Mortality from cervical cancer is ten times less in females who have had access to cytologic examinations.

6. CERVICAL CARCINOMA IN EL SALVADOR

N. Díaz-Bazán

I. GEOGRAPHICAL CANCER PATHOLOGY

I.A. Latin-American countries

Studies of the geographical pathology throughout the world have demonstrated that the incidence and characteristics of uterine carcinoma change according to different geographical zones, different countries and ethnic groups. Some Latin-American countries have similar characteristics in incidence, prevalence, age, and obstetrical history, to name a few.

I.B. Central American countries

Countries in Central America have similar geographical, racial, socio-economic, nutritional, climatic and religious factors related to geographical cancer pathology. In all Central American countries, for example (with the exception of Costa Rica), cervical carcinoma represents the most predominant type of neoplasia, relating also to age incidence, obstetrical history and histopathological types.

I.C. Republic of El Salvador, C.A.

Despite similar population and living conditions in Central America, there are difinite local differences found in El Salvador in relation to regional pa-

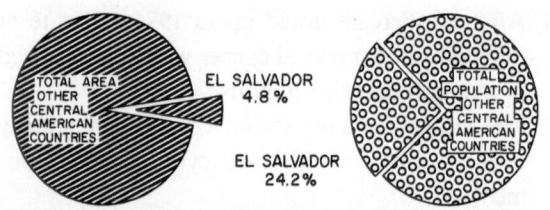

Figure 1. Comparison of area and population of El Salvador with other Central American countries. El Salvador represents only 4.8% of the total Central American area and 24.2% of the total population.

thology. This chapter will describe the very high incidence of cervical carcinoma associated with pregnancy, as well as the extraordinary and unexplained incidence of cervical carcinoma associated with procidentia (Díaz- Bazán 1964; Díaz-Bazán 1965).

II. GEOGRAPHICAL CHARACTERISTICS

II.A. Central American countries

The population of Central America has two ethnological origins: the native and Spanish, which represents a mixed population of Spanish-American. There are certain differences however, as the Caribbean area received black immigration from the Antilles.

II.B. El Salvador

El Salvador is located in the center of Central America, with a border coastline to the Pacific Ocean. This is the smallest and most densely populated country in Central America. As of 1978, the population was estimated at 4,435,000, representing 210 inhabitants per square kilometer. The Bureau of Statistics and Census calculated a 3.2% increase in population from 1976 to 1977. El Salvador represents just 4.8% of the total Central American area and 24.2% of the total Central American population (Figure 1).

The total female population over 25 years of age represents 55.2% of the total population. A definite and progressive decrease in the possible susceptibility of cervical carcinoma can be observed in each successive five-year age group (Figure 2).

Hafez, E.S.E., Smith, J.P. (eds.), Carcinoma of the Cervix: Biology and Diagnosis. ISBN-13: 978-94-009-7487-6
© 1982, Martinus Nijhoff Publishers, The Hague/Boston/London.

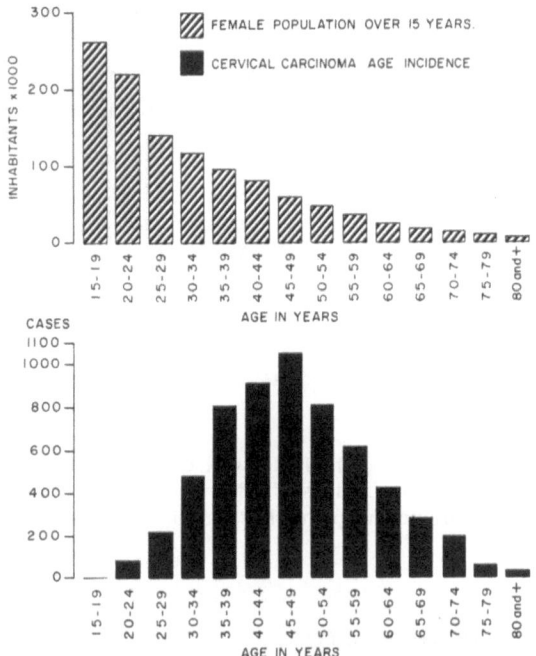

Figure 2. Republic of El Salvador, C.A. *Upper:* Female population over 15 years of age susceptible to cervical carcinoma. *Lower:* Cervical carcinoma age incidence, analysis of 6,158 cases. Ratio per population in age groups.

III. INCIDENCE OF CERVICAL CARCINOMA

Cervical carcinoma is the predominant type of neoplastic disease and ranks highest in incidence throughout most Central American countries. In El Salvador, the predominant type of malignant disease is the gynecological cancer representing 46% of all cancer localization. The cervical localization is highly predominant, representing 40% of cancer in general, 62% of cancer in women and 88.5% of gynecological cancer (Díaz-Bazán 1964; Infante-Díaz 1964; Astacio 1960; Sosa 1954).

In El Salvador, 11,680 cases of cervical carcinoma were detected between 1963–1977. From this series, 7,859 cases (67%) corresponded to invasive carcinoma and 3,821 (33%) to carcinoma *in situ.* Due to the progressive cancer detection program, there has been a significant improvement in the statistical data in detecting the increase of carcinoma *in situ* cases and their relationship to invasive carcinoma (Figure 3).

Concerning invasive cervical carcinoma only, an incidence of 25.5 × 100,000 exists in relation to the total female population, whereas 46.3 × 100,000

exists in relation to the population over 15 years of age. From two groups of women in the United States, the rate of incidence varies from a low 3.6 × 100,000 in Jewish women to a high of 97.6 × 100,000 for Puerto Rico women (Novak et al. 1976).

IV. AGE INCIDENCE

Invasive cervical carcinoma in the United States and other countries is a disease of advanced age – the peak incidence occurring between the ages of 45 to 55 years (Gusberg and Frick 1970; Ackermann and Del Regato 1970; Novak et al. 1976; Parsons and Sommers 1978). In the United Kingdom, the occurrence is more frequent between the age of 40 and 60 years (Way 1951). Cervical carcinoma is infrequently found in young women and there are few cases reporting an incidence occurring in women younger than 20 years of age. In the United States, however, cervical carcinoma has been detected in more women in their twenties (Parsons and Sommers 1978). Out of 2,568 patients studied in El Salvador, 148 (5.3%) cases were found in the 20–29 years age group (Díaz-Bazán 1965).

From 1969–1975, there were 6,158 cases of cervical carcinoma reviewed, showing a peak incidence occurring in the 45–49 year age group (1,090 cases, 17%). The incidence decreased with every decrease in age group (Figure 2). For instance, there were 510 cases found in women aged 30–34 years and 300 cases in the 20–29 year age group. From this series, 59% of the total incidence corresponded to the 20–49

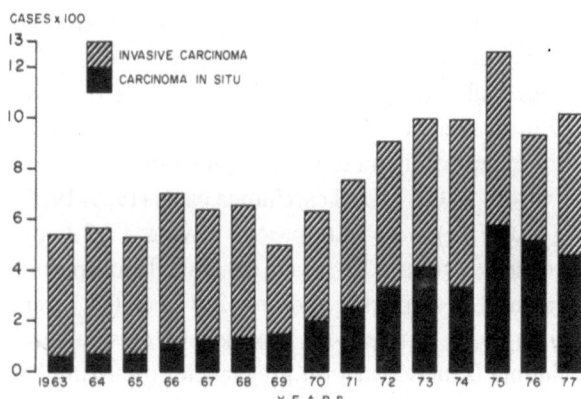

Figure 3. Cervical carcinoma in El Salvador, C.A. Study of 11,680 cases (1963–1977). Comparison of proportion of carcinoma *in situ* with invasive carcinoma.

year age group and 41% to the 50 year and over age group. There are more younger incidences in El Salvador as compared to other countries in Latin America.

V. MARITAL STATUS AND OBSTETRICAL HISTORY

There is a correlation between the incidence of cervical carcinoma with early marriage, sexual activities and number of pregnancies.

V.A. Marriage and sexual relations

Over 50% of patients with cervical carcinoma married before the age of 20 years (Lombard and Potter 1950; Ackerman and Del Regato 1970). The most demonstrative evidence to the relationship of sexual activity and carcinoma is a study from Canada where 13,000 death certificates of nuns showed no single case of cervical carcinoma (Gagnon 1950, 1952). Whereas, one report on the prisons in the United States, showed a high incidence of cervical carcinoma among women who have lived in promiscuity (Pereyra 1961). Evidence is similarly shown on the high incidence in prostitutes (Raven 1958). In El Salvador, one study on 1,835 cases having cervical carcinoma, showed that 1,373 cases (75%) were between the ages of 12–19 years.

V.B. Obstetrical history and age of first delivery

Cervical carcinoma represents a high incidence in multiparous women and is relatively rare in nulliparous (Ackerman and Del Regato 1970). In the United Kingdom, a representative series showed 93.3% incidence were multiparous and only 6.7% were nulliparous (Way 1951). In most Latin and Central American countries, cervical carcinoma is highly predominant in multiparous women.

From 5,809 cervical carcinoma cases (1969–1975), 4,450 (77%) were multiparous having 4–12 + deliveries; 960 cases (17%) were controlled multiparous having 1–3 deliveries; and only 238 cases (4%) were nulliparous (Figure 4). The risk of cervical carcinoma is increased with pregnancies occurring before the age of 20 years. Cervical carcinoma cases in El Salvador showed a 70% incidence when the first delivery took place in women under 21 years of age.

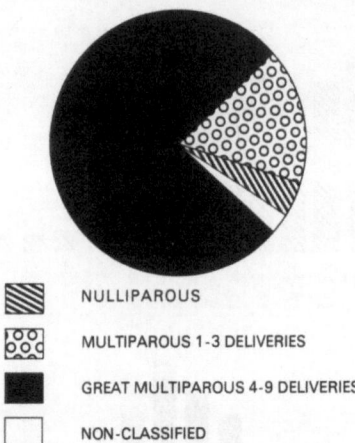

	NULLIPAROUS
	MULTIPAROUS 1-3 DELIVERIES
	GREAT MULTIPAROUS 4-9 DELIVERIES
	NON-CLASSIFIED

Figure 4. Republic of El Salvador, C.A. Cervical carcinoma and obstetrical history, analysis of 5,809 cases: great multiparous 76.6%; controlled multiparous 16.8%; nulliparous 4%, non-classified 2.6%.

VI. PATHOLOGICAL TYPES

Two pathological types of cervical carcinoma correspond to the two types of epithelium of the cervix: (1) epidermoid carcinoma or squamous cell carcinoma, and (2) adenocarcinoma. The average frequency is 95% epidermoid carcinoma and 5% adenocarcinoa (Gusberg and Frick 1970; Ackermann and Del Regato 1970). There were 2,857 cases of invasive cervical carcinoma pathologically analyzed, showing a 97% incidence of epidermoid carcinoma and 3% adenocarcinoma. In the epidermoid group, the following proportions were found: spinal cell – 36%, transitional – 36%, indifferentiated – 19%, and non-classified – 8.5%.

All studies reviewing the Salvadorean bibliography from various authors were found consistent (Díaz-Bazán 1965; Sosa 1954; Astacio 1964; Infante-Díaz 1964). From a Central American survey, histopathological types of cervical carcinoma showed that epidermoid carcinoma ranged between 93 to 98% and adenocarcinoma was between 1 to 3%.

VII. INTERNATIONAL CLINICAL CLASSIFICATION

Between 1969–1975, a series of 5,205 cases of cervical carcinoma were analyzed by the International Clinical Classification system. There were 1,915 cases (37%) of carcinoma *in situ*, Stage 0° detected and 3,290 cases of invasive carcinoma (63%). The different stages of invasive carcinoma showed the following: 510 cases were found in Stage I (15.5%), 1,350 cases in Stage II (41%), 1,250 cases in Stage III (38%) and 180 cases in Stage IV (5,5%). These results were determined strictly by clinical examination only.

VIII. SOCIOECONOMIC AND ETIOLOGICAL FACTORS

VIII.A. Socioeconomic groups

Epidemiological factors emphasize the socioeconomic status comparing to the tendency to marry early and have children before the age of 20 years. In the United States, as in other countries of similar positions, cervical carcinoma has been shown more frequently in black population, perhaps being due to a less favorable economic condition, poor obstetrical practice and inadequate hygiene. The incidence apparently decreases among blacks as their economic status improves (Parsons and Sommers 1978).

VIII.B. Other etiological factors

In 1964, statistical data of Latin American countries proved that highest incidence of carcinoma of the uterine cervix occurs in the lowest socioeconomic population. A study from Boston found that the incidence of cancer was 3 per 1000 patients attending a private hospital, compared to 10 per 1000 patients admitted to Boston City Hospital which cares for low socioeconomic populations (Marchant 1969). Comparing different health centers in El Salvador, a very high incidence of cervical carcinoma was detected in charity hospitals, while a very marked decrease of incidence was shown in social security and other semi-private hospitals. The lowest incidence was shown in private health centers.

Promiscuity is a very important factor according to studies on prostitutes and prisoners where the frequency of cervical cancer is four times greater when compared with other groups of patients (Pereyra 1961; Raven 1958), for instance, cervical carcinoma is practically unknown in virgins (Gagnon 1950).

In El Salvador, cervical carcinoma is a very predominant type of neoplastic localization, representing 40% of all cancers in general. Cervical carcinoma is highly predominant in the lowest socioeconomic group, precisely where the following conditions coincided: (a) precocious sexual intercourse, (b) pregnancies occurring at age 20 or less, (c) no control of natality, (d) multiple deliveries, (e) promiscuity, (f) inadequate hygiene, (g) bad nutrition, (h) no systematic medical examination, and (i) lack of sufficient study in the incidence of carcinoma of the penis.

There have been 20 cases of carcinoma of the penis reported giving an incidence of $2.6 \times 100,000$ inhabitants (Levy Van Severen 1947). A review of the National Cancer Statistics report carcinoma of the penis in 146 cases from 1945–1962, representing 1.8% of all cancer localizations (Infante-Díaz 1964).

IX. INCIDENCE OF CERVICAL CARCINOMA IN RELATION TO ENDOMETRIAL CARCINOMA

Statistical data from the United States and some European countries has reported a progressive increase in the incidence of endometrial carcinoma (Novak et al. 1976; Gusberg and Frick 1970; Parsons and Sommers 1978). The ratio of occurrence of carcinoma of the endometrium to carcinoma of the cervix has undergone a considerable change in the past three decades: from 1×2.5 to 1×1.4.

In most Latin American countries, the proportion of cervical carcinoma to endometrial carcinoma is quite different. In El Salvador (1945–1966), 130 cases of endometrial carcinoma were found, contrasting with 3,459 cases of cervical carcinoma, representing an incidence of 1×25 (Díaz-Bazán 1964, 1979). These findings are comparable to other Latin American studies (Contreras et al. 1964; Grosmann-Siegert 1964). When epidemiologically comparing statistical data from Latin American countries were different geographic zones have such variance (Mexico connecting with North America, Central America and South America on the completely opposite side of the globe), a greater significance is placed on socioeconomic and living conditions rather than on geographical zones.

X. CERVICAL CARCINOMA ASSOCIATED WITH PROCIDENTIA

Cervical carcinoma in complete prolapse-procidentia is very rare. A prolapse uterus has generally an immunity to carcinoma. There is little on the subject emphasizing the rarity of this condition. A review of world literature indicates 184 proven cases, including the series of 35 cases from El Salvador, representing the highest incidence throughout the world (Figure 5) (Díaz-Bazán 1964; Novak et al. 1976).

XI. CONCLUDING REMARKS

Important epidemiological characteristics in El Salvador include: cervical carcinoma represents 40% of all cancer localizations; 62% of all cancer is found in the female and 89% constitute gynecological cancer. The proportion of endometrial carcinoma in relation to cervical carcinoma is 1 × 25, whereas the proportion of uterine sarcoma in relation to uterine carcinoma is 1 × 100. There is a definite association between the high incidence of cervical carcinoma with pregnancy (1 carcinoma × 830 obstetrical patients). Finally, there is an exceptional and unexplained incidence of carcinoma associated with procidentia which requires further investigative research.

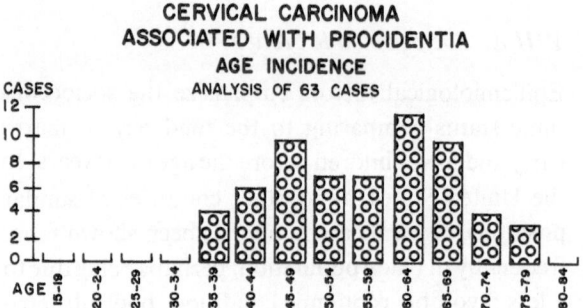

Figure 5. Comparative age incidence in cervical carcinoma associated with procidentia.

REFERENCES

Ackerman LV, Del Regato JA: Cancer, Diagnosis, Treatment & Prognosis. C.V. Mosby Co, 4th ed, 169 pp, 1970.

Astacio Julio: Contribución al Estudio del Cáncer. Tésis Doctoral, Escuela de Medicina, Universidad de El Salvador, San Salvador, El Salvador, C.A., 48 pp, 1960.

Astacio JN: Carcinoma del Cuello Uterino. Consideraciones Anatomo-Patológicas. Arch Colegio Médico de El Salvador 17: 72–79, 1964.

Contreras R, Vásquez-Rinza E, Lastro-Garrido N: Patología Geográfica del Cáncer del Utero en México. Symposium de Epidemiologia del Cáncer del Utero, U.I.C.C., La Prensa Médica, Ed. Argentina, 73–75, 1964.

Díaz-Bazán N: Patología Geográfica del Cáncer del Utero en Centro América. Symposium sobre Epidemiología del Cáncer del Utero, U.I.C.C., México, D.F., La Prensa Médica, Ed. Argentina, 47–53, 1964.

Díaz-Bazán N: Aspectos Epidemiológicos del Cáncer del Utero en El Salvador y Centro América. Arch Col Médico de El Salvador 18: 1–23, 1965. Abstract published The Year Book. Obst & Gyn Greenhill JP, 1965–1966) 508.

Diaz-Bazán N: Cervical Cancer with Procidentia in El Salvador. Report of 10 New Cases. Obstetrics and Gynecology 23: 281–288, 1964.

Gagnon F: Contribution to the Study of the Etiology and Prevention of Cancer of the Cervix of the Uterus. Am J Obst & Gynec 60: 516–522, 1950.

Gagnon F: Lack of Occurrence of Cervical Carcinoma in Nuns. Proc Second Nat Cancer Conference I: 625, 1952.

Grossman-Siegert E: Patología Geográfica del Cáncer del Utero en Venezuela. Symposium sobre Epidemiología del Cáncer del Utero, U.I.C.C., La Prensa Médica, Ed. Argentina, 93–96, 1964.

Gusberg SB, Frick II, HC: Corscaden Gynecological Cancer. The Williams & Wilkins Co., 4th ed, 176 pp, 1970.

Infants-Díaz S: Cáncer en El Salvador. Editorial Ministerio de Educación, San Salvador, El Salvador, C.A. 251 pp, 1964.

Levy Van Severen H: Consideraciones sobre 20 casos de Cáncer del Pene. Gaceta Médica de Occidente, El Salvador, C.A. 55: 1899, 1947.

Lombard HL, Potter EA: Epidemiological Aspects of Cancer of the Cervix, Hereditary and Environmental Factors. Cancer 3: 960, 1950.

Marchant DJ: Current Concepts, Cancer of the Cervix. New England Med 281: 602, 1969.

Novak ER, Jones GS, Jones HW: Novak's Text Book of Gynecology. The Williams & Wilkins Co., 9th ed. Carcinoma of the Cervix, pp 246. Cervical Carcinoma with Prolapse, pp 310, 1976.

Parsons L, Sommers SC: Gynecology. 2nd ed. W.B. Saunders Co., Chapter 59 Cancer of the Cervix, pp 1300–1312, 1978.

Pereyra AJ: The Relationship of Sexual Activity to Cervical Cancer. Obst & Gynec 17: 154–159, 1961.

Raven RW: Cancer. Vol. 3. London: Butterworth Co., 256–259, 1958.

Sosa M: Cáncer en El Salvador, Estudio Analítico de 1750 Casos. Tésis Doctoral, Universidad de El Salvador, El Salvador, C.A. pp 6, 1954.

Way S: Malignant Disease of the Female Genital Tract. Philadelphia: The Blackinston Co., pp 239, 1950.

7. CERVICAL CARCINOMA IN KUWAIT

H. Hathout, S. Motawy and S. Hassan

Kuwait is an Arab Moslem country with a rapidly growing population that increased from one third of a million in 1961 to one and one third million in 1980. The Kuwaiti population constitutes less than half of the total inhabitants, as the remainder represents imported – mainly Arab – labor. The way of life of the society reflects on the magnitude of the cervical cancer problem, being devoid of some of the currently established socio-etiologic factors (Abel 1973). Sexual conservatism is prevalent, and the incidence of premarital sex is unacceptable. Religious dictates also include male circumcision, meticulous genital hygiene in both sexes and a ritual bath after intercourse, menstruation and the puerperium.

I. INCIDENCE

The extent of cervical carcinoma in Kuwait is small. Between 1971–1978 inclusive, 144 cases of cervical carcinoma were received, apart from 2 cases of leiomyosarcoma in cervical fibroids. Of these 144 patients, 58 came from neighboring countries for the purpose of receiving treatment, leaving only 86 who were residents of Kuwait, of whom 29 were Kuwaities and 57 non-Kuwaities. Concerning carcinoma of the cervix, the principal beneficiaries of the Radiotherapy-Oncology Service (1969), are patients from neighboring countries lacking such facilities.

Considering only patients residing in Kuwait, the average number of cases of cervical carcinoma was 10.8 per year. Relating to the average annual number of the female population the relative frequency of cervical carcinoma was around 2.4 cases per 100,000 females. The relative frequency for non-Kuwaities was 3.3 per 100,000 females, and for Kuwaities only 1.5. The figure for non-Kuwaities might entail some underestimation for they are a labile group and many foreigners do not spend all their life-span in Kuwait. The figure for Kuwaities is quite low, much lower than the 4.2 per 100,000 Jewish women in Israel (Menczer et al. 1978).

There is only one gynecologic pathology laboratory and one oncology center in the country. This incidence depicts mainly invasive carcinoma. Only 4 cases had pre-invasive cancer when diagnosed, and in the absence of a regular panpopulation screening program, there is no clue as to the number of *in situ's* that could have been discovered. Such a program has not been deemed feasible by the authorities due to the low incidence, especially since those women at highest risk would be the least likely to participate in such a program (Wakefield 1971; Scaiffe 1972). Inspite of the availability of an adequate cytology service supporting the hospital gynecology clinics, only 7 patients were diagnosed after routine screening cytology. Although the majority of patients attending the gynecologic clinic are cytologically examined, the same does not apply to pregnant women.

II. PATIENT CHARACTERISTICS

Many nationalities were represented in the patient population, but the large majority were Arabs. Ethnic groups included 122 Arabs, 12 Indians, 4 Europeans, 3 Iranians and 3 miscellaneous. Religion was Islam in 124, Christianity in 15 and Hinduism in 5. Marital status denoted 106 married, 28 widowed, 7 divorced and 3 single. The age (Figure 1) ranged between 23 and 82 years, with maximal concentration in the 40–49 and 50–59 age groups. It is hoped that with female education now

Hafez, E.S.E., Smith, J.P. (eds.), Carcinoma of the Cervix: Biology and Diagnosis. ISBN-13: 978-94-009-7487-6

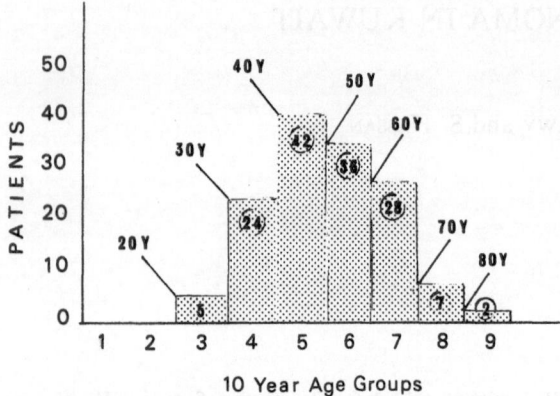

Figure 1. Age distribution in 10-year age groups amongst 144 cases of cervical carcinoma in Kuwait, 1971–78.

in progress, public awareness and motivation will result in earlier diagnosis at an earlier age.

Presently there are more females than males at the University of Kuwait, and it is becoming more common to see women coming to the gynecology clinics only for a 'Pap smear' check-up without having gynecologic complaints. It is this growing demand that will stimulate the authorities to reinforce the cytology services. Government health facilities in Kuwait, including cytology, are open to everyone free of charge, so that the financial factor is not a deterrent to the individual, nor does it pose an appreciable taxation over a wealthy state like Kuwait.

The majority of the patients in this series (76) were postmenopausal when diagnosed. The postmenopausal period ranged between 1 and 25 years, the mean being 15–19 years. Again, earlier diagnosis might alter this pattern in the future. Obstetric history denoted previous deliveries ranging between 0–15 with an average of 6.2 deliveries per patient. Abortions (usually spontaneous, due to the restrictive abortion policy) varies from 0–24 per patient with an average of 1 abortion. Total gravidity ranged between 0–32 with an average of 7.2 pregnancies per patient. These figures express high parity and early age of sexual activity (i.e. by marriage in this society), but this does not vary from the general population at large. It is known that in Kuwait, women marry at an early age and attain high parity (Kuwait, having one of the highest birth rates in the world); neither of which seems to be

incompatible with that of low incidence of cervical carcinoma.

III. PRESENTATION

The majority of patients (125) were presented with the usual symptom of abnormal bleeding and/or leucorrhoea. A minority were presented with pain (6), urinary symptoms (2) or cachexia (2). In two, the diagnosis was incidental during histology of the removed unsuspicious uterus. Two were diagnosed coinciding with other illnesses, while 7 were detected by cytology check-up without having any complaint. Three cases were pregnant. Two were aborted for the sake of treatment while the third remained undiagnosed until delivered by cesarean section for antepartum bleeding and cervical dystocia. Associated malignancy was noted in 2 cases, one with concomitant thyroid carcinoma and the other with radical mastectomy for breast cancer 4 years previously.

This series shows a regrettable delay in diagnosis (Table 1). Esthetic reasons or fear tend to prolong the patients' tolerance of their symptoms. The prevalence of Stages II and III lags behind the modern trends (Campos 1971; Roman and Latour 1967). Education, motivation and extension of cytology services are the hope for a better future in Kuwait.

IV. PATHOLOGY PATTERNS

To ensure meaningful comparison with other communities the currently recognized classifications were adopted. Invasive cancer was classified into

Table 1. Relative proportions of various stages of cervical carcinoma when first diagnosed.

Stage at diagnosis	No.	%
Intraepithelial	4	2.8
Microinvasive	4	2.8
Stage I	18	12.5
II	67	46.5
III	31	21.5
IV	20	13.9
Total	144	100.0

Table 2. Proportion of various histopathologic patterns of cervical carcinoma in Kuwait, 1971–1978 (144 cases).

Epidermoid invasive	124	
microinvasive	4	91.7%
intraepithelial	4	
Adenocarcinoma	8	5.5%
Muco-epidermoid	2	
Adenosquamous	2	2.8%

epidermoid, glandular and reserve cell types (Abel 1973) and the degree of differentiation was noted (Ferenczy 1977). In epidermoid carcinoma, the international histologic typing as large cell keratinizing, large cell nonkeratinizing and small cell nonkeratinizing was followed (Poulsen et al. 1975). For microinvasive epidermoid carcinoma the maximal limit for stromal invasion was 3 mm from the highest basal lamina. Intraepithelial carcinoma with or without glandular filling was diagnosed on cone biopsy. Histologic patterns appeared similar to most published series (Table 2). In 124 invasive epidermoid carcinomas, tumor differentiation was moderate in 108, good in 8 and poor in 8. Adenocarcinomas were mostly well differentiated.

V. CONCLUDING REMARKS

Various attempts have been made to define groups of women who are at low risk or at high risk of cervical cancer (Novak et al. 1971), and several etiologic factors are being extensively studied. There is little doubt that sexual activity correlates to cervical cancer, although there is no justification that this type of cancer is of monofactorial etiology. The Kuwaiti society exhibits the interesting association of extreme sexual conservatism and meticulous personal hygiene with a very low incidence of carcinoma of the cervix, inspite of low age at marriage and high parity.

REFERENCES

Abel MR: Invasive carcinomas of uterine cervix. *In* Norris H, Hertig A, Abell M (eds): The Uterus. International Academy of Pathology Monograph. Baltimore: Williams & Wilkins, 1973, pp 41.

Campos JL: Mortality trends in carcinoma of the cervix uteri. J Chronic Dis 24: 701, 1971.

Ferenczy A: Carcinoma and other malignant tumors of the cervix. *In* Blaustein A (ed): Pathology of the Female Genital Tract. New York: Springer-Verlag, 1977, 180.

Menczer J, Modan B, Oelsner G, Sharon Z, Steintiz R, Sampson

S: Adenocarcinoma of the uterine cervix in Jewish women. A distinct epidemiological entity. Cancer 41: 2464, 1978.

Novak E, Jones G, Jones H: *In:* Gynecology (condensed from Novak's). Baltimore: Williams & Wilkins, 1971, 101.

Poulson HE, Taylor CW, Sobin LH: Histological Typing of Female Genital Tract Tumors. Geneva: WHO, 1975, 51.

Roman TN, Latour JPA: The effect of early diagnosis on survival statistics in carcinoma of the uterine cercix. Am J Obstet Gynecol 97: 739, 1967.

Scaiffe B: A survey of cervical cytology in general practice. B Med J 3: 200, 1972.

Makefield J: The family doctor and cervical cytology. A study of 38,741 women. Health Trends 3: 25, 1971.

8. ABNORMAL CERVICAL CYTOLOGY IN JAMAICA

J.St.E. Hall

I. CERVICAL CYTOLOGY

Proper management of the abnormal Papanicolaou smear is of the greatest importance in clinical practice. Cancer of the cervix may well be a preventable disease and much of the credit for recognising this belongs to G.N. Papanicolaou whose definitive studies on vaginal and cervical cytology at the Cornell Medical College, New York proved the usefulness of exfoliative cytology in dectecting cervical cancer in its incipiency – a stage which can be completely removed or cured by simple forms of treatment. Papanicolaou's work ranks as one of the greatest contributions to science and the report on his studies is now one of the classics in medical literature (Papanicolaou and Trout 1943). Notable contributions to the development of this diagnostic tool have been made by Ruth Graham and associates (1948), Earnst Ayre (1954) in the United States, and by Watchel and Plester (1954) and Anderson (1959) in the United Kingdom. From the nature of the cells seen and the general pattern of the smear a trained cytoligst can confidently differentiate between cervical dysplasia, carcinoma *in situ* and invasive cancer (Papanicolaou and Trout 1943; Reagan et al. 1957; Koss and Durfee 1961). A review of the false negative rate for cervical cytology in nine published series shows a range of from 2.4 to 18 per cent. This argues a strong place for repeat Pap smears in certain cases, for periodic screening and follow-up.

I.A. Screening programmes

One of the earliest screening programmes in the United States began in Toledo, Ohio in 1947. By 1964 about 100,000 of the city's 160,000 women had been screened cytologically. In Memphis, Tennessee intensive publicity campaigns supported the programme, resulting in a satisfactory participation by the public. In this project, during the period 1952 to 1957 cytology smears were taken at least once from 151,000 women who represented 67.3 per cent of the white population and 57.3 per cent of the negro population aged 20 years and over (Kaiser et al. 1960). Among many other mass cytology screening programmes reported on are that of British Columbia, Canada (Fidler et al. 1968) and that in Aberdeen, Scotland (MacGregor 1967). It is claimed that as a result of the British Columbia screening programme there has been a decline in the incidence of clinical cancer from 28.4 per 100,000 in 1955 to 13.6 per 100,000 in 1966, that is, a 48 per cent decrease in 12 years. A fall in mortality rate was also reported from 11 to 7.8 per 100,000 per annum. Other screening programmes in different parts of the world show roughly similar results. Despite these claims we are really not in a position to conclude that cervical cytology screening is solely responsible for this decline in the incidence of cervical cancer. Other changing factors in community health would have made some contribution and not least among these are the increasing facilities for precise diagnosis with colposcopy and effective treatment of precancerous lesions with cryosurgery.

I.B. Prevalence rates for carcinoma in situ

Prevalence rates for preclinical cancer in different countries will vary because of certain variable factors such as the method of obtaining the smear, the age of the group screened, the type of smear (initial or repeat) whether or not there is biopsy confirmation and the efficiency of taking and preparing the smear.

Hafez, E.S.E., Smith, J.P. (eds.), Carcinoma of the Cervix: Biology and Diagnosis. ISBN-13: 978-94-009-7487-6
© 1982, Martinus Nijhoff Publishers, The Hague/Boston/London.

Carcinoma *in situ* in British Columbia, Canada was found to begin most commonly in the age group 25–29 years (Boyes et al. 1962). Similar findings were reported from the San Diego (Dunn 1966) and Memphis (Kaiser et al. 1960) screening programmes. The highest prevalence rate was observed in the age group 35–39 years. Prevalences of carcinoma *in situ* as reported from large-scale screening programmes range from 3.7 per 1,000 (Christopherson et al. 1962), in the United States to 7.2 per 1,000 (MacGregor 1967) in Scotland. The 18-year survey (1949–1966) in British Columbia (Fidler et al. 1968) showed a prevalence rate of 4.3 per 1,000 for carcinoma *in situ*. The study in Memphis, Tennessee referred to above showed a higher prevalence in the negro (4.0 per 1,000) than in the white population (3.1 per 1,000). On the other hand, in Columbia, South America with one of the highest incidence rates for carcinoma of the cervix in the world, the prevalence rates reported for preclinical cancer are 50 per 1,000 in the age group 25–34 years and 35 per 1,000 in women aged 35–44 years. The patients screened were from low income communities of apparently healthy women.

II. CERVICAL INTRAEPITHELIAL NEOPLASIA (CIN)

II.A. The concept

In the natural history of cervical cancer the disease begins as an intraepithelial lesion at the squamo-columnar junction of the transformation zone, contiguous to the native portio epithelium. This has been established by colpomicroscopic studies of cervical intraepithelial neoplasia (Richart 1966) and by serial conization reconstruction studies (Przybora and Plurtowa 1959; Takeuchi and McKay 1960). The lesion usually begins as a single cell event: this was indicated by glucose-6-phosphate dehydrogenase marker studies (Smith et al. 1971; Park and Jones 1968). Progression from this single cell event to invasive cancer occurs as a series of random events and the usual course of the disease is that of a continuing process described by the term Cervical Intraepithelial Neoplasia (CIN). One stage of the continuum merges imperceptibly into the next. The concept of a continuum (CIN) has become widely accepted as it makes the approach to

both diagnosis and therapy more logical and coherent when they are based on the lesion's distribution and ease of eradication rather than on its histological diagnosis. The use of the traditional terms dysplasia and carcinoma *in situ* tends to indicate a two-stage disease calling for different lines of management. With the substitution of the term Cervical Intraepithelial Neoplasia to embrace all grades of dysplasia and carcinoma *in situ* as CIN 1, CIN 2, CIN 3 the idea of a single disease process obligates the clinician to individualise therapy basing it more on the patient's characteristics – age, parity, size of lesion – than on fine histological features. The pathologist has to distinguish metaplastic and reparative processes from intraepithelial neoplasia. This distinction is based largely upon an assessment of the organizational pattern and differentiation of the cells in histological sections and upon their cytology. Important features of the cytology include alterations in chromatin distribution pattern, nuclear enlargement, hyperchromaticity, irregularities in the nuclear membrane, mitotic abnormality and the presence of aneuploidy.

The pathologist's impression must be communicated to the clinician in simple meaningful terms which can indicate appropriate therapy.

II.B. The natural history of Cervical Intraepithelial Neoplasia (CIN)

Progression from 'dysplasia' to carcinoma *in situ* occurs in about 50 per cent of the study populations in ten years. Patients with cervical dysplasia diagnosed only by cytology and colpomicroscopy have been followed without biopsy or therapy of any kind at intervals from one to four months with repeat Papanicolaou smears and repeat colpomicroscopy (Richart and Barron 1969). By certain statistical analyses it was possible to estimate the mean time spent in each stage of dysplasia. It was found that the progression rate increased with increasing grade of CIN and that the transit time to carcinoma *in situ* was approximately 85 months for mild dysplasia, 38 months for moderate dysplasia, 12 months for severe dysplasia and 44 months for all the dysplasias taken together. Other studies have revealed that in large populations, CIN grade I will fail to progress to the next higher stage during a ten year period in some 40 to 50 per cent of the

38

patients whereas CIN grade III will fail to progress to the next higher stage in only 10 to 20 per cent of the patients. These progression rates are statistical entities pointing to trends in large numbers of patients grouped in a study project. They can have no specific application in clinical practice to an individual patient. Progression rates are not uniform and they are higher in the later stages of the continuum than in the earlier stages. Spontaneous regressions occurring in the absence of biopsy or other types of therapy are rare. At present there are no means of predicting which lesion will regress, which will remain static or which will progress and at what rate. The behaviour of a particular CIN lesion in an individual patient is unpredictable. For example, a moderate dysplasia, CIN grade II, in one patient may progress to invasive cancer sooner than does carcinoma *in situ*, CIN III, in another patient. This underlines the necessity for definitive treatment of every CIN lesion. The line of management will largely depend upon colposcopic evaluation of the lesion – its size and grade. The lesion may be eradicated by one of the following means: colposcopic biopsies, cone biopsy, cryosurgery, electrocautery or hysterectomy depending on the patient's characteristics and the skills of the gynecologist.

As long as the lesion is intraepithelial, histological grade is therapeutically not so important. The next stage beyond carcinoma *in situ* is microinvasion, the diagnosis of which implies that nowhere in the cervix is the lesion more advanced. This means that thorough evaluation of a cone biopsy has been made. Beyond microinvasion is invasive cancer, the diagnosis and treatment of which has no dependence on its precursor lesion. Although the field theory of carcinogenesis is operative in the lower genital tract, it appears not to be applicable to the uterine cervix. This has important implications in the treatment of CIN, since the total removal or destruction of a single lesion is expected to produce a cure and new independent foci would only rarely be expected to appear. This is the experience of many who have followed up treated patients over 10 to 15 years. In general, small CIN lesions treated by cryosurgery have high cure rates regardless of histological grade while larger lesions are more difficult to cure regardless of histological grade. In other words, the size of a CIN lesion (on col-

poscopy) is an important prognostic factor. Treatment will only be effective if it removes the entire lesion. This makes it important to perform a curettage of the endocervical canal as part of the routine diagnostic procedure. Only then can the limits of the lesion be ascertained. If conization is performed the surgical limits on the cervix should lie outside the limits of the transformation zone thus ensuring that neoplastic epithelium will not remain following incomplete removal. Recurrences of CIN are rare in those patients whose lesions are completely removed and whose transformation zone has been destroyed. The new squamous epithelium which replaces it has a very low potential for reproducing another CIN lesion.

Any patient with a diagnosis of cervical neoplasia must be followed carefully for new lesions occurring elsewhere in the squamous epithelium of the lower genital tract. When such vaginal or vulval lesions occur – rare as they are – they generally occur as independent multifocal lesions and not usually as extensions from the cervix. At the time of colposcopic examination of the cervix, an inspection of the vaginal fornices is made in cases where multiple or large CIN lesions are evident on the cervix. If a patient has CIN and there is no demonstrable lesion in the vaginal fornices it is questionable whether removal of a vaginal cuff at the time of hysterectomy for CIN has any merit. The extended operation certainly carries some morbidity and does not produce better results on follow-up of the patients. In 580 colposcopically diagnosed cases of carcinoma *in situ* treated by conization or simple hysterectomy follow-up has not detected a single case of recurrent carcinoma *in situ* at the vaginal vault (Coppleston et al. 1971).

III. CORRELATION BETWEEN CYTOLOGY, COLPOSCOPY
AND CONIZATION

The following outlines a Jamaican experience in a situation which the author feels is prevalent in many developing countries with scarce medical resources and a high incidence of cervix cancer. At the Jamaica Cancer Society the clinic screens about 5,000 women per year mainly from the low income groups of Kingston and St. Andrew with a population of nearly 700,000 people. Of the number screened about two-thirds are new cases while the remainder are follow-up cases.

Previous to 1976 when a change of medical staff at the clinic occurred, colposcopy was performed on patients with suspicious and positive cytology (Classes III to V) and directed punch biopsies taken: superficial electrocautery or electrodiathermy (without anaesthesia) was then used for the treatment of cervical erosions, cervical dysplasias and even carcinoma *in situ*.

Whereas some cases were lost to follow-up, many others were seen for years with repeat cytology and colposcopy. The change of medical staff brought a change of approach. Colposcopy was employed for the assessment of cases with abnormal cytology or macroscopically suspicious cervices. At the same time, cone biopsy of the cervix was strongly favoured for all cases of repeated abnormal cytology regardless of negative colposcopy findings. Prior to 1976 cone biopsy was rarely employed as a diagnostic tool mainly because of scarce hospital facilities and medical personnel.

These circumstances provided an opportunity to evaluate the efficacy of previous conservative management of cervical lesions including dysplasias and carcinoma *in situ*. It was also an opportunity to evaluate the usefulness of cone biopsy of the cervix in the given situation.

Over 300 cone biopsies were performed on patients with any of the following features: (a) macroscopically suspicious cervix; (b) repeated abnormal cytology (Class III to V); (c) a colposcopic examination regarded as unsatisfactory; (d) reports on colposcopic biopsies showing carcinoma *in situ* or severe dysplasia; (e) an endocervical smear report showing suspicious or malignant cells; (f) a cytology report in advance of the colposcopic biopsy report; (g) a long history of 'Pap' smears varying between Class I to IIIB – all of whom had undergone previous treatment with cautery or cryosurgery.

Colposcopy was performed by the standard procedure after application of three per cent acetic acid to the cervix. Endorcervical curettage was routinely taken with a Kevorkian curette; Schiller's test was used on selected cases. In some instances up to three directed biopsies were taken to obtain sufficient material for adequate diagnosis. All colposcopic examinations were performed by the author and all cytological studies and histology on the colposcopic and cone biopsy specimens were carried out in the same laboratory. The cone biopsies carried out with this liberal policy should be described as 'limited' cones as the depth of tissue was limited to 4–5 mm, to minimize or avoid bleeding complications and cut down the hospitalization stay to two days – a matter of great importance in a developing country. The limits of these cones were in some cases determined by previous colposcopic examination and in others by the application of Schiller's iodine at the time of coning.

III.A. Repeat cytology

An appreciable difference was noted between the reports on 'Pap' smears taken at the first visit and that taken later at colposcopic examination after an interval of around eight weeks (Table 1). From 202 patients with Class III Pap smear reports referred for colposcopic evaluation the repeat smear at colposcopy showed reports as follows: 18 in Class I, 32 in Class II, 134 in Class IIIA-B, 18 in Class IV. That is, there was consistency in 134 cases or roughly 66 per cent. In 18 cases (roughly nine per

Table 1. A detailed comparison of the original 'Pap' smear and the repeated smear at colposcopy – usually six weeks later.

Cytology report	Original smear	Repeat smear at colposcopy				
		Class I	Class II	Class III-AB	Class IV	Class V
Class I	18	8	7	3	0	0
Class II	120	28	77	11	4	0
Class III A,B	202	18	32	134	18	0
Class IV	46	0	6	10	26	4
Class V	14	0	0	0	5	9
Total	400	54	122	158	53	13

Table 2. A correlation of histology reports on colposcopic punch biopsy specimens with Pap smear reports – 400 cases.

Cytology report	Number	Histology reports – colposcopic punch biopsies			
		Non-specific cervicitis	Dysplasia	Carcinoma *in situ*	Invasive cancer
Class I	18	11	5	2	0
Class II	120	84	28	8	0
Class III A,B	202	15	129	43	15
Class IV	46	4	12	22	8
Class V	14	0	0	4	10
Total	400	114	174	79	33

cent) the repeat smear was more advanced and in 50 cases (roughly 25 per cent) was less advanced than the original. In 46 cases of Class IV smears the repeat smear was confirmatory in 26 cases or 56 per cent. This argues a strong place for early follow-up of all cases with Class IIIA-B reports. Further support for this comes from an earlier Jamaican study showing that 80 per cent of 43 patients with suspicious smears (Class IIIA-B) proved to have malignancy in the biopsy material. Over the past three years Class IIIA-B smears occurred with a prevalence of 36 per 1,000.

III.B. Cytology and colposcopy

Histology reports on colposcopic biopsies are correlated with the most advanced smear report (Table 2). The colposcope revealed eight cases of carcinoma *in situ* from 120 Class II smears, 15 cases of invasive cancer from 202 Class III smears. Of 14 Class V smears, 10 were confirmed as invasive and four downgraded to carcinoma *in situ*. In our laboratory, Class III is applied to a suspicious smear, Class IV to a smear suggesting carcinoma *in situ* and Class V suggests invasive cancer.

The overall assessment of results in this study

show a false negative rate in cytology of 17 per cent and a false positive rate of four per cent. A review of the literature shows a false negative rate varying from six to 28 per cent in some large series.

III.C. Colposcopy and conization

During the study, 734 colposcopic examinations were performed and of these 151 (18 per cent) were considered unsatisfactory. Colposcopic and cone biopsies performed on the same patients are reported on (Table 3). In 252 patients out of 300 (roughly 83 per cent) the reports on colposcopic and conization biopsies are in agreement. Conization revealed two cases of carcinoma *in situ* and two cases of invasive cancer from a group of 85 cases colposcopically diagnosed as non-specific cervicitis; also 11 of these cases were upgraded to dysplasia – CIN I and II. Similarly, more advanced lesions were revealed from some colposcopic reports of dysplasia and carcinoma *in situ*.

In one case out of the 25 cases diagnosed by colposcopy as invasive, the cone biopsy revealed a less severe lesion. This may be explained if the punch biopsy had previously removed the sinister portions of the cervix.

Table 3. Comparison of colposcopic biopsies and conizations – 300 cases.

Colposcopic biopsy	Number	Conizations			
		Non-specific cervicitis	Dysplasia	Carcinoma *in situ*	Invasive cancer
Non-specific cervicitis	85	70	11	2	2
Dysplasia	131	7	110	11	3
Ca *in situ*	59	0	4	48	7
Invasive	25	0	0	1	24
Total	300	77	125	62	36

The 'failure rate' of colposcopy will depend on the training and skill of the colposcopist. Hence the figures reported above must be interpreted with caution as the early part of the work was a learning experience. There are reports, however, of cases of invasive cancer detected on conization that had been missed by colposcopic biopsy carried out by expert hands.

This experience indicates that 'limited' cone biopsy is a valuable adjunct to cytology and colposcopy in following up patients with CIN. The age pattern of the patients on whom cone biopsy was performed is shown in Figure 1.

IV. DIAGNOSTIC PROCEDURES – AN APPRAISAL

IV.A Schiller's test

In this test, normal squamous epithelium, unlike early metaplastic squamous epithelium stains a dark brown color with Schiller's iodine solution. The active or 'bad areas' of the cervix lack glycogen and will not take up iodine and hence remain as pale areas. Clinicians differ on their assessment of

the reliability of the test. On occasions, sharply limited iodine negative areas (pale areas) small or large, single or multiple are revealed which show no atypical features on colposcopic examination or on histological study. The colposcopist who sees no abnormality will not take a biopsy. Many innocent cervical lesions including typical transformation zones fail to stain with iodine. The greatest advocate for the iodine test (Younge 1964) found it positive in 82 per cent of cases with carcinoma *in situ*. On the other hand, in one study, 28 per cent of carcinoma *in situ* failed to take the stain (Richart 1964).

IV.B. Colposcopy

The colposcope gives a small scale stereoscopic magnification of the cervix of between 6 and 40 times. Through it, one can see epithelial characteristics not visible to the naked eye and from which it is possible to forecast histological findings with a fair amount of accuracy. Colposcopically guided biopsies are taken from what appears to be the worst areas on the cervix for histological study. The accuracy of screening for cervical intraepithelial

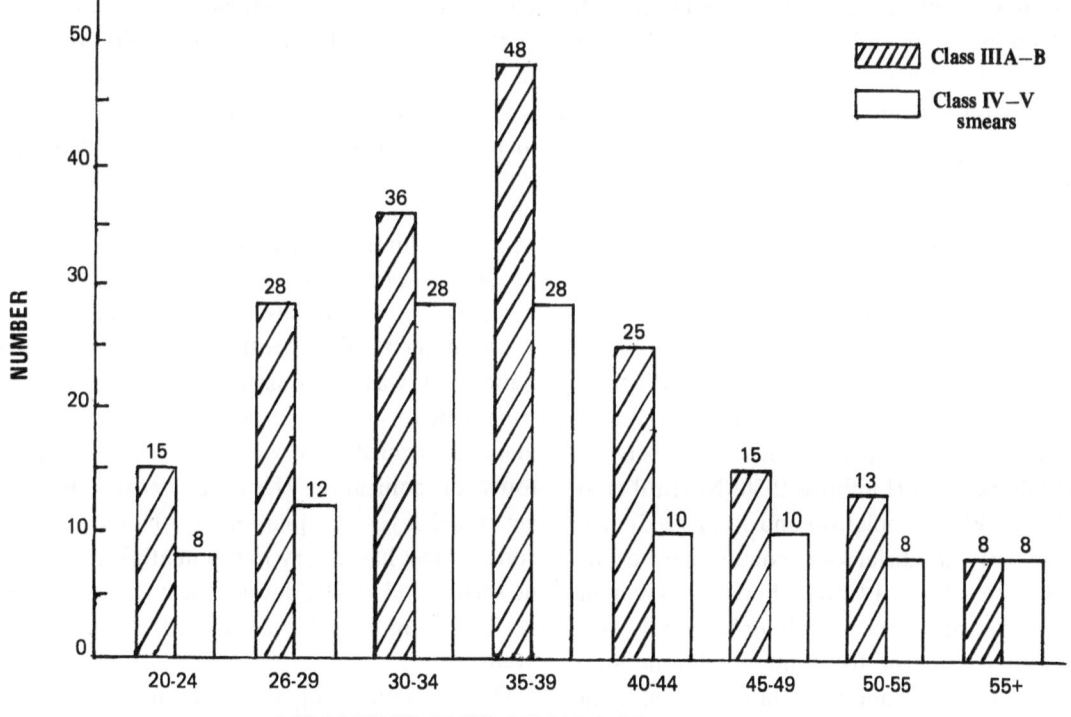

AGE PATTERN OF THE 300 PATIENTS HAVING CONE BIOPSIES.

Figure 1. Age pattern of the 300 patients having cone biopsies.

neoplasia (CIN) by cytology alone is variably reported at from 70 to 90 per cent.

In a series of 55,000 patients among whom there were 838 cases of cervical carcinoma, it was found that 87 per cent of the neoplastic lesions were diagnosed cytologically and 79 per cent were detected colposcopically (Navratil et al. 1958). With the simultaneous use of both methods, 98.8 per cent of cases were recognised on initial examination. Similar findings have been reported by other authors (Limburg 1958; Trace et al. 1959). It is now generally agreed that cytology and colposcopy may be used to complement each other and that for technical reasons cytology remains the principal method for screening programmes. The main value of colposcopy is in the evaluation of patients with abnormal cytologic findings: it is possible to recognise the lesion, determine its extent and sample it for histology. In skilled hands colposcopy is accurate in differentiating between invasive and non-invasive lesions and between inflammatory atypias and neoplasia. In a report on 1206 patients, with abnormal cytology the colposcopic impression and directed biopsies were accurate in 85 per cent of cases; in 11.7 per cent the neoplasia was less advanced than expected and in 3.3 per cent of the patients, it was more advanced (Stafl and Mattingly 1973). Colposcopy is really not complete without an endocervical curettage. In another study curettage was positive for malignant cells in 31 of 301 patients – 11.5 per cent (Treadway and Townsend 1972). Another series shows that in 32 per cent of 310 patients with CIN, the lesion extended from the portio into the cervical canal (Hollyock and Channer 1972). Treatment of CIN can never be complete if endocervical lesions are missed.

It must be admitted however that a number of dysplastic and even frankly invasive lesions can be missed by the colposcope. The reported incidence of false negative colposcopic findings varies between five and 40 per cent (Limburg 1958; Navratil et al. 1958; Gray 1964; Coppleston and Reid 1967). The frequency of unsatisfactory colposcopic examinations at the Jamaica Cancer Society's screening clinic was around 18 per cent. In order to rely on a colposcopic biopsy the following conditions must be satisfied: (a) An abnormality must be seen in the face of an abnormal 'Pap' smear; (b) The colposcopic biopsy must satisfactorily explain the abnormal smear; (c) The entire squamo-columnar junction must be visible colposcopically: the entire lesion must be seen; (d) If micro-invasion is found on a colposcopic biopsy conization is necessary to rule out frank invasion.

When the squamo-columnar junction is fully visible, the false negative rate of colposcopy is very low – a rate of 0.3 per cent (Stafl and Mattingly 1973).

IV.C. Cone biopsy of the cervix

Many gynecologists favor cone biopsy of the cervix as the diagnostic procedure of choice when there is repeated abnormal or positive smears. The advocates of cone biopsy point to the known limitations of colposcopy and to the false negative rate in colposcopic findings.

In the past cone biopsy was not popular because there were many complications to consider, immediate and late. In addition to the need for hospitalization there are the postoperative complications of haemorrhage and cervical stenosis, with possible later effects on fertility and cervical function in labour. The author considers that these complications belong to the time when extensive cone biopsies were performed. The author has performed limited cone biopsies with the aid of Schiller's test and the colposcope, without troublesome bleeding. Ninety-four per cent of the specimens were adequate for histological diagnosis as reported by the pathologist. Tissue was usually obtained to a depth of 4–5 mm at the level of the squamo-columnar junction and to a level half way up the cervical canal. The solid advantages of conization are its reliable diagnostic potential and its simultaneous therapeutic effect. In a series of 438 patients it was demonstrated that the results of treatment of carcinoma *in situ* of the cervix were identical regardless of whether it was by hysterectomy or conization (Kolstad 1970). The newly generated layer of squamous epithelium following cone biopsy has a very low potential for initiating neoplasia and so the development of invasive cancer following cone biopsy for CIN is a very rare event.

Once a cone biopsy has been done and the histological report describes an intraepithelial lesion the clinician can reassure his patient that her lesion has been eradicated – has been cured – and that the chances of recurrence are minimal. Follow-up can safely be at relatively longer intervals than would be appropriate for colposcopic punch biopsies and this must have a good psychological effect on the patient. As it is technically difficult to remove all the suspicious area in some cervical lesions, it would seem sensible to prefer cone biopsy for those cases seen on colposcopy to cover a large part of the cervix. It has been pointed out that the treatment of such cases by cryosurgery has a high failure rate.

REFERENCES

Anderson AF: The Management of the Cytology Test. J Obstet Gynec Brit Emp 66, 239, 1959.

Ayre JE: Frequency of early cancer of cervix: results of cytologic screening in private physician's office. Obstet Gynec 3: 111, 1954.

Boyes DA, Fidler HK, Lock DR: Significance of in situ Carcinoma of the Uterine Cercix. Brit Med J 1: 203, 1962.

Christopherson WM, Parker JE, Drye JC: Control of Cervical Cancer: Preliminary Report on Community Programme. J Amer Med Ass 182: 179, 1962.

Coppleston H, Reid B: Preclinical Carcinoma of the Cervix Uteri. Oxford, Pergamon Press: 1967.

Coppleston M, Reid B: Colposcopy. Springfield, Illinois: Charles C. Thomas, 1971.

Dunn JE, Jr: The Presymptomatic Diagnosis of Cancer with special Reference to Cervical Cancer. roc Roy Soc Med 59: 1198, 1966.

Fidler HK, Boyes DA, Worth AJ: Cervical Cancer detection in British Columbia. J Obstet Gynec Brit Cwlth 75: 392, 1968.

Graham RM, Sturgis SH, McGraw: A comparison of the accuracy in diagnosis of the vaginal smear and the biopsy in Carcinoma of the Cervix. Amer J Obstet Gynec 55: 303, 1948.

Gray LA: Carcinoma in situ and Microinvasive Carcinoma of the Cervix Uteri. Springfield, Illinois: Charles C. Thomas, 1964.

Hollyock VE, Chanen W: The use of the Colposcope in the Selection of patients for Cervical cone biopsy. Am J Obstet Gynecol 114: 185, 1972.

Kaiser RF, Erickson CC, Bennett EE, Gilliam AG, Graves LM, Walton M, Sprunt DH: J Nat Cancer Inst 25: 863, 1960.

Kolstad P: Diagnosis and Management of Precancerous lesions of the Cervix Uteri. Int J Gynecol Obstet 8: 551, 1970.

Koss LG, Durfee GR: Diagnostic Cytology and its Histopathologic Bases. Philadelphia: Lippencott, 1961.

Limburg H: Comparison between Cytology and Colposcopy in the diagnosis of early Cervical Carcinoma. Am J Obstet Gynecol 75: 1298, 1958.

MacGregor JE: Cervical Carcinoma. Lancet 2: 1296, 1967.

Navratil E, Burghardt E, Bajardi F, Nash W: Simultaneous Colposcopy and Cytology used in screening for Carcinoma of the Cervix. Am J Obstet Gynecol 75: 1292, 1958.

Papanicolaou GN, Trout HF: Diagnosis of Uterine Cancer by the vaginal smear. London, Oxford and New York: The Commonwealth Fund, 1943.

Park IJ, Jones HW: Glucose6-phosphate Dehydrogenase and the Histogenesis of Epidermoid Carcinoma of the Cervix. Am J Obstet Gynecol 102: 106, 1968.

Przybora LA, Plutowa A: Histological Topography of Carcinoma in situ of the Cervix Uteri. Cancer 12: 263, 1959.

Reagan JW, Hamonic MJ, Wentz WB: Analytical Study of the Cells in Cervical Squamous-cell Cancer. Lab Invest 6: 241, 1957.

Richart RM: A radioautographic analysis of cellular proliferation in dysplasia and carcinoma in situ of the uterine cervix. Am J Obstet Gynec 86: 925, 1963.

Richart RM: Colpomicroscopic Studies of Cervical Intraepithelial Neoplasia Cancer 19: 396, 1966.

Richart RM, Barron BA: A Follow-up Study of Patients with Cervical Dysplasia. Am J Obstet Gynec 105: 386, 1969.

Stafl A, Mattingly RF: Colposcopic diagnosis of Cervical Neoplasia. Obstet Gynecol 41: 168, 1973.

Smith JW: Genetic variants of Glucose-6-phosphate Dehydrogenase in the study of Carcinoma of the Cervix. Cancer 28: 529, 1971.

Takeuchi, McKay DB: The area of the cervix involved by Carcinoma in situ and Anaplasia (Atypical Hyperplasia). Obstet & Gynecol 15: 134, 1960.

Trace RJ, Brew BA, Rollins JH, McCall ML: Preliminary report on Colposcopy in Gynecology and Obstetrics. Surgical Forum 10: 736, 1959.

Treadway DR, Townsend DE: Colposcopy and Cryosurgery in Cervical Intraepithelial Neoplasia. Am J Obstet Gynecol 114: 185, 1972.

Watchel E, Plester JA: Hormonal assessment by vaginal cytology. J Obstet Gynaec Brit Emp 61: 155, 1954.

Younge PH: Dysplasia, Carcinoma in situ and Microinvasive Carcinoma of the Cervix. Springfield, Illinois: Charles C. Thomas, 1964.

II. GROWTH PATTERNS, STRUCTURE AND ULTRASTRUCTURE

9. GROWTH PATTERNS OF MICROINVASIVE CARCINOMA OF THE CERVIX

J.C. SESKI and W.A. SCHMIDT

The ideal definition for microinvasive squamous carcinoma of the cervix characterizes the lesions at a transition from dysplasia or carcinoma *in situ* to frank invasion. By morphological criteria, the microinvasive lesion is clearly invasive, but it lacks the more aggressive biologic characteristics of cancer and is, therefore, amenable to conservative therapy.

A number of definitions for microinvasion are currently in usage, which vary substantially in content. In 1974 the Society of Gynecologic Oncologists proposed a definition for microinvasion that limited the depth of stromal invasion to 3 mm below the base of the epithelium and excluded cases of lymphatic or blood vascular invasion. In July, 1976, the International Federation of Obstetrics and Gynecology classified microinvasion as stage IA carcinoma of the cervix, without establishing exact histologic criteria for microinvasion. To date a standard definition has not been adopted and consequently there is no consensus regarding the most appropriate treatment.

Much of the confusion about microinvasion has been brought about by the proliferation of terms used to describe the lesion itself. Incipient microinvasion (Przybora 1953; Morton 1964; Marcuse 1971), microcarcinoma (Mestwerdt 1953), early stromal invasion (Hamperl 1959; Burghardt 1973), advanced stromal invasion (Hamperl 1959; Burghardt 1973), superficial invasion (Dillworth and Maxwell 1962), and carcinoma *in situ* with early invasion (Fennell 1955; Kottmeier 1965) are used more or less interchangeably by different authors to describe identical lesions. There is also considerable uncertainty about the clinical significance of the various microinvasive growth patterns such as fingerlike, drop invasion, confluence, bulky outgrowth, advanced bulky outgrowth and reticular or network invasion.

Most of the disagreement about microinvasion centers around two important criteria: the depth of stromal invasion and whether or not cases with lymphatic or vascular involvement should be excluded. Opinions regarding the extent to which stromal invasion has progressed from the surface epithelium vary from 1 mm (Averette et al. 1976), to 3–4 mm (Ullery et al. 1965; Creasman and Parker 1973), to 5 mm (Frick et al. 1963; Christopherson and Parker 1964) depending on the author. Data on the significance of microvascular invasion with respect to lymph node metastases are conflicting (Mattingly 1970).

It is clear that microinvasive carcinoma and its treatment will remain controversial until the descriptive nomenclature is standardized, microinvasive growth patterns are clearly defined and the clinical significance of depth of invasion and vascular infiltration understood.

I. DIAGNOSIS OF MICROINVASION

The diagnosis of microinvasion can be made only when all the criteria establishing a lesion as microinvasive are fulfilled and when sufficient cervical tissue is available to exclude the presence of invasive carcinoma in the cervix. Cervical biopsy with or without colposcopic guidance may be useful in the preliminary diagnosis of microinvasion. However, because of the limited size of the tissue specimen returned by cervical biopsy, it cannot be relied upon to assess either the depth of microinvasion or, more importantly, the presence of lymphatic or blood vascular invasion.

Cervical conization prior to hysterectomy was performed in 41 of 54 cases of microinvasion (Seski et al. 1977). Cone biopsy disclosed the most signifi-

Hafez, E.S.E., Smith, J.P. (eds.), Carcinoma of the Cervix: Biology and Diagnosis. ISBN-13: 978-94-009-7487-6
© 1982, Martinus Nijhoff Publishers, The Hague/Boston/London.

cant lesion i.e. greatest depth of invasion, in 34 of 41 cases when compared to the hysterectomy specimen. This represents a diagnostic accuracy of 83%. However, cone biopsy did not disclose the area of deepest invasion in 2 cases and completely failed to show microinvasion in 5 other instances. In these 7 cases the margins of the cone biopsy showed carcinoma *in situ* or microinvasion.

If the diagnosis of microinvasion is to be made on the basis of cervical cone biopsy, an ample specimen sampling the entire transformation zone should be obtained. This should include a portion of the ectocervix, external cervical os and endocervical canal. All margins of the cone need to be free of dysplasia and curettage of the remaining endocervical canal should not show residual dysplasia or a more advanced lesion high in the endocervical canal may be overlooked.

II. PREPARATION OF THE CONE BIOPSY

The cervical conization specimen demands great care from both the surgeon and pathologist, particularly in the search and documentation of microinvasion. Maximizing the information obtained from the specimen requires close cooperation between these two parties. A variety of methods are available to describe the gross and microscopic features of such specimens (Blaustein 1977; Silverberg 1977; McInroy et al. 1976). We recommend a series of easily remembered and simple steps (X).

1. The specimen should have a suture marking the anterior lip at 12 o'clock and should be transported immediately to the pathologist in such a way as to prevent drying.

2. While taking great care to avoid touching epithelial surfaces the weight, length and diameter are measured – some recommend volume determination as well – cones less than 1.0 cm long and 2.5 cm³ in volume are more likely to contain atypical epithelium at resection margins (Rubio et al. 1975; Rubio et al. 1978); other grossly identifiable features are recorded.

3. The ecto- and endocervical epithelial resection lines are marked with India ink (Blaustein 1977) or silver nitrate (Christopherson 1977).

4. The cone is opened at 3 o'clock and pinned, mucosa uppermost, to a cork board or paraffin block; the pins may not be placed through the epithelium (Christopherson 1977; Silverberg 1977; Blaustein 1977); photography may be taken at this point, before and/or after exercising the option of pouring Lugol's solution on the specimen.

5. Fixation is by immersion in formalin or Bouin's solution for 3–36 hours (Kennedy 1977).

6. Whether fresh or fixed, cones should be cut only with numerous fresh blades (Silverberg 1977; Sanerkin and Fraser 1975); the sections are made at 0.1–0.3 cm intervals extending from one end to the other, throughout the entire specimen; all sections must be exactly perpendicular to the epithelial surface to allow accurate micrometer measurement of depth of invasion on the subsequent microscopic slide; all blocks are marked on corresponding faces with India ink so that facing surfaces of adjacent blocks are never sectioned (Blaustein 1977, Silverberg 1977); each block so marked is submitted in a single cassette.

7. One or more sections from each block are placed on a single slide; level sections are obtained later as needed; in this way the location of lesions may be determined within 0.1–0.2 cm.

III. MEASUREMENT OF STROMAL INVASION

The measurement of depth of stromal invasion is most critical when assessing the microinvasive lesion. More than any other parameter, depth of stromal invasion correlates best with the likely clinical behavior of the microinvasive lesion. This is the criterion which clinicians singularly heed when deciding treatment. Such measurements must be made with an ocular micrometer which has been calibrated at all magnifications. Holding a glass slide up to the light and attempting to measure depth of invasion with a ruler is inaccurate.

The boundaries for the measurements extend from the point of origin of invasion to the furthest extent of stromal penetration. The limits of the measurement should always be specified as originating from either the top or base of the surface epithelium since this practice varies among examiners. A more accurate recording is obtained when measurements are taken from the base rather than the surface of the epithelium because variations in measurements caused by differences in epithelial thickness are eliminated. Such variations seem insignificant especially when dealing with a nearly normal epithelium where the thickness differs only from 0.2 mm to 0.3 mm. With markedly dysplastic or hyperkeratotic epithelia however, the potential error becomes more significant and the variations here may exceed 0.5 mm (Averette et al. 1976).

When microinvasion originates from a cervical gland lying free in the stroma it is important to take the measurement from the point of origin of invasion. In this case it would be from the epithelium within the gland and not from the surface epithelium. At the same time there should be absolute certainty that one is dealing with invasion from a gland and not with a tangential section through the tip of a deep projection of invasive cancer. Serial step sections will be helpful in such instances.

IV. ORIGIN OF MICROINVASION

Microinvasion most frequently begins as an outgrowth from carcinoma *in situ*, although it may originate from the basal layer of a dysplastic epithelium (Figure 1). A completely normal epithelium never seems to give rise to microinvasion but sometimes a microinvasive focus is found beneath a completely normal epithelium. Such instances represent an artifact; serial sections will invariably confirm that the microinvasive focus has its origin in an area of abnormal epithelium at some distance away and has invaded the stroma horizontally beneath the normal epithelium.

Microinvasive lesions are located predominantly in the transformation zone where they may originate from the surface epithelium or from within cervical glands where the native columnar cells have been replaced by dysplastic squamous epithelium (Figure 2). Microinvasion may arise simultaneously from the surface and endocervical glands. This multifocal origin is most frequently seen when carcinoma *in situ* is present throughout the cervix with extensive endocervical gland involvement.

The most obvious misinterpretation of microinvasion is over-diagnosis, particularly when carcinoma *in situ* extends into and fills endocervical

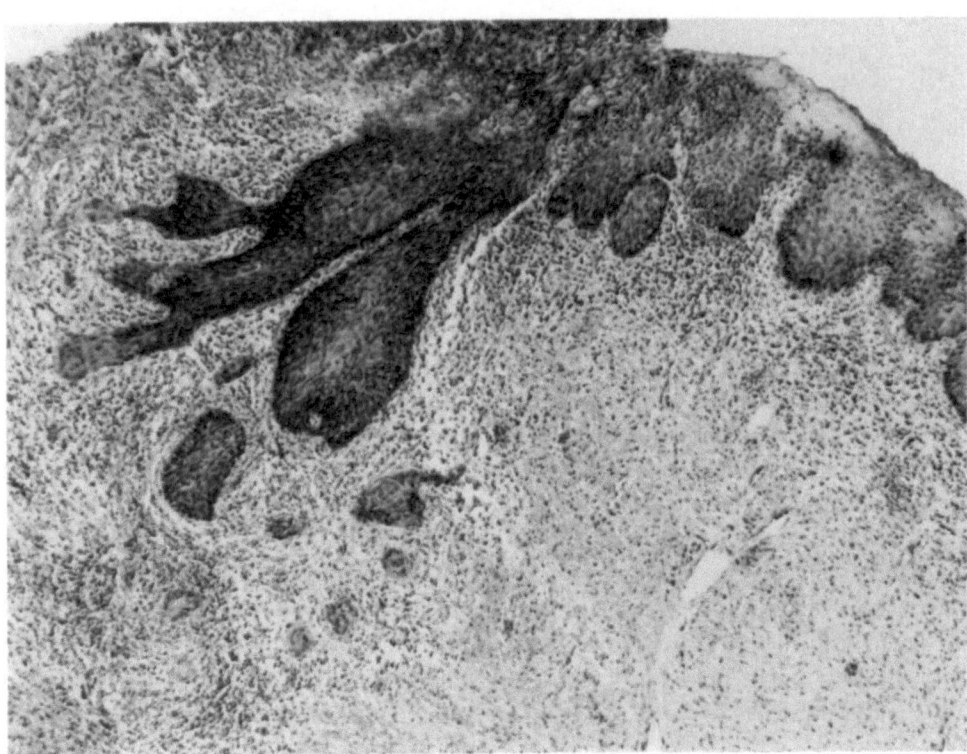

Figure 1. Non-confluent, finger-like microinvasion streams out from carcinoma *in situ*. Drop-like foci are scattered in the stroma. Squamous differentiation is present at the tips of the projections. A loose stromal reaction and inflammatory cell infiltrate is noted (From: Seski et al. (1977).

48

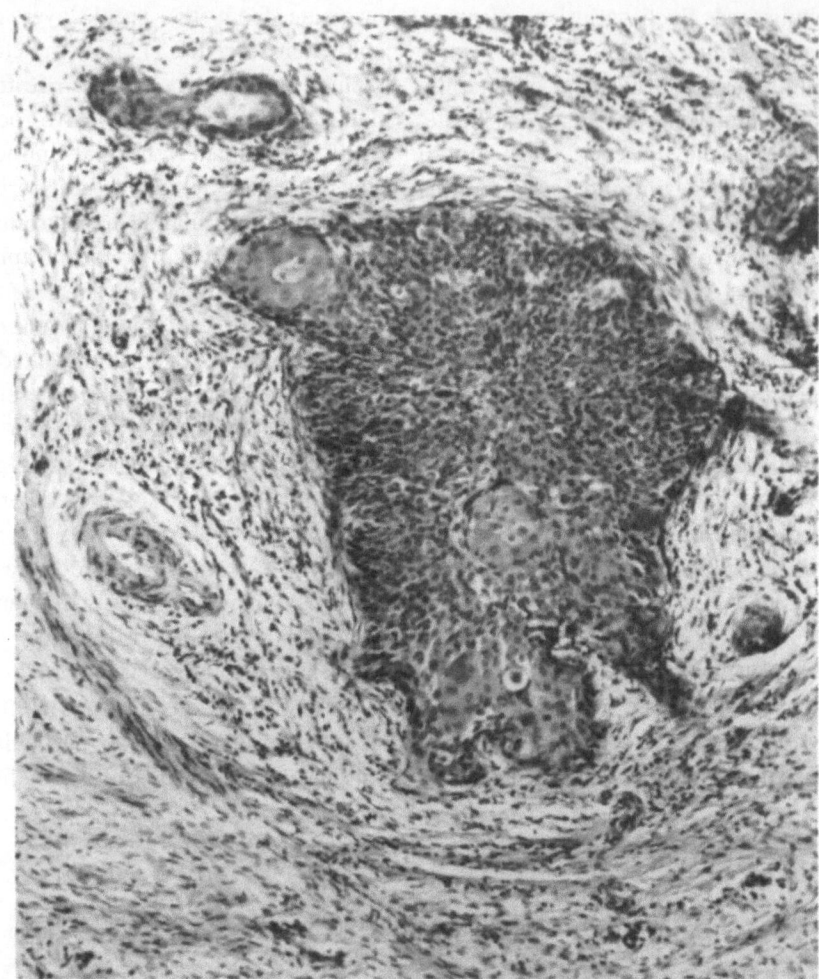

Figure 2. Non-confluent microinvasion with squamous differentiation arising from carcinoma *in situ* within an endocervical gland. Note the stromal edema and round cell infiltrate.

glands which appear separated from the surface epithelium and isolated in the stroma. This problem is usually resolved by carefully examining serial sections and tracing the isolated focus back to the surface epithelium. The finding of an admixture of columnar and squamous epithelium in the questionable invasive focus will correctly identify it as a cervical gland. An architectural arrangement characteristic of gland involvement is usually recognizable at low power. Nonetheless, it can be most difficult to distinguish microinvasion from gland involvement, especially in the presence of a heavy inflammatory cell infiltrate.

V. CELLULAR MORPHOLOGIC CHANGES OF MICROINVASION

The histologic appearance of the microinvasive lesion can be recognized by architectural changes or growth patterns of microinvasion and by morphologic changes occurring within the individual neoplastic cells.

Microinvasion begins when isolated pegs or prongs of malignant cells penetrate through the basement membrane into the stroma. The individual cells within these microinvasive foci tend to orient and align themselves along the longitudinal axis of the microinvasive projection giving the appearance of cells actually streaming out into the stroma (Figure 1). Alternatively, the cells lose their orientation and appear to be extruded out into the

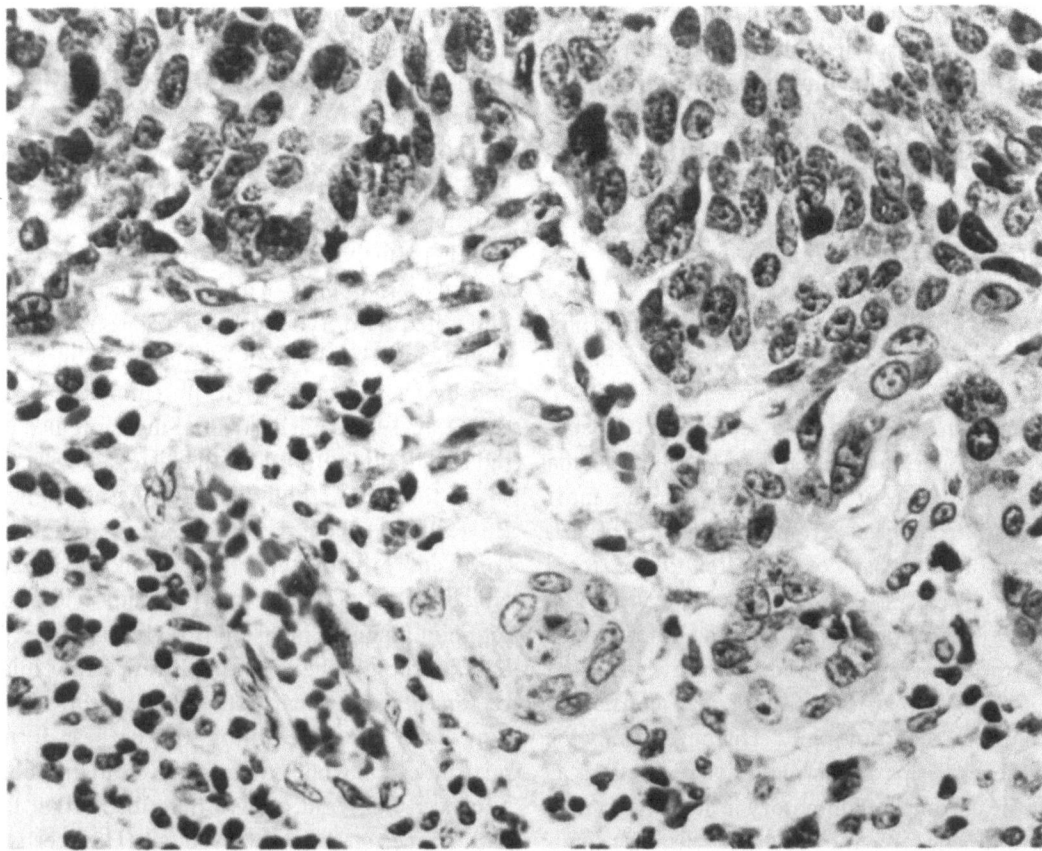

Figure 3. A small clump of squamous carcinoma cells has broken through the basement membrane beneath carcinoma *in situ.* The cells are large and pleomorphic with pale cytoplasm and plump, round nuclei. There is some differentiation towards a squamous appearance. Lymphocytes and plasma cells make up the inflammatory infiltrate.

stroma as if under pressure from some unseen force within the epithelium itself.

The individual cells within microinvasive foci appear large and plump when compared to those of carcinoma *in situ* (Figures 1–3). Their cytoplasm is abundant and strikingly eosinophilic. The nuclei are larger and more rounded than those in carcinoma *in situ* which are smaller, darker and oval in shape (Figure 3). The nucleoli are prominent but mitotic figures, are infrequent and when present often have bizarre configurations. Generally, the cells of microinvasion are pleomorphic and suggest maturation towards keratin production, whereas the cells of carcinoma *in situ* are undifferentiated and strikingly uniform. Far less commonly microinvasive carcinoma occurs as an undifferentiated small cell type. Such cases of microinvasion arise from an undifferentiated small cell carcinoma *in situ* and adopt the characteristics of a keratinizing carcinoma with advanced stromal invasion.

Epithelial pseudopearls, seen as a whorl of clumped eosinophilic cells with shrunken and pyknotic nuclei, are a feature often associated with differentiated microinvasive lesions. This finding is not pathognomonic of microinvasion, for pseudopearls are also seen in normal and dysplastic epithelia and invasive keratinizing carcinoma.

The basement membrane, seen with considerable difficulty by light microscopy in hematoxilin and eosin stained sections is a fine hyaline structure located between the epithelium and stroma representing the first anatomic boundary disrupted by microinvasion. The absence of the basement membrane, however, may not be unequivocal evidence of microinvasion because it is commonly obscured in the presence of chronic inflammation. Furthermore, the basement membrane may almost appear to be intact in certain cases of microinvasion where a bulky, broad down-growth of tumor pushes into and compresses the stroma at its leading edge.

Nevertheless, the integrity of the basement membrane in areas of suspected microinvasion is a useful criterion when assessing microinvasion. Disruption of the basement membrane, when demonstrable, may be considered a hallmark of microinvasion.

VI. STROMAL REACTIONS TO MICROINVASION

The stroma in the immediate vicinity of microinvasive lesions reacts to the presence of the malignant cells with characteristic changes (Figures 1–3). A loosening up of the stroma reflected in a separation and obscuring of reticulin fibers, local edema and an inflammatory cell infiltrate is the most consistently recognized stromal reaction. The cellular infiltrate consists of an often dense focal collection of plasma cells and lymphocytes. Occasionally eosinophils are found interspersed among the lymphocytes and plasma cells, and rarely the inflammatory infiltrate may consist almost entirely of eosinophils. Histocytes may be present near the tips of microinvasive projections as part of the chronic inflammatory infiltrate and may form prominent foreign body giant cells. The significance of the cellular infiltrate is unknown although it presumably represents an immunologic response to the malignant squamous epithelium.

The inflammatory cell infiltrate may also reflect a nonspecific reaction and is not diagnostic of invasion. When decidedly focal it is, however, a feature helpful in distinguishing between microinvasion and carcinoma *in situ* with questionable invasion. The presence of an isolated focus of inflammatory cells with local stromal edema beneath a dysplastic epithelium should arouse the suspicion that invasion may be present. Such an inflammatory focus may simply represent a lymphoid follicle in an area of chronic inflammation, however, serial step sections of the immediate area are warranted and not infrequently will reveal a focus of microinvasion.

VII. MICROINVASIVE GROWTH PATTERNS

Numerous authors have attempted to characterize microinvasive carcinoma by its pattern of stromal invasion. A multitude of confusing terms and complex classifications have been employed to describe these growth patterns. Stoddard (1952), Fennell (1954, 1955), Bajardi and Burghardt (1957) initially described the entity known as microinvasion. They recognized the essential features of the lesion: its origin, typical cellular changes, stromal reactions, and growth patterns. In retrospect, these descriptions are strikingly similar.

Others further characterized the lesion according to its pattern of growth and behavior. Some authors illustrated two types of early stromal invasion, namely invasion by buds of well-differentiated cells and by prongs of poorly-differentiated cells (Friedell et al. 1958). Early stromal invasion also occurred as a 'flaking-off' of small clusters of cells and by sharp tongues or bulbous outgrowths (Fidler and Boyes 1959). These patterns were separate from the confluent growth typical of frank invasion. Incipient cervical cancer was also subdivided into a pinpoint and area invasion (Przybora 1965). One of the most comprehensive classifications for microinvasion categorized early stromal invasion and bulky outgrowth as representing the earliest forms of microinvasion while advanced stromal invasion and advanced bulky outgrowth described larger lesions with deeper stromal involvement (Hamperl 1959).

Hamperl's scheme was expanded to include drop infiltration, bulky infiltration, early stromal erosion and invasion, and network infiltration (Fettig 1964). The term microcarcinoma was added to describe the more advanced forms of microinvasion with deeper stromal penetration (Mestwerdt 1953). Strict morphologic criteria alone were utilized to characterize an incipient and advanced form of microinvasion (Marcuse 1971). One of the best descriptions stated that early stromal invasion developed in a pattern of finger-like and bulky outgrowth while advanced bulky outgrowth and network pattern occurred with progressive invasion (Burghardt 1973). Later only four patterns were recognized: drop, finger-like, bulky and confluent invasion (Sugimore et al. 1979). While some have reduced the classification to three patterns: finger-like, confluent and mixed types (Alan et al. 1969; Roche and Norris 1975; Leman et al. 1976) others include the mixed types together with confluent lesions and describe only two growth patterns, confluent and non-confluent (Seski et al. 1977).

The growth patterns of microinvasive carcinoma can be subdivided into two broad categories of

51

confluent and non-confluent. The non-confluent pattern of microinvasion consists of small intrusive foci penetrating the stroma as either narrow, finger-like prongs or broad, bulky projections. With progression these individual microinvasive foci (finger-like or bulky) branch extensively, coalesce and anastomose to form the confluent growth pattern. This transition from one pattern to another and progression from intraepithelial neoplasia to frank invasion is illustrated in Figure 4. Although these individual growth patterns of microinvasion may be classified separately for descriptive purposes, no finite distinction between the patterns is evident. Rather, the growth of microinvasion represents a spectrum of change whereby one pattern blends with another as invasion develops.

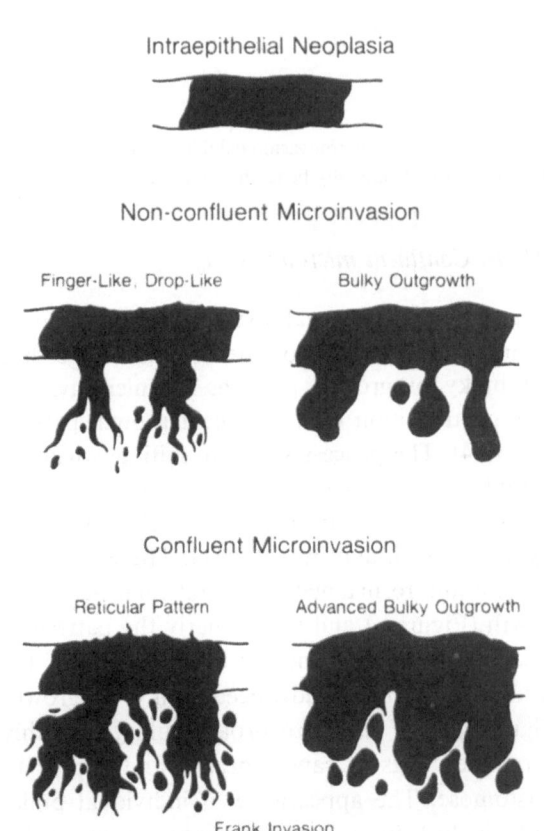

Intraepithelial Neoplasia

Non-confluent Microinvasion

Finger-Like, Drop-Like   Bulky Outgrowth

Confluent Microinvasion

Reticular Pattern   Advanced Bulky Outgrowth

Frank Invasion

Figure 4. Microinvasive carcinoma represents a transition from intraepithelial neoplasia to frank invasion. The non-confluent growth pattern consists of a finger-like or bulky outgrowth. With progressive invasion the individual foci anastomose together forming confluent growth seen as a reticular pattern or advanced bulky outgrowth.

VII. A. Non-confluent microinvasion

One of the earliest forms of non-confluent microinvasion begins when individual neoplastic epithelial cells penetrate the basement membrane and invade the stroma (Figure 3). These foci initially give the appearance of individual cells trickling down into the stroma. As cell aggregates become larger they form small tongues surrounded on three sides by stroma. With further growth the tongues taper and branch forming pointed and forked finger-like projections – hence the name finger-like microinvasion (Figures 1 and 4).

The cells in these early finger-like prongs are undifferentiated and similar to cells of carcinoma *in situ*. Although it is uncommon, these tumor cells may continue to invade into the stroma for a short distance and retain their undifferentiated appearance. Maturation usually occurs soon after the initial invasion of the stroma and is most evident at the tips of the microinvasion projections (Figures 1 and 2). Squamous differentiation may occasionally occur simultaneously with basement membrane penetration.

A second recognizable non-confluent microinvasive pattern is characterized as the bulky outgrowth pattern. Herein microinvasion occurs as a down growth of bulky, broad pegs that extend into the stroma across a wide front (Figures 4 and 5). These microinvasive foci are nodular and massive in comparison with the fine pointed projections of the finger-like pattern. Usually the cells in the bulky down growths are undifferentiated although differentiation and maturation do occur with deeper stromal invasion. A mixed pattern of growth is evident when finger-like projections secondarily bud from the edges of bulky pegs.

Disassociated epithelial nests are frequently scattered around the tips of either finger-like or bulky microinvasive projections (Figures 1 and 4). These clusters seem to lack direct continuity with the microinvasive foci and appear to grow autonomously and to lie free in the stroma. Actually these drop-like foci do not represent metastases to the stroma. Rather serial sections reveal them as an artifact caused by tangential sections taken through the tips of either finger-like or bulky prongs. These drop-like foci actually communicate directly with the invasive projections and with the surface epithelium.

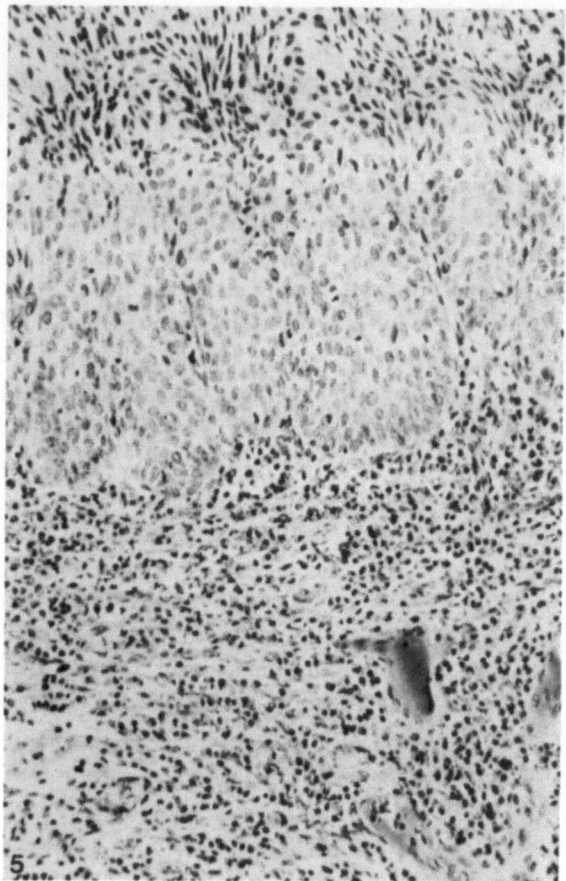

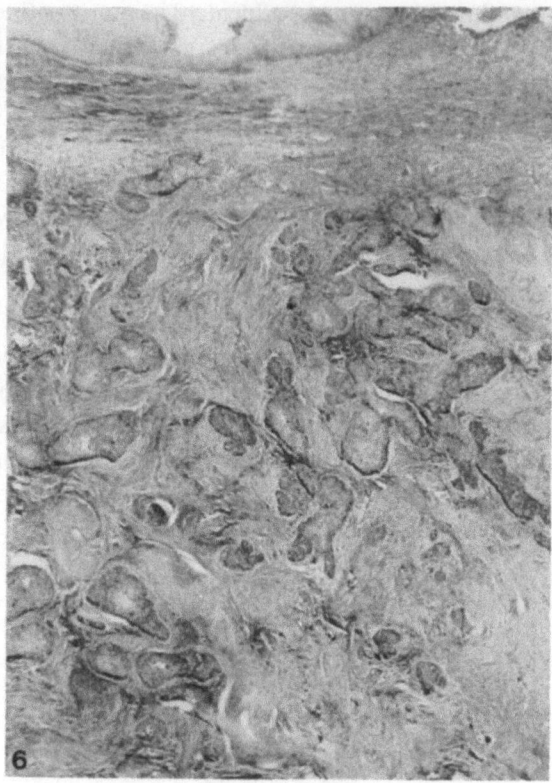

Figure 6. Confluent microinvasion exhibiting a reticular pattern of growth extends laterally beneath a normal epithelium.

Figure 5. Early bulky outgrowth pushes into the stroma across a broad front. Note the characteristic cellular changes with squamous differentiation.

The neoplastic cells within the drop-like lesions usually show maturation; less commonly they remain in an undifferentiated form. This appearance depends on whether the microinvasive focus from which they derived is differentiated or undifferentiated.

Tangential sections through the tip of an undifferentiated broad down growth of microinvasion will appear as undifferentiated isolates surrounded on all sides by stroma. Such a lesion can be difficult to distinguish from carcinoma *in situ* within a cervical gland. The status of the basement membrane, presence of inflammatory infiltrate and stromal reaction may aid in confirming the presence of invasion. Examining the area around the suspicious focus for other glands containing carcinoma *in situ*, their spatial arrangement and location in the stroma is helpful. Serial step sections may give further insight into whether gland involvement by carcinoma *in situ* or microinvasion is present.

VII. B. Confluent microinvasion

With progressive stromal invasion and corresponding increase in tumor volume both the finger-like and bulky outgrowth patterns of microinvasion undergo transition to a confluent growth pattern (Figure 4). The process seems to initiate when the multiple invasive prongs of the finger-like pattern that form narrow strands located close together begin to branch and interconnect. These extensive ramifications form a network or reticular pattern of growth (Figures 4 and 6). Similarly the pattern of bulky outgrowth expands into the depths of the stroma to form an advanced bulky outgrowth (Figures 4 and 7). These broad, bulky, smoothly marginated pegs of cancer branch and appear to anastomose. The appearance of individual bulky cords is lost in a jumbled arrangement of interconnecting, anastomosing epithelial formations. The distinction between the reticular pattern and advanced bulky down-growth becomes more highly subjective with deeper more advanced degrees of stromal penetration. Frequently, both patterns of

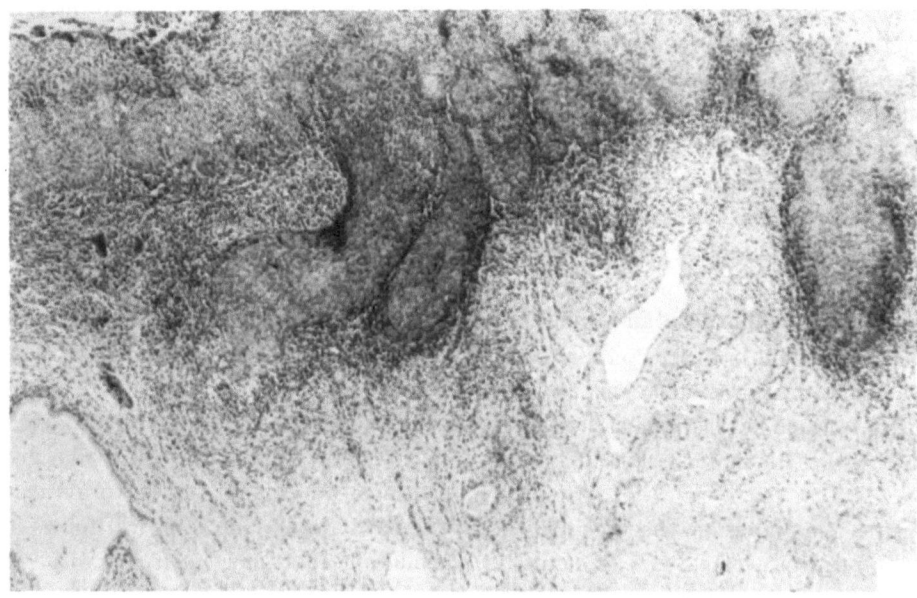

Figure 7. Microinvasion demonstrating advanced bulky outgrowth. Bulky cords appear to anastomose and merge together forming confluent growth.

growth are present in the same specimen. This is particularly evident when the bulky outgrowths develop secondary excrescences (Figure 7). These secondary extensions appear as finger-like projections that bud from the margins of the bulky outgrowths and independently begin to invade the stroma.

With further stromal invasion, particularly beyond 3 to 5 mm, differences in growth patterns become less distinct and quite arbitrary. Under such conditions carcinoma extends in broad sheets throughout the cervical stroma. Traces of the original fine reticular pattern or bulky outgrowth may persist along the periphery of advanced invasion, but often a clear distinction between patterns can not be made in the presence of frank invasion.

VII. C. Growth patterns and depth of stromal invasion

The growth pattern of microinvasion, whether confluent or non-confluent, is generally related to the depth of stromal invasion. The non-confluent pattern is the earliest form of invasion and is seen most commonly when penetration into the stroma is less than 1 mm in depth, and rarely occurs beyond a depth of 2 to 3 mm before confluence appears. Confluence represents a more advanced invasion

both in depth of stromal penetration and lateral extent or width. Hence, confluent invasion is less common with stromal penetration less than 1 mm, and is invariably the predominant pattern with deeper stromal invasion (2 to 3 mm).

In an analysis of 54 cases of microinvasion limited to 3 mm in depth without lymphatic or blood vascular involvement (Seski et al. 1977), confluence of microinvasion was seen in 33 of 54 cases (61%). As the depth of microinvasion increased lesions were more often confluent in nature while virtually all non-confluent invasion was 1 mm or less in depth (Table 1). Only 3 cases of non-confluent invasion beyond 1 mm were seen and in each invasion extended less than 2 mm. Conversely all lesions with invasion beyond 2 mm were confluent. This finding was confirmed in another study of 135 cases of microinvasion (Hasumi et al. 1980). None of these cases with invasion up to 1 mm had a

Table 1. Confluence and depth of microinvasive carcinoma.

Depth of invasion (mm)	Confluent	Non-confluent
0–1	8	18
1–2	12	3
2–3	13	0

From: Seski et al. 1977.

confluent pattern whereas 25 of 45 (55%) with invasion from 1 to 3 mm had a confluent pattern. All 29 patients with invasion beyond 3 mm had the confluent pattern.

An analysis of 115 cases of microinvasive carcinoma found that 71 invaded less than 1 mm and 96% were non-confluent. The 44 cases that invaded beyond 2 mm showed a confluent pattern in 39% (Ruch et al. 1976).

When microinvasion is multifocal in origin with varying depths of invasion, both the confluent and non-confluent pattern may be noted. This mixture of growth patterns should be classified as confluent since the term describes the more advanced form of microinvasion.

Definitions for microinvasion that exclude lesions with a confluent growth pattern are actually restricting the depth of stromal invasion, since the non-confluent pattern seldom invades beyond 2 mm. Conversely, definitions that limit the depth of stromal invasion to 1 mm exclude most confluent lesions which are more characteristic of deeper stromal penetration.

VIII. LYMPHATIC AND BLOOD VASCULAR INVASION

Invasion into lymphatic or blood vascular channels can occur with any degree of stromal invasion but the significance of vascular invasion with microinvasive carcinoma has yet to be determined. Since the ideal definition for microinvasion attempts to characterize the lesion as having virtually no potential for regional metastases, it seems logical to exclude any case where vascular invasion is noted. It is recognized that invasive cervical lesions of larger size have a higher incidence of regional metastases when lymphatic or blood vascular invasion is present (Friedell and Parsons 1962) and even when the regional lymph nodes are free of metastases, tumors with vascular invasion have a worse prognosis (Morley and Seski 1976).

Scientific data to support the concept that vascular invasion worsens the prognosis for microinvasive cancer is lacking. In fact, some authors have shown that vascular invasion is found frequently with microinvasion and is not associated with lymph node metastases. Fifty-one cases of microinvasion were reported in which microvascular in-

vasion was noted in 24% and no lymph node metastases were found (Leman et al. 1976). Micro lymphatic involvement was present in 57% of 30 cases of microinvasion but there was no evidence of lymph node metastases (Roche and Norris 1975). Conversely, other investigators cite cases of microinvasion with regional metastases that are associated with vascular invasion (Bohm et al. 1976; Seski et al. 1977; Lohe et al. 1978). At the present time it would seem that microinvasion with regional metastases is frequently associated with vascular invasion but vascular invasion is not invariably associated with lymph node metastases.

Though the significance of vascular invasion with microinvasion remains unknown its recognition is important. Most clinicians will follow the recommendation that microinvasion with vascular in-

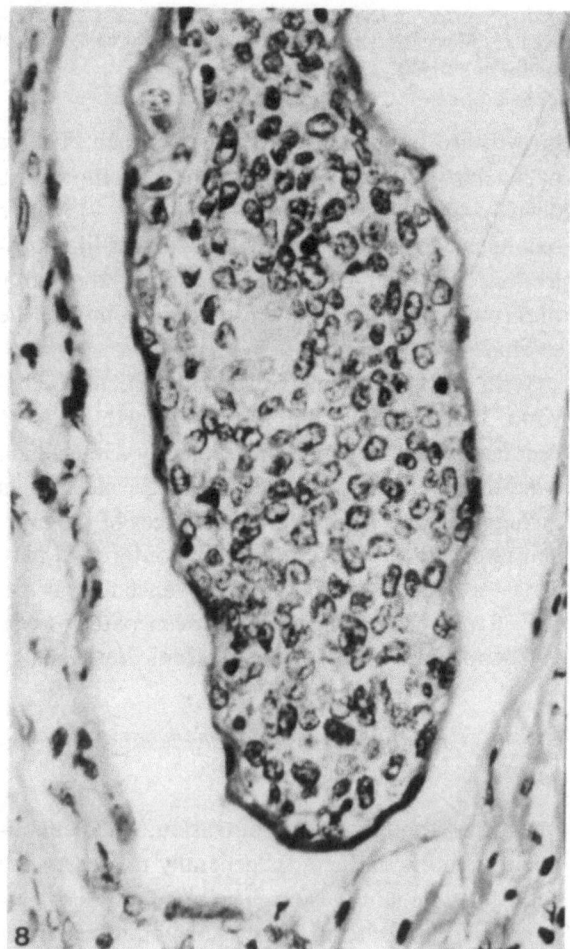

Figure 8. A focus of squamous carcinoma lying within a distended vascular channel. The vessel exhibits a continuous lining of endothelial cells. In this case confluent microinvasion invaded the stroma to a depth of 3 mm.

volvement should be treated in a more aggressive fashion regardless of the depth of invasion (Mattingly 1979).

An unequivocal diagnosis of microvascular invasion can only be made when carcinoma is found within endothelial lined spaces (Figure 8). The distinction between invasion of a lymphatic or small vein is difficult if not impossible and only when erythrocytes or lymphocytes alone are found within the lumen can the distinction be made with any degree of certainty. This has prompted some authors to designate any endothelial lined cavity as a capillary-like space and to avoid the separation of lymphatics from venules (Roche and Norris 1975).

Most of the confusion about capillary-like invasion occurs in distinguishing it from the artifact caused by tissue shrinkage. Shrinkage occurs when fixation and processing cause the edematous stroma around a cancer focus to retract, leaving a free space. This can be differentiated from true vascular invasion by the absence of endothelial cells lining the stromal pseudo-cavities. Compressed stromal cells with pyknotic nuclei may have the appearance of endothelial cells but they seldom extend around the entire circumference of the lumen. Further, the borders of the lumen caused by shrinkage closely match the irregular contours of the invasive focus and when multiple shrinkage artifacts are present throughout a microscopic field one must doubt a diagnosis of vascular invasion. Serial sections through a questionable area may help demonstrate vascular involvement by showing progressive invasion from the stroma into an obvious vessel or by clearly demonstrating an intact endothelial lining.

Finally, the presence of erythrocytes or lymphocytes within a suspected lumen, although uncommon, is diagnostic of lymphatic or blood vascular invasion.

Vascular invasion can be found with larger lesions and microinvasive lesions that have limited degrees of stromal invasion. Most frequently it occurs with stromal invasion deeper than 1 mm (Leman et al. 1976). Vascular invasion can be found with either the finger-like or confluent growth pattern. Differences in conflicting opinions regarding the association of vascular invasion with various growth patterns may be explained in part by the highly subjective interpretation of what constitutes a confluent or non-confluent growth pattern.

IX. CONCLUDING REMARKS

Microinvasive squamous carcinoma represents a spectrum of changes that illustrates the transition from intraepithelial neoplasia to frank invasion. The various microinvasive growth patterns in themselves demonstrate this continuum of changes. Categorization of the different patterns is useful to characterize and understand the evolution of squamous carcinoma but this separation is artificial and has little clinical significance. There is no doubt that microinvasive carcinoma as an entity exists and that such a lesion is amenable to conservative therapy. The task of clarifying the salient points that characterize the lesion, such as depth of invasion and vascular involvement, remains unfinished.

REFERENCES

Alan BP, Ng MB, Reagan JW: Microinvasive carcinoma of the uterine cervix. AM J Clin Path 52: 511, 1969.

Averette HE, Nelson JH, Ng ABP, et al.: Diagnosis and management of microinvasive (stage IA) carcinoma of the uterine cervix. Cancer 38: 414, 1976.

Bjardi F, Burghardt E: Ergebnisse von histologischen serienschnittuntersuchungen beim. Carcinoma Colli O Arch Gynaelcol 189: 392, 1975.

Blaustein A: Gross description and processing of obstetric and gynecologic tissue. In Blaustein A (ed): Pathology of the Female Genital Tract. New York: Springer-Verlag, 1977.

Bohm JW, Krupp PJ, Lee FYL, et al.: Lymph node metastasis in microinvasive epidermoid cancer of the cervix. Obstet Gynecol 48: 65, 1976.

Burghardt E: Early histological diagnosis of cervical cancer. Philadelphia: W.B. Saunders, 1973, 259.

Christopherson WM, Parker JE: Microinvasive carcinoma of the cervix: A clinical pathological study. Cancer 17: 1125, 1964.

Christopherson WM: Dysplasia, carcinoma in situ, and microinvasive carcinoma of the uterine cervix. Hum Path 8: 489, 1977.

Creasman WT, Parker RT: Microinvasive carcinoma of the cervix. Clin Obstet gynecol 16: 261, 1973.

Dillworth EE, Maxwell GE: Superficial invasive carcinoma and carcinoma in situ of the cervix. Am J Obstet Gynec 84: 83, 1962.

56

Fazzini E, et al.: A Manual for Surgical Pathologists. Springfield: C.C. Thomas, 1972.

Fennell RH: Morphologic aspects of the transition from intraepithelial to invasive carcinoma of the uterine cervix. Am J Pathol 30: 623, 1954.

Fennell RH: Carcinoma in situ of the cervix with early invasive changes. Cancer 8: 302, 1955.

Fettig O: Zur morphologischen und klinischen problematik des mikrocarcinomas (Collum carcinoma stadium 1a). Arch Gynaekol 199: 571, 1964.

Fidler HK, Boyes DA: Patterns of early invasion from intraepithelial carcinoma of the cervix. Cancer 12: 673, 1959.

Foote FW, Jr, Stuart FW: The anatomical distribution of intraepithelial epidermoid carcinoma of the cervix. Cancer 1: 431, 1948.

Frick HC, Janovski NA, Gusbert SB, et al.: Early invasive cancer of the cervix. Amer J Obstet Gynec 85: 926, 1963.

Friedell GH, Hertig AT, Younge PA: The problem of early stromal invasion in carcinoma in situ of the uterine cervix. Arch Path 66: 494, 1958.

Friedell GH, Parsons L: Blood vessel invasion in cancer of the cervix. Cancer 15: 1269, 1962.

Friedell GH: Cancer of the cervix – A selective review. In: Somers SC (ed): Genital and Mammary Pathology Decennial. New York: Appleton-Century-Crofts, 1975, 2953.

Hamperl H: Definition and classification of the so called carcinoma in situ. In: Cancer of the Cervix. Ciba Foundation study group No. 3. London: Churchill, 1959, 2.

Hasumi K, Sokamoto A, Sugono H: Microinvasive carcinoma of the uterine cervix. Cancer 45: 928, 1980.

Hertig AT, Gore H: Tumors of the female sex organs, part 2. In: Tumors of the Vulva, Vagina and Uterus. Washington: Armed Forces Institute of Pathology, 1960.

Kennedy A: Basic Techniques in Diagnostic Histopathology. New York: Churchill Livingstone, 1977.

Kottmeier HL: Questionable early stromal invasion and minimal invasive cervical carcinoma. J Int Fed Gynoec Obstet 3: 3, 1965.

Leman MH, Jr, Benson WL, Kurman RJ, et al.: Microinvasive carcinoma of the cervix. Obstet Gynec 48: 571, 1976.

Lohe KJ, Burghardt E, Hillemanns HG, et al.: Early squamous cell carcinoma of the uterine cervix: II Clinical results of a cooperative study in the management of 419 patient with early stromal invasion and microcarcinoma. Gynecol Oncol 6: 31, 1978.

Marcuse PM: Incipient microinvasive carcinoma of the uterine cervix. Obstet Gynecol 37: 360, 1971.

Mattingly R: Panel on microinvasive carcinoma: Moderator's Summary. Third World Congress of Cervical Pathology and Colposcopy. Obstet Gynecol Survey 34 (11): 841, 1979.

McInroy RA et al.: Cone biopsy histology report. J Clin Path 29: 167, 1976.

Mestwerdt G: Atlas der Kolposkopie. Jena: Fischer, 1953.

Morley GW, Seski JC: Radical pelvic surgery versus radiation therapy for stage I carcinoma of the cervix (exclusive of microcarcinoma). Am J Obstet Gynecol 126: 785, 1976.

Morton DG: Incipient carcinoma of the cervix. Amer J Obstet Gynec 90: 64, 1964.

Przybora LA: Incipient invasion of cervical cancer: Morphologic aspects of carcinogenesis in 74 cases. Gynecolog 160: 69, 1965.

Roche WD, Norris HJ: Microinvasive carcinoma of the cervix: The significance of lymphatic invasion and confluent patterns of stromal growth. Cancer 36: 180, 1975.

Rubio CA et al.: Influence of the size of cone specimens on postoperative hemorrhage. Amer J Obst Gyn 122: 939, 1975.

Rubio C et al.: Big cones and little cones. Histopath 2: 133, 1978.

Ruch RM, Pitcock JA, Ruch WA, Jr: Microinvasive carcinoma of the cervix. Am J Obstet Gynecol 125: 87, 1976.

Sanerkin NG, Fraser JMR: A technique for the orientation of blocks and sections from unbisected cervical cones. J Clin Path 28: 202, 1975.

Seski JC, Abell MR, Morley GW: Microinvasive squamous carcinoma of the cervix: Definition, histologic analysis, late results of treatment. Obstet Gynecol 50: 4, 1977.

Silverberg SG: Surgical Pathology of the Uterus. New York: J Wiley and Sons, 1977.

Stoddard LD: The problem of carcinoma in situ with reference to the human cervix uteri. In: McManus (ed): Progress in Fundamental Medicine. Philadelphia: Lea & Febiger, 1952, 203.

Sugimore H, Matsoyama T, Kashimura M, et al.: Histological study of microinvasive carcinoma of the uterine cervix. Gynecol Oncol 7: 153, 1979.

Telinde RW, Mattingly RF: Operative Gynecology (4th ed). Philadelphia: Lippincott, 1970, 739.

Ullery JC, Boutselis JG, Botschner AC: Microinvasive carcinoma of the cervix. Obstet Gynec 26: 866, 1965.

10. GROWTH, SPREAD AND GRADING IN SQUAMOUS CELL CARCINOMA OF THE UTERINE CERVIX

J. Baltzer, K.J. Lohe and J. Zander

Kundrat (1903), Brunet (1905) and Scheib (1909) have already presented meticulous histological studies of surgical specimens of patients who had been operated on for cervical carcinoma. The results obtained in these surgical specimens indicated that squamous cell carcinoma of the uterine cervix spreads to the parametrial tissue at an early stage, and leads to regional lymph node metastases on the wall of the pelvis.

Studies by Ober et al. (1961), Ober and Huhn (1962), Kindermann and Ober (1972) provided new information on the spreading of cervical carcinoma. These observations made it evident that squamous cell carcinoma of the cervix affects the lymph nodes on the wall of the pelvis discontinuously before it has infiltrated the parametrial tissue. These investigations were based on special histological work-up of the surgical specimens as well as preparation of systematic large surface sections (Schneppenheim et al. 1958; Matuschka 1962).

I. METHODOLOGY

The study of 718 surgical specimens from patients with squamous cell carcinoma of the uterine cervix presented here are based on a standardized histological work-up. The investigations were carried out in the framework of a collaborative study at four University Departments of Gynecology and Obstetrics (Cologne 1958–1974, Erlangen 1963–1974, Heidelberg 1965–1970, Munich I 1970–1974) with regard to tumor growth, spread and grading.

The fresh surgical specimens were stretched unfixed on a cork frame immediately after its removal from the abdominal cavity in order to prevent distortion or shrinkage of the parametrial tissue. After fixation for 24 hours in a formalin-acetic acid mixture a 5 mm thick sagittal tissue slice was first cut from the middle of the cervix. The lateral cervical wall with the attached parametrial tissue is cut into consecutively numbered tissue slices. Further tissue blocks are cut from the corpus uteri and the adnexae (Figure 1).

The lymph nodes and fatty tissue from the same anatomical location were kept together and placed in different bottles of Bouin solution according to the side of removal. This solution stains lymphatic tissue but not fat (bride yellow). The prepared lymph nodes are counted, lamellated into slices one to two mm thick and embedded. Four serial sections at an interval of 150 μ are first prepared from each lymph node block. If no tumor metastases were found, all lymph node blocks were completely worked up.

Large surface sections were prepared from all tissue blocks and stained with iron-hematoxylin and eosin. The factors tumor grading, growth and spread are additionally correlated with the age of the patients. The women operated on are divided into age groups of 16–30, 31–40, 41–50, 51–70 years old in order to ensure comparable class compositions. The data were put on to punch cards.

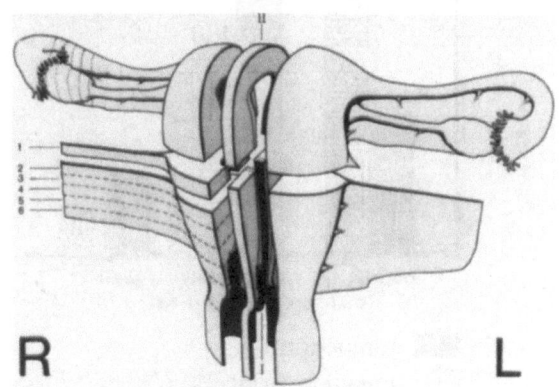

Figure 1. Sectioning technique of the surgical specimen.

Hafez, E.S.E., Smith, J.P. (eds.), Carcinoma of the Cervix: Biology and Diagnosis. ISBN-13: 978-94-009-7487-6
© 1982, Martinus Nijhoff Publishers, The Hague/Boston/London.

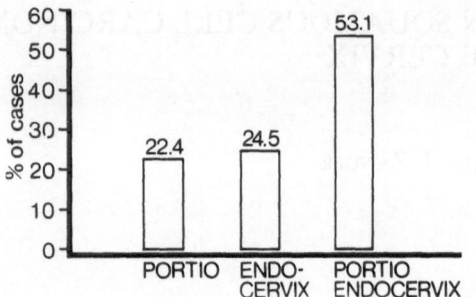

Figure 2. Tumor localization (*n* = 718 squamous cell carcinoma).

Statistical evaluation was carried out using the SAVOD dialog system for interactive processing and evaluation of medical data (Selbmann and Raab 1976). All findings are statistically significant at the 1% level.

II. RESULTS

II.A. Tumor localization and tumor growth

Among the 718 carcinomas the tumor is localized on the portio in 22.4% and endocervically in 24.5%. Tumors which have affected both the portio and the endocervix are most frequent (53.1%) (Figure 2). Taking into account the kind of tumor growth, there is a mainly exophytically growing carcinoma in 12.7% and a chiefly endophytically growing carcinoma in 60.2%. 27.1% of tumors are growing both exophytically and endophytically.

II.B. Tumor grading

According to the degree of maturation the carcinomas are subdivided into poorly, moderately and well-differentiated tumors. This grading is made more difficult by differences in the same tumor. In order to enable a better evaluation, the tumor center and the invasion front of the carcinoma are evaluated separately (Figure 3). In 56.7% there are moderately, in 16.6% well and in 26.7% poorly differentiated carcinomas in the tumor center. On the other hand, for the invasion front a poorly differentiated carcinoma is registered in 52.1%, a moderately in 43.3% and a well-differentiated carcinoma in only 4.6%. The tendency to increasing immaturity of the carcinoma in the direction of the invasion front becomes evident.

II.C. Tumor dissociation

A pronounced dissociating tumor growth is registered in 24.3%, a slightly dissociating tumor growth in 52.5%. A tumor dissociation is absent in 24.2%. These findings indicate that in contrast to other carcinomas (e.g. breast cancer) the squamous cell carcinoma of the cervix mainly grows in closed and solid formations.

II.D. Tumor spread

Consideration of the factors tumor localization and tumor growth makes it evident that mainly exophytic carcinomas are present on the portio, whereas the majority of endophytically growing tumors is observed endocervically (Figure 4). The carcinomas

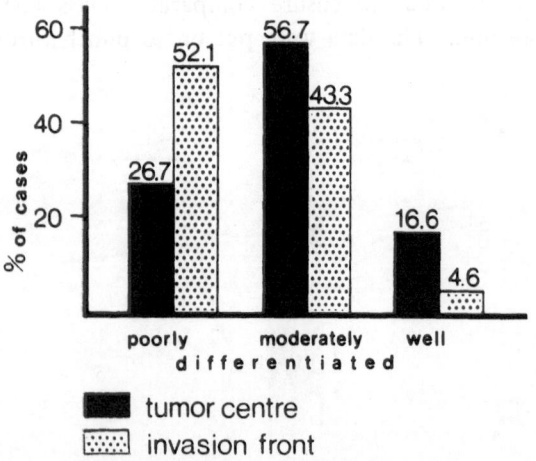

Figure 3. Tumor grading (*n* = 718 squamous cell carcinoma).

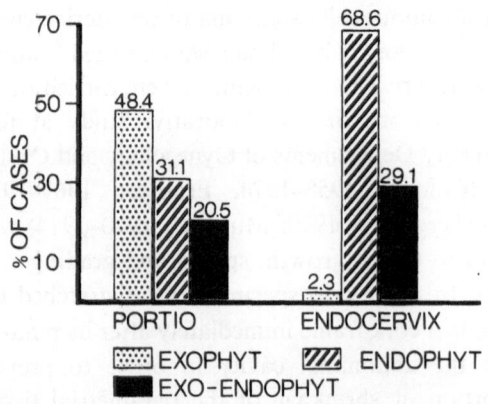

Figure 4. Tumor localization / tumor growth (*n* = 718).

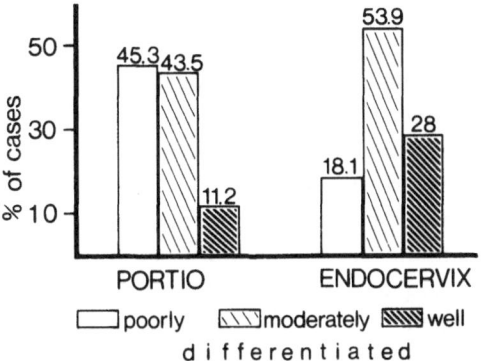

Figure 5. Tumor localization / dissociating tumor growth (*n* = 718).

localized in the region of the portio reveal a highly pronounced dissociating growth in only 11.2%, whereas the endocervically situated tumors display this morphological appearance in 28% (Figure 5).

With regard to the continuous tumor spreading in the direction of the parametrium, it becomes evident that involvement of the parametrium is present in only 2% of cases in which the carcinomas are localized on the portio, whereas it is present in 17.2% of the endocervically situated carcinomas.

There are also distinct correlations between tumor growth and tumor grading. The exophytic carcinomas display the lowest percentage of poorly differentiated carcinomas (23.1%) and the endophytic carcinomas the lowest percentage of well-differentiated carcinomas (10.5%). The exophytic and the exo-endophytic carcinomas have the highest proportion of well-differentiated carcinomas (25.3% and 26.1% respectively) (Figure 6).

A pronounced dissociating tumor growth is observed more frequently in the endophytic (31.7%) than in the exophytic carcinomas (7.7%).

II.E. Vascular invasion

A tumor invasion into lymphatic vessels is registered in more than half of the cases (56.8%). Tumor infiltration into blood vessels is present in 9.6% of the cases. The degree of maturity of the carcinoma is significant for the tumor invasion into vessels. Thus a tumor infiltration into lymphatic vessels is present in 65.2% of the poorly differentiated carcinomas, and in 45.5% of the well-differentiated carcinomas. A tumor infiltration into blood vessels is registered in 14.7% of poorly differentiated carcinomas, but never in well-differentiated tumors.

II.F. Age-dependent factors

Correlations can also be detected between the age of the patient and the tumor growth. In the 16–30 year old patients, the proportion of endocervical carcinomas is 67.3% (Figure 7). With increasing age of the patient, there is a preponderance of endocervically situated carcinomas. The proportion of these carcinomas is 87.3% in the 51–70 year old patients. Carcinomas localized on the portio are registered in 32.7% of young women and in 12.7% of old women.

If one considers the tumor growth the percentage of 21.8% exophytic carcinomas in young women is striking. This percentage falls with increasing age to 6.4%. On the other hand, the proportion of exophytic carcinomas rises from 41.8% in young women to 72.8% in old women. Tumor spread is also age dependent. Whereas a tumor involvement of the parametrium is registered in only 11.3% of the

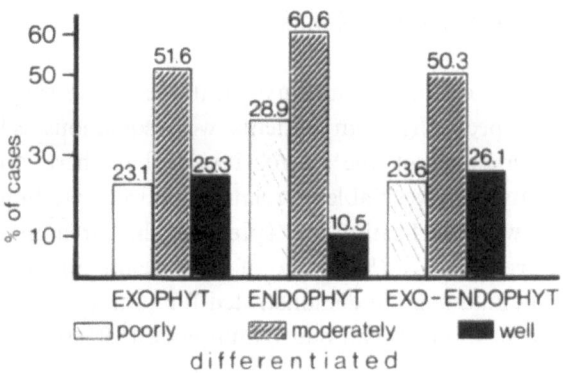

Figure 6. Tumor growth / tumor grading (*n* = 718).

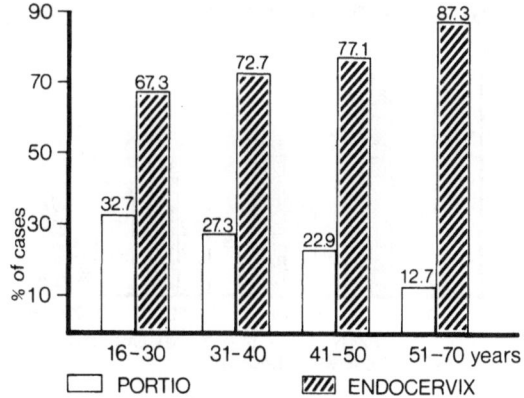

Figure 7. Tumor localization / patient's age (*n* = 718).

16–30 year old women, the percentage is 22.1% in the 51–70 year old women.

It is noticeable that statistically verifiable differences cannot be demonstrated in the individual age groups taking into account the tumor grading. There are also no age-specific differences for tumor infiltration of blood and lymphatic vessels.

However, age-dependent differences can be demonstrated in the analysis of the lymph node findings. Whereas the carcinoma has metastasized into the regional lymph nodes in 16–30 year old women in 54.5%, metastases are observed in only 31.2% of the 51–70 year old women. In the evaluation of the lymph node morphology a hyperergic reaction is registered in 67.9% in the 16–30 year olds whereas this reaction is only present in 22.5% of the 51–70 year old (Figure 8). Atrophic lymph nodes are present in only 1.9% of the patients in the first group, whereas they are present in 29.9% of the patients in the second group.

III. DISCUSSION

In the study presented, correlations between growth, spread and grading of squamous cell carcinomas of the uterine cervix are investigated. Determination of the tumor localization revealed predominantly endocervically situated tumors. In terms of their growth form, more than half of the cases involve endophytically growing carcinomas. Similar observations have been presented by Gusberg et al. (1953), who investigated 91 surgical preparations for localization and growth of the carcinoma.

It is illuminating that the high proportion of exophytic mature carcinomas with dissociative growth and rare involvement of the parametrium is typical for carcinomas localized on the portio. On the other hand, the endocervically situated tumors are characterized by a higher proportion of endophytic immature carcinomas with more dissociative growth and with more frequent involvement of the parametrium. It also becomes evident that with increasing immaturity of the carcinoma a more frequent tumor infiltration into lymphatic and blood vessels is registered.

It could be shown with regard to the age of the patients that there are relations between age and tumor localization, growth and spread for carcinoma *in situ* (Schneppenheim et al. 1958; Ober 1958; Ober and Bontke 1959; Burghardt 1963; Hillemans 1964; Burghardt and Holzer 1970). Thus, exophytically growing carcinomas predominantly localized on the portio which had infiltrated more rarely into the parametrial tissue were involved in young women. With increasing age, the percentage of endocervically situated endophytically growing carcinomas rises, and the parametria are affected more frequently.

Lymph node metastases are registered more frequently in young than in old women. Sidhu et al. (1970) have also observed lymph node metastases more frequently in younger women than in older women. The lymph node alterations with predominance of a hyperergic reaction in young women and predominance of atrophic lymph nodes in old women were also typical. The significance of lymph node morphology in cervical carcinoma has also been pointed out by Tsakraklides et al. (1973), Kozlowski and Hrabowska (1975) and Van Nagell et al. (1977).

IV. CONCLUDING REMARKS

Systematic histological investigations on 718 surgical specimens from patients with squamous cell carcinomas of the cervix reveal that there are statistically verifiable correlations between grading, growth, localization and spread of the carcinoma. Correlations with the age of the patients operated on could also be demonstrated for tumor growth, localization, spread and lymph node metastases.

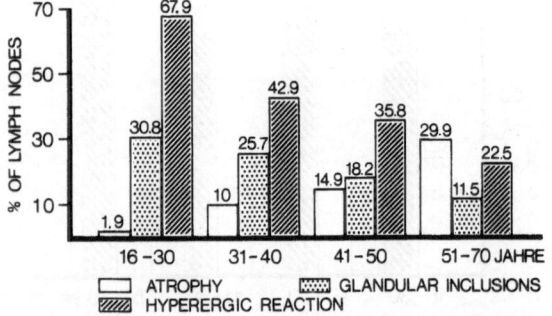

Figure 8. Morphology of the lymph nodes / patient's age (*n* = 718).

ACKNOWLEDGEMENTS

Statistical analysis was performed in cooperation with Dr. W. Koepcke, Institute of Medical Information Processing, Statistics and Biomathematics, University of Munich (Prof. K. Ueberla). The financial support of the Deutsche Forschungsgemeinschaft (Bonn) is gratefully acknowledged.

REFERENCES

Brunet G: Ergebnisse der abdominalen Radikaloperation des Gebärmutter-Scheiden-Krebses mittels Laparotomia hypogastrica. II. Pathologisch-anatomischer Teil. Z Geburtsh Gynäk 56: 1–87, 1905.

Burghardt E: Die diagnostische Konisation der Portio vaginalis uteri. Operationstechnik, histologische Diagnostik und klinische Ergebnisse. Geburtsh u Frauenheilk 23: 1–30, 1963.

Burghardt E, Holzer E: Die Lokalisation des pathologischen Zervixepithels. I. Carcinomata in situ, Dysplasien und abnormes Epithel. Arch Gynäk 209: 305–330, 1970.

Gusberg SB, Fish SA, Wang YY: Growth Pattern of Cervical Cancer. Obstet and Gynec 2: 557–561, 1953.

Hillemanns HG: Entstehung und Wachstum des Zervixkarzinoms. Basel: Karger, 1964.

Kindermann G, Ober KG: Ausbreitung des Zervixkrebses. In: Käser O, Friedberg V, Ober KG, Thomsen K, Zander J (eds): Gynäkologie und Geburtshilfe, Band III. Stuttgart: Thieme, 1972.

Kozlowski H, Hrabowska M: Types of Reaction in the Regional Lymph Nodes in Non-metastatic and Minute Metastatic Carcinoma of the Uterine Cervix. Arch Geschwulstforsch 45: 658–669, 1975.

Kundrat R: Über die Ausbreitung des Karzinoms im parametranen Gewebe bei Krebs des Collum uteri. Arch Gynäk 69: 355–409, 1903.

Matuschka M: Unsere histologische Technik zur Aufarbeitung von Konisationen, ganzen Uteri und Uteri mit anhängenden Parametrien. Geburtsh u Frauenheilk 22: 498–505, 1962.

Ober KG: Cervix uteri und Lebensalter. Die Bedeutung der Formwandlung der Zervix für die Krebsdiagnostik und die Frage der sogenannten Portioerosion. Dtsch med Wschr 83: 1661–1672, 1958.

Ober KG, Bontke E: Sitz und Ausdehnung der Carcinomata in situ und der beginnenden Krebse der Zervix. Arch Gynäk 192: 55–68, 1959.

Ober KG, Huhn FO: Die Ausbreitung des Zervixkrebses auf die Parametrien und die Lymphknoten der Beckenwand. Arch Gynäk 197: 262–290, 1962.

Scheib A: Klinische und anatomische Beiträge zur operativen Behandlung des Uteruscarcinoms. Arch Gynäk 87: 1–66, 233–285, 1909.

Schneppenheim P, Hamperl H, Kaufmann C, Ober KG: Die Beziehungen des Schleimepithels zum Plattenepithel an der Cervix uteri im Lebenslauf der Frau. Arch Gynäk 190: 303–345, 1958.

Selbmann HK, Raab A: SAVOD-Q. Benützerhandbuch. Technischer Bericht. 3. ISB München, 1976.

Sidhu AS, Koss LG, Barber KRK: Relation of Histologic Factors to the Response of Stage I Epidermoid-carcinoma of the Cervix to Surgical Treatment. Obstet and Gynec 35: 329–338, 1970.

Tsakraklides V, Anastassiades OT, Kersey JH: Prognostic Significance of Regional Lymph Node Histology in Uterine Cervical Cancer. Cancer 31: 860–868, 1973.

Van Nagell JR, Donaldson ES, Parker JC, van Dyke AH, Wood EG: The Prognostic Significance of Pelvic Lymph Node Morphology in Carcinoma of the Uterine Cervix. Cancer 39: 2624–2632, 1977.

11. MICROINVASIVE CARCINOMA OF THE CERVIX: DEFINITION AND BEHAVIOR

G.R. Schrodt and W.M. Christopherson

In simple morphologic terms microinvasive squamous carcinoma of the uterine cervix (MIC) defines those lesions with limited invasion of the cervical stroma. In biologic terms (MIC) refers to those lesions with limited potential for metastases.

There is however no universally acceptable definition. The American Joint Committee for Cancer Staging and End Results Reporting (1978) defines Stage IA as microinvasive carcinoma (early stromal invasion). According to that staging system which is identical to that of the International Federation of Gynecology & Obstetrics (FIGO) microinvasive carcinoma 'represents those cases of epithelial abnormalities in which histologic evidence of early stromal invasion is unambiguous. The diagnosis is based upon microscopic examination of tissue removed by biopsy, conization, portio amputation or on removal of the uterus.' The Society of Gynecologic Oncologists has accepted the following definition: viz., one in which the neoplastic epithelium invades the stroma in one or more places to a depth of 3 mm or less below the basement membrane, and lymphatic or vascular involvement is not demonstrated. Stromal invasion to a depth of 5 mm and capillary-like space involvement are features acceptable to some (Christopherson et al. 1976). Tumors invading no deeper than 5 mm but extending greater than 10 mm in length and/or 10 mm in width are sometimes considered frankly invasive carcinomas (Lohe 1978).

As a corollary, there is no uniformly acceptable treatment for MIC despite the efforts of investigators for the past twenty years to arrive at a formula for optimum therapy.

I. HISTORICAL

Limited stromal invasion by squamous carcinomas of the cervix has been recognized for many years. In one of the earliest reports (Rubin 1910) three cases of incipient carcinoma of the uterus are discussed. The pathologic examination of the hysterectomy specimens must have been quite complete. Plate drawings served as illustrations. By today's standard the lesions might well be interpreted as demonstrating surface and glandular involvement without clear evidence of stromal invasion. It is of interest, however, that Rubin described in one case lymphatic spread but also mentioned that no tumor was found in the lymph nodes removed at surgery. One of the first reports in which an early carcinoma of the cervix was measured is that of (Martzloff 1922). In his case report a lesion had invaded 2 mm into the stroma and invaded lymphatic channels. The patient underwent a modified Wertheim hysterectomy and was doing well at time of the report although a follow-up time was not given. No mention was made of presence or absence of metastases in the removed lymph nodes. In another of the early papers (Schiller 1933) 'early cancer' is discussed without quantitation of the lesion. It is of note that Figure 9 of this rather lengthy article depicts *in situ* carcinoma or dysplasia. Schiller claimed that this particular lesion recurred. These reports are important from a historical viewpoint but for the most part did not attempt to define MIC in strict morphologic terms.

Concerted efforts to define squamous microinvasive carcinoma of the uterine cervix in morphological and biological terms began about 20 years ago. During this time period an increased number of cases of *in situ* squamous cell carcinoma of the cervix and of microinvasive carcinoma have

Hafez, E.S.E., Smith, J.P. (eds.), Carcinoma of the Cervix: Biology and Diagnosis. ISBN-13: 978-94-009-7487-6
© 1982, Martinus Nijhoff Publishers, The Hague/Boston/London.

been detected primarily as the result of increased utilization of cervical cytological screening. Literally scores of investigators have presented their experience in the diagnosis of early cervical cancer and recommendations for treatment.

II. CLINICAL FEATURES OF MICROINVASIVE CARCINOMA

MIC is most frequently detected in patients between the ages of 40 and 50 years. The mean age has been variously reported as 48.3 years (Mussey et al. 1969), 46±12.7 years (Ng and Reagan 1969; Christopherson et al. 1976).

The majority of patients are asymptomatic. Elicted complaints include vaginal discharge, bleeding and pain.

Diagnosis is most often suspected following cervical cytology studies. In most cases the cervix by clinical examination appears normal or else exhibits abnormalities such as cervicitis or erosions. Colposcopy has improved the clinical detection rate (Kolstad 1969).

III. MORPHOLOGIC FEATURES OF MIC

The qualitative histologic features of (MIC) have been adequately described (Ng and Reagan 1969; Averette et al. 1976; Leman et al. 1976; Lohe 1978) and are generally recognized. An occasional lesion exhibiting questionable stromal invasion is best regarded as an example of *in situ* carcinoma. MIC most typically originates from an abnormal surface epithelium. The earliest lesions, which may be single or multifocal consist of irregular finger-like or tongue-like extensions into the stroma. Customarily the cells at the advancing edges mature as evidenced by increasing cytoplasmic eosinophilia and kerati-

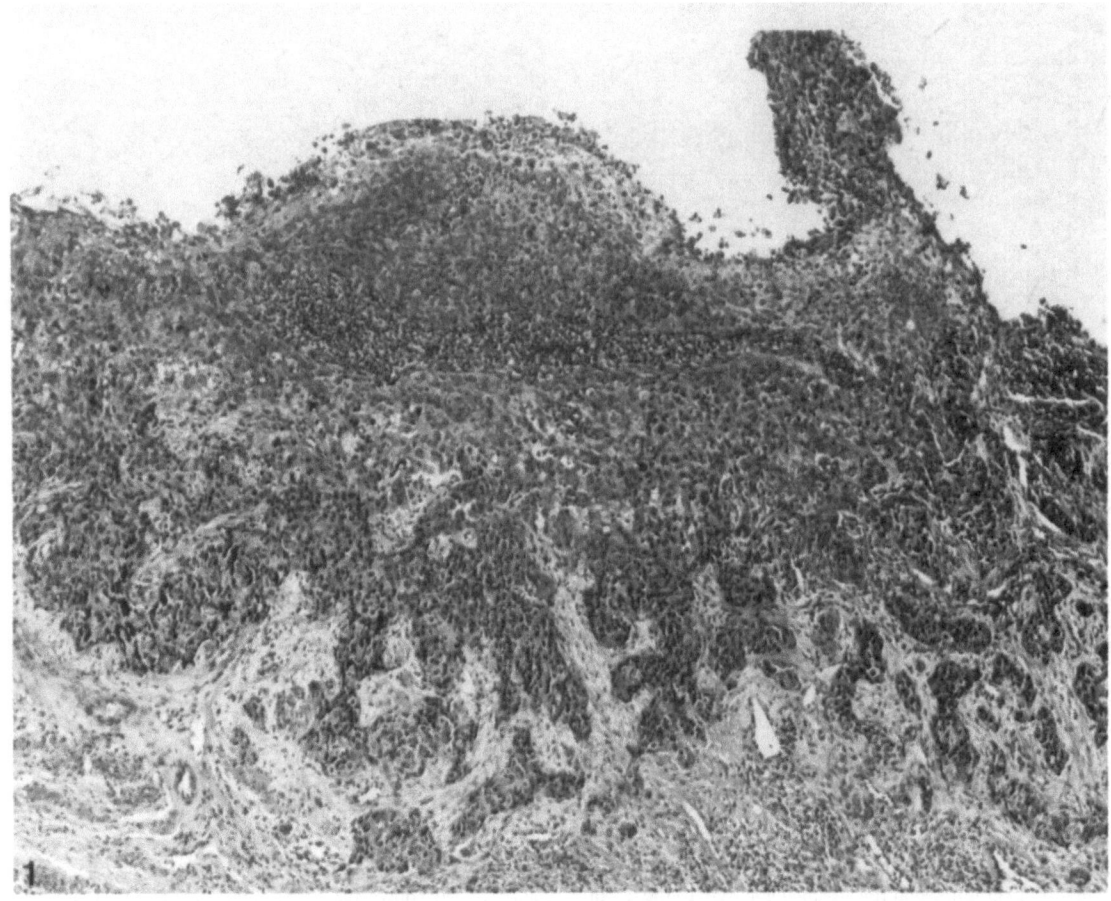

Figure 1. Microinvasive carcinoma of the cervix. Tongue-like projections of tumor have invaded the stroma, × 92.

64

nization. Lymphocytes, plasma cells and occasional neutrophils may be found in variable numbers at the advancing margins of the tumor (Figure 1).

While the above qualitative histologic criteria are generally acceptable there are additional qualitative and quantitative features which remain controversial. These include (1) acceptable depth of invasion; (2) significance of the so-called confluent growth pattern (Figure 2); (3) significance of capillary-like space involvement by the tumor (Figures 2 and 3); (4) acceptable extent of the tumor in length and width; and (5) significance of tumor present at the margins of a conization specimen.

Depth of invasion has most often been measured from the basement membrane of the surface epithelium or an involved gland adjacent to the point or points of invasion. More recently depth of invasion has been measured from the surface of the epithelium at the site of invasion (Roche et al. 1975; Christopherson et al. 1976). It probably matters

little which measurement is used since the surface epithelium is only 1/3 to 1/4 mm thick.

Permissible depth of stromal invasion for MIC is variously established between one and five millimeters. In many reported series three millimeters of stromal invasion is acceptable (Bohm et al. 1976; Creasman and Weed 1979; Foushee et al. 1969; Yajima and Noda 1979). Invasion to a depth of 5 mm is acceptable to others (Boutselis et al. 1971; Iverson et al. 1979; Lohe 1978; Leman et al. 1976). Paradoxically, in one recent review (Roche et al. 1975) lesions with less than two millimeters of invasion were excluded from consideration.

While some evidence has been published that the likelihood of lymph node metastases is directly proportional to depth of invasion, lesions invading to less than 3 mm may rarely have metastases (Hasumi 1980).

Two general patterns of stromal invasion have been described in MIC, viz., finger-like and con-

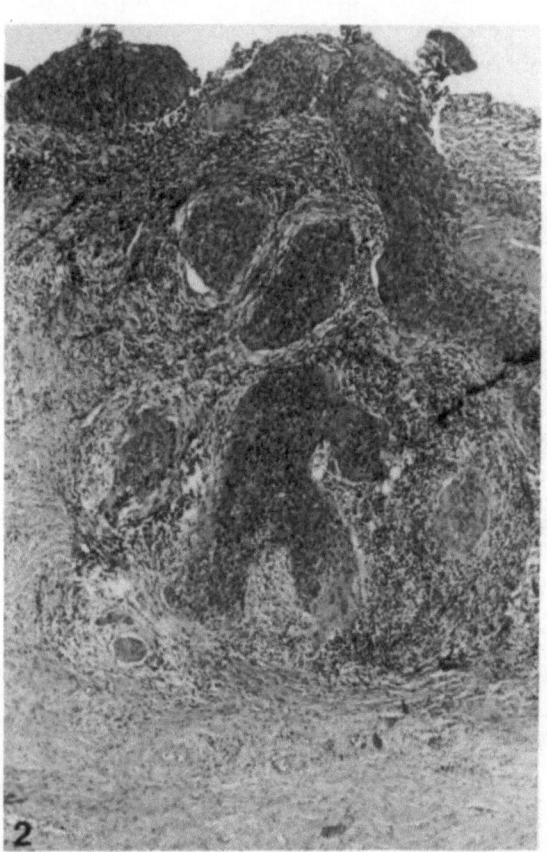

Figure 2. Microinvasive carcinoma with so-called confluent growth pattern. There is a moderate lymphocyte infiltrate. CL space involvement is noted at the advancing margin to the left of center, × 55.

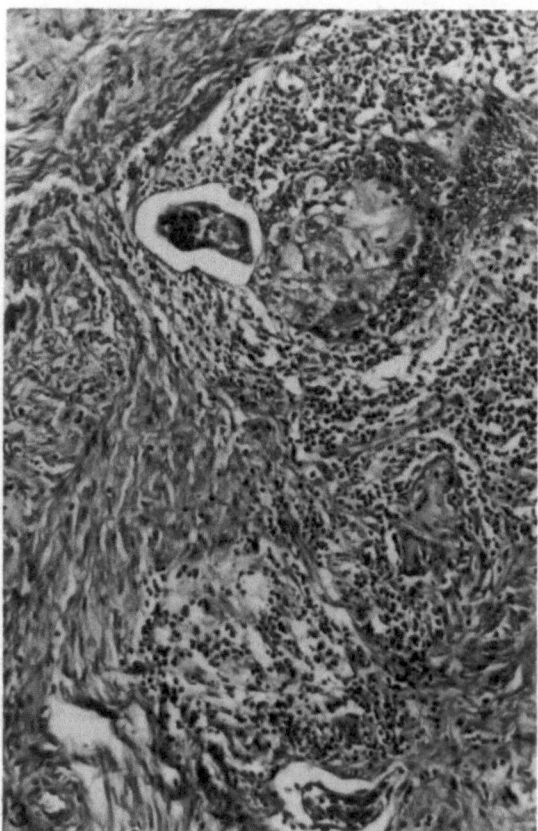

Figure 3. Microinvasive carcinoma. Two capillary-like spaces contain tumor cells, × 130.

fluent. Mixtures of the two patterns are common. Confluence of growth, which might be regarded as fusion of smaller aggregates of neoplastic cells, is more prominent in the more deeply invasive lesions. A confluent growth pattern, according to the criteria of some investigators (Savage 1972; Yajima and Noda 1979) excludes the lesion from consideration as MIC. At times lesions exhibiting a confluent pattern are included as examples of MIC for statistical purposes; the finding, however, is regarded as an indication for more aggressive therapy. In more recent published reports, less significance is placed on growth pattern as evidence accumulates that the pattern of growth has little relationship to biologic behavior of this tumor (Hasumi 1980; Roche and Norris 1975).

Involvement or invasion of vascular spaces in MIC has been widely recognized and variously interpreted. For many (Averette et al. 1976; Creasman and Weed 1979; Mussey et al. 1969; Foushee et al. 1969; Sedlis et al. 1979) only to name a few – the demonstration of vascular space involvement in a given tumor excludes that tumor as an example of MIC, or else demands extended therapy. Recently it has been suggested (Roche and Norris 1975; Leman et al. 1976) that the so-called vascular spaces be termed CL spaces (capillary-like spaces). Regardless of the term employed there is little evidence that involvement of these CL spaces correlates with the presence of metastases to regional lymph nodes. Lymph node metastases have been observed in cases with capillary space involvement, but metastases have also been identified in lesions in which capillary-like space involvement has not been observed (Bohm et al. 1976). In a study of 30 cases (Roche and Norris 1975) capillary-like space involvement was demonstrated in 57% of cases and in none of these were lymph node metastases demonstrated. Lemans study of 51 cases provides similar findings. In his series capillary-like space involvement was demonstrated in 24% of the patients; metastases were not found in any of the lymph nodes removed at surgery, and all cases in both studies had lymph node dissection.

A morphologic parameter given little consideration until recently is tumor length and width (Lohe 1978). In his elaborate analysis of a large series of cases Lohe defines early invasive cervical carcinoma into two categories, viz., those with early

stromal invasion and microcarcinomas. Microcarcinomas are lesions with greater stromal involvement but are limited to maximum depth of invasion of 5 mm and maximum lateral extent to 10 mm in length and/or width. The figure of 10 mm was arbitrarily chosen since in larger lesions regional lymph node metastases were occasionally found.

Contrary to the American Joint Committee – FIGO staging rules MIC cannot be diagnosed by biopsy, but rather requires at least a cold knife conization specimen, serially blocked and adequately sectioned. Of what significance is microinvasive carcinoma at the cone margins? More extensive therapy has been recommended in those cases where the cone margins are incomplete (Sedlis et al. 1979;Leman et al. 1976). Conversely there is evidence that incomplete margins in MIC do not adversely affect outcome (Christopherson et al. 1976).

In summary, there is no consensus of the histologic definition of microinvasive carcinoma of the cervix. However, it might be emphasized that several organizations including the Society of Gynecologic Oncologists have established a definition which includes limited invasion of stroma to no more than 3 mm measured from the base of the epithelium and excluding examples with lymphatic or vascular involvement. One might assume that the majority members of the society believe that lesions invading from 3 to 5 mm in depth are biologically more aggressive than those invading to a depth of 3 mm or less. To arrive at this conclusion one must interpret the available published data differently from those who believe that the biologic behavior of invasive lesions less than 3 mm is no different from those invading to a depth of 3 to 5 mm.

IV. CLINICAL-PATHOLOGICAL CORRELATES

There are certain clinical-pathologic correlates regarding microinvasive carcinoma of the cervix *which are more or less generally accepted.* These would include: (1) Diagnosis is optimally based on histologic examination of the entire cervix, the specimen preferably obtained by cold knife conization. Under optimal conditions the cone specimen is opened fresh, pinned to an appropriate anchor such as a cork board and fixed. Twelve to twenty blocks are readily obtained from an adequate cone. Step sections of the individual blocks may be indicated, but at least one section from each tissue block must be examined. Further, the pathologist should employ an ocular micrometer, properly calibrated, to adequately measure the lesions. (2) Microinvasive carcinoma may on rare occasion metastasize to regional lymph nodes. Metastases may derive from lesions invading to one millimeter or less. (3) Involvement of capillary-like spaces may occur in up to 57% of cases. Involvement of CL spaces rarely results in demonstrable lymph node metastases. Furthermore, lymph node metastases may occur in the absence of demonstrable CL space involvement. (4) Lesions with very minimal stromal invasion without a confluent growth pattern or involvement of CL spaces may be treated by simple hysterectomy.

V. THE LOUISVILLE EXPERIENCE

The data on MIC derived from the University of Louisville are essentially those developed by Christopherson and co-workers (Christopherson and Parker 1964; Christopherson et al. 1976). A position, liberal in terms of the extent of the lesion which may be treated by less than so-called radical means, has been presented, and has gained much support in the past few years. Our present definition of microinvasive carcinoma would include lesions invading to a depth of 5 mm measured from the epithelial surface at the origin of the lesion, including cases with confluence of growth and capillary-like space involvement.

Between the years 1953 and 1973, one hundred and eleven cases of MIC were evaluated. In every

Table 1. Method of treatment.

Cone only	3
Excision of cervical stump	2
Simple hysterectomy	79
Cone + irradiation	14
Hysterectomy + irradiation	3
Radical hysterectomy	10
Total	111

Reproduced by permission of the authors and publisher. Table 1. Christopherson, W.M., Gray, L.A. and Parker, J.E. Microinvasive Carcinoma of the Uterine Cervix. Cancer 38: 630, 1976. Courtesy J.B. Lippincott Co., Philadelphia, PA.

Table 2. Follow-up by method of treatment.

	Alive 5 yr	Dead 5 yr	Alive 10 yr	Dead 10 yr
Cone only	2	0	2	0
Excision of cervical stump	2	0	2	0
Simple hysterectomy[a]	60	2	50	3
Cone + irradiation	12	2[b]	7	6[b]
Hysterectomy + irradiation	3	0	3	0
Radical hysterectomy	7	1	6	1
Total	86	5	70	10

[a]One patient lost to follow-up at 5.5 years.
[b]Death certificate attributed death to cervix cancer for one patient at 2 years, 7 months, and one at 8 years.

Reproduced by permission of the authors and publisher. Table 2. Christopherson, W.M., Gray, L.A. and Parker, J.E. Microinvasive Carcinoma of the Uterine Cervix. Cancer 38: 630, 1976. Courtesy J.B. Lippincott Co., Philadelphia, PA.

case the diagnosis was established by serial block examination of a cervical cone or the entire cervix. The method of treatment is outlined in Table 1. It should be noted that approximately twenty-five percent of the patients were treated by less than radical methods.

Follow-up data is summarized in Table 2. It can be noted that two deaths were attributed to cervical cancer. In each case the death certificate was signed by a non-physician coroner's assistant and autopsy was not performed. Of significance is the fact that the tumor in one patient had invaded to a maximum depth of 1 mm and in the other to a maximum depth of 1.1 mm. Both patients were treated by conization plus irradiation, and in neither was there evidence of death from disease. One patient was actually seen the day prior to death in the GYN tumor clinic. Her pelvic examination was negative and she was in severe heart failure.

VI. THERAPY OUTCOME

A final test to measure effectiveness of therapy is that which compares outcome with alternate modes of therapy for lesions of comparable biologic behavior. The biologic behavior of MIC can be assessed by determining the likelihood of nodal metastases, frequency of recurrence and most important, survival rate. Additionally the morbidity and mortality associated with the various modalities must be considered. In effect, the optimum treatment is directly proportional to the survival rate and indirectly proportional to the adverse effects of therapy.

Reported frequency of regional lymph node metastases derived from tumors invading to 5 mm or less have been variously reported as being from 0% to 20%. A recent and most comprehensive review places the frequency at about 1% (Lohe 1978). There is some evidence that the likelihood of nodal metastases is directly related to the depth of invasion (Hasumi 1980). However, nodal metastases may result from lesions with very limited stromal invasion (Hasumi 1980; Christopherson et al. 1976).

The 5-year survival rate for MIC in most reported series ranges between 95% and 100%. It has been suggested that the more deeply invasive tumors, 3 mm to 5 mm have a higher 5 year mortality. Of 1180 patients with early stromal invasion reviewed by (Lohe 1980), 4 with tumor recurrence subsequently died of their tumor. In this same article 17 deaths (from a group of 569) were *attributed* to recurrent microcarcinoma, with 11 deaths recorded in 1 series (Boyes et al. 1970). Analysis of Boyes' paper, however, reveals that the tumors in question were actually categorized as occult invasive carcinomas. Over one-half the lesions exceeded 1 cm in extent; furthermore, the depth of invasion was not recorded.

In a recent summary report of *in situ* carcinoma with microscopic foci of invasion 353 cases have been followed for 5 years with only 1 patient dead of disease. No additional deaths have occurred in 249 patients which have been followed for 10 years (Boyes 1980).

Most of the published reports on MIC fail to discuss therapy complications; there are however some notable exceptions. (Bohm et al. 1976) stated that there were no operative deaths in a group of 56 patients with MIC who were treated by radical hysterectomy and lymphadenectomy. Conversely (Foushee et al. 1969) reported a 14% complication rate in radical hysterectomy – lymphadenectomy patients resulting in permanent disability or requiring surgical correction. (Leman et al. 1976) recorded in his series of 51 patients who received radical surgery 13 minor complications and seven major, including pulmonary embolus, small bowel obstruction and wound evisceration.

A final note can be made when comparing mortality data with treatment regimens for MIC. Perhaps as many as 50% of all deaths attributed to these lesions have occurred in (Boyes et al. 1970; Lohe 1980) patients who received radical therapy. Stated in different fashion there is no 100% assurance that radical therapy will result in a favorable outcome, even in lesions with early stromal invasion and absence of demonstrable capillary space involvement.

It might appear therefore that a more liberal definition of microinvasive carcinoma of the cervix is justified and that less than radical therapy for this lesion is warranted.

REFERENCES

Averette HE, Nelson JH, Jr, Ng ABP, Hoskins WJ, Boyce JG, Ford JH, Jr: Diagnosis and management of microinvasive (Stage IA) carcinoma of the uterine cervix. Cancer 38: 414, 1976.

Bohm JW, Krupp PJ, Lee FY, Batson HWK: Lymph node metastasis in microinvasive epidermoid cancer of thE cervix. Obstet and Gynecol 48: 64, 1976.

Boutselis JG, Ullery JC, Charme L: Diagnosis and management of Stage IA (microinvasive) carcinoma of the cervix. Amer J Obstet Gynec 110: 984, 1971.

Boyes DA, Worth AJ, Fidler HK:·The results of treatment of 4389 cases of pre-clinical cervical squamous carcinoma. The J of Obstet and Gynecol of the British Commonwealth 77: 769, 1970.

Boyes DA: Personal communication.

Christopherson WM, Parker JE: Microinvasive carcinoma of the uterine cervix, A clinical-pathological study. Cancer 17: 1123, 1964.

Christopherson WM, Gray LA, Parker JE: Microinvasive carcinoma of the uterine cervix. Cancer 38: 629, 1976.

Creasman WT, Weed JC, Jr: Microinvasive cancer vs occult cancer. Int J Radiation Oncology Biol Phys 5: 1871, 1979.

Foushee JHS, Greiss FC, Lock FR: Stage IA squamous cell carcinoma of the uterine cervix. Am J Obst & Gynec 105: 46, 1969.

Hasumi K, Sakamoto A, Sugano H: Microinvasive carcinoma of the uterine cervix. Cancer 45: 928, 1980.

Iversen T, Abeler V, Kjorstad KE: Factors influencing the treatment of patients with stage IA carcinoma of the cervix. British J of Obstet and Gynecol 86: 593, 1979.

Kolstad P: Carcinoma of the cervix Stage IA. Am J Obst & Gynec 104: 1015, 1969.

Leman MH, Jr, Benson WL, Kurman RJ, Park RC: Microinvasive carcinoma of the cervix. Obstet and Gynecol 48: 571, 1976.

Lohe KJ: Early squamous cell carcinoma of the uterine cervix: Definition and histology. Gynecologic Oncology 6: 10, 1978.

Lohe KJ, Burghardt E, Hillemans HG, Kaufmann C, Ober KG, Zander J: Early squamous cell carcinoma of the uterine cervix: Clinical results of a cooperative study in the management of 419 patients with early stromal invasion and microcarcinoma. Gynecologic Oncology 6: 31, 1978.

Lohe KJ: Early squamous cell carcinoma of the uterine cervix: Frequency of lymph node metastases. Gynecologic Oncology 6: 51, 1978.

Martzloff KH: Carcinoma of the cervix uteri: A very early case. Johns Hopkins Hosp Bull 33: 221, 1922.

Mussey E, Soule EH, Welch JS: Microinvasive carcinoma of the cervix. Am J Obst & Gynec 104: 738, 1969.

Ng ABP, Reagan JW: Microinvasive carcinoma of the uterine cervix. Amer J Clin Path 52: 511, 1969.

Roche WD, Norris HJ: Microinvasive carcinoma of the cervix: The significance of lymphatic invasion and confluent patterns of stromal growth. Cancer 36: 180, 1975.

Rubin IC: The pathological diagnosis of *incipient* carcinoma of the uterus. Amer J of Obstet and Dis of Women and Children 62: 668, 1910.

Savage EW: Microinvasive carcinoma of the cervix. Am J Obstet Gynecol 113: 708, 1972.

Schiller W: Early diagnosis of carcinoma of the cervix. Surgery, Gynecology and Obstetrics 56: 210, 1933.

Sedlis A, Sall S, Tsukada Y, Park R, Mangan C, Shingleton H, Bless JA: Microinvasive carcinoma of the uterine cervix: A clinical-pathologic study. Am J Obstet Gynecol 133: 64, 1979.

Yajima A, Noda K: The results of treatment of microinvasive carcinoma (Stage IA) of the uterine cervix by means of simple and extended hysterectomy. Am J Obstet Gynecol 135: 685, 1979.

12. HYPERKERATOTIC CERVICAL DYSPLASIA

R.A. KOMOROWSKI and E.J. WILKINSON

The concepts of cervical dysplasia, carcinoma *in situ*, and invasive carcinoma are now generally accepted. The histologic evaluation of the typical cervical dysplastic processes are standardized. There is general agreement on the grading of cervical dysplasia as mild, moderate or severe depending on the ratio of the thickness of the abnormal cervical epithelium compared to its full thickness. Carcinoma *in situ* is a full thickness replacement of normal epithelium with abnormal dysplastic epithelium, while invasion is present when there is penetration of the basement membrane by the carcinoma. No such standard approach is available, however, to evaluate and grade the significance of variants of cervical dysplasia. One variant of cervical dysplasia is hyperkeratotic cervical dysplasia and is defined as cervical dysplasia with a granular layer and a keratotic surface. This particular variant provides the pathologist with a challenge in grading, whether one uses the standard grading of cervical dysplasia or one of the proposed newer classifications (Richart 1973).

When reviewing cervical dysplasia and carcinoma, the diagnosis of a hyperkeratotic lesion may vary among pathologists from dysplasia to carcinoma. Such a lesion would be considered cancer if located on the pars vaginalis but only dysplasia if the lesion occurred in the endocervical canal (Christopherson 1977). No evidence or criteria supported the divergent diagnoses. Another problem associated with these lesions is the possibility of false negative cytologic diagnosis (Lambert and Woodruff 1963). Atypical epithelial cells may not readily shed because of the hyperkeratotic surface.

Hyperkeratotic dysplasia and carcinoma have been recognized in the past as a variant of cervical neoplasia (Koss et al. 1963) and hyperkeratotic lesions have been described as histologic accompaniments of leukoplakia and uterine prolapse. However, even experts in gynecologic pathology recognize the difficulty in precisely categorizing and grading these lesions.

The histology, cytology and long-term prognosis of this variant of cervical dysplasia was systematically studied. All cervical surgical specimens diagnosed as dysplasia or carcinoma *in situ* over the period 1956 to 1976 were reviewed. Multiple step sections were available on almost all specimens. Additional sections were obtained where deemed necessary. Biopsies in which the cervical epithelium had both a granular layer and a keratotic surface became the basis of the study. Excluded were cases with only surface keratinization without a granular layer and cases with only individual cell keratination or surface parakeratosis.

Dysplasia was graded as mild, moderate or severe. Dysplastic cells were those which were hyperchromatic with increased nuclear-cytoplasmic ratios. They showed poor orientation with increased mitoses and in some cases abnormal mitoses. Some cells also showed hypermaturation characterized by deep pink cytoplasm and even individual cell keratinization. The dysplasia was graded mild if these changes were limited to the lower one third of the epithelial layer, moderate if limited to the lower two-thirds. The process was graded severe if the upper third of the epithelium showed dysplastic changes with normal surface maturation. The granular layer was considered the surface for grading purposes. Thus, a full thickness alteration of epithelial cells from basement membrane to the granular layer would be diagnosed as carcinoma *in situ*.

Hafez, E.S.E., Smith, J.P. (eds.), Carcinoma of the Cervix: Biology and Diagnosis. ISBN-13: 978-94-009-7487-6

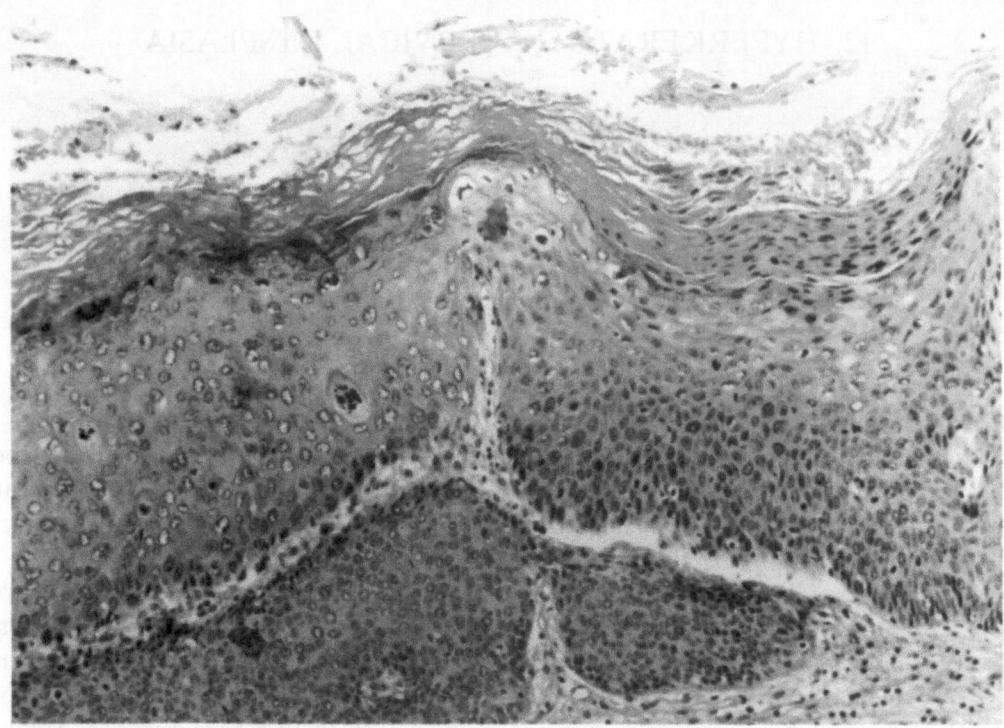

Figure 1. Dysplastic cervical epithelium has a thick granule layer with a hyperkeratotic surface on left. Right has surface parakeratosis. Focal abnormal cells give a Bowenoid appearance, HE × 160.

I. CLINICAL FEATURES

A total of 46 patients (48 of 1556 biopsies) had hyperkeratotic cervical dysplasia (Figures 1 and 2) or carcinoma (Figure 2b). This change was seen in 3.1% of the total number of biopsies examined (Table 1). Patients ranged in age from 20 to 86 years. Of the 46 patients, 35 were less than 50 years of age. Also, 35 patients had either severe dysplasia or carcinoma *in situ*. Six of the patients with carcinoma *in situ* had microinvasion to a depth of 3 mm or less measured from the basement membrane of the surface epithelium. All patients with carcinoma *in situ* or carcinoma *in situ* with microinvasion were treated by hysterectomy. None have

had recurrence with follow-ups of between 7 and 10 years (average 7.6 years).

Women with hyperkeratotic cervical dysplasia tended to have the hyperkeratotic process persist if the dysplasia persisted. A number of women have had such lesions over 9 years. In addition, with resolution of the dysplastic process, the hyperkeratosis resolved in all but one patient.

II. HISTOLOGIC FEATURES

A number of histologic features were commonly seen in the cases of hyperkeratotic cervical dysplasia. The epithelial surface was often irregular

Table 1. Grade of keratinizing dysplasia vs patient age; age range: 20–86.

Histology	Less than (years) 21	21–30	31–40	41–50	51–60	61–70	71–80	81–90	Total
Mild dysplasia	1	1	3						5
Moderate dysplasia		3		3					6
Severe dysplasia	2	6	4	6	1	1	1	1	22
Carcinoma *in situ*		2	5	2	3	1			13
Total	3	12	12	11	4	2	1	1	46

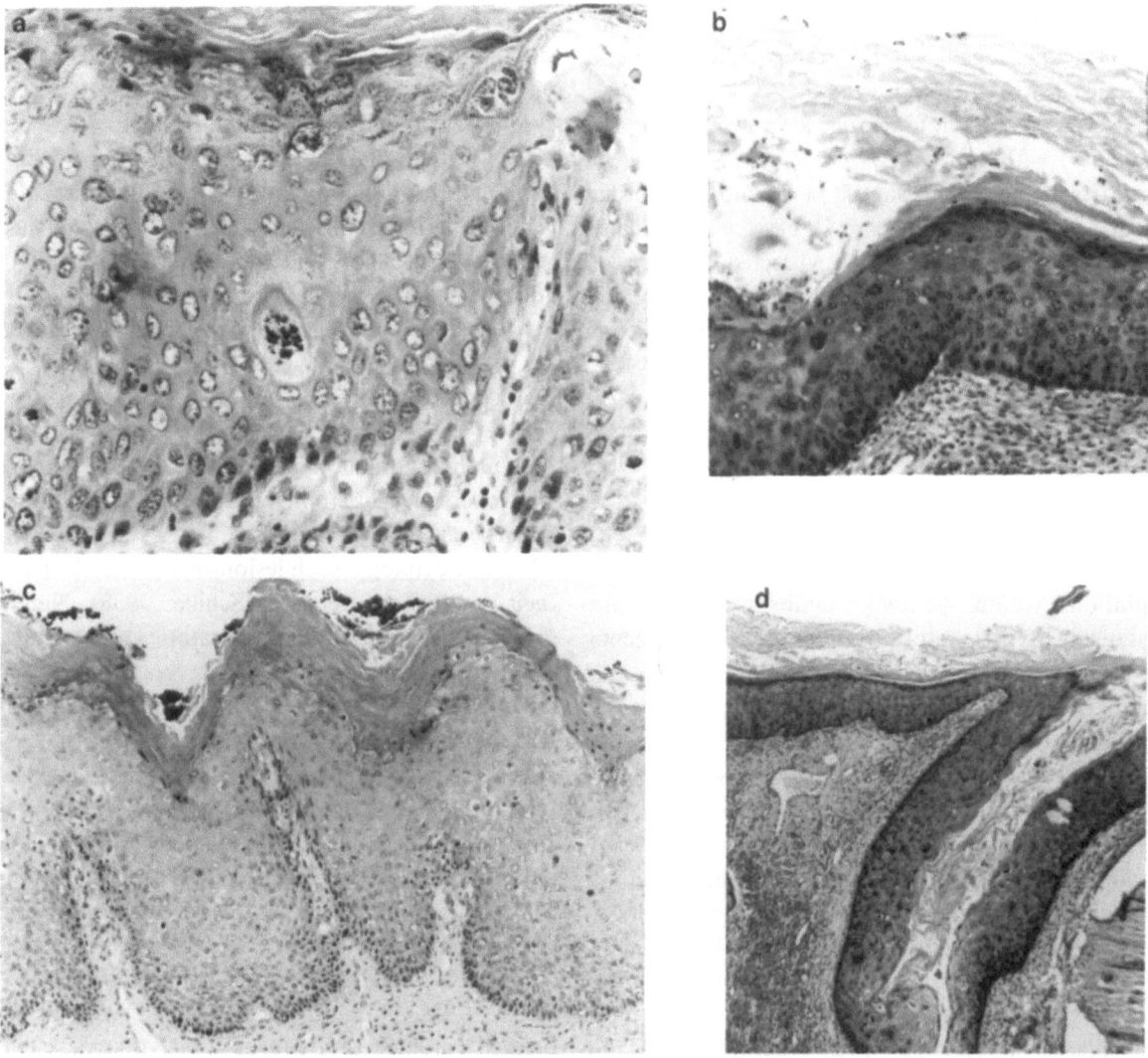

Figure 2.(a) Higher magnification of Fig. 1 showing abnormal maturation of epithelium and prominent granular layer with hyperkeratotic surface, HE × 200. *(b)* Epithelium shows lack of maturation which extends to the granular layer. Such change would be graded as carcinoma *in situ.* HE × 160. *(c)* Surface of cervix is irregular giving it a verracous appearance. Epithelium is moderately dysplastic, HE × 120. *(d)* Hyperkeratotic cervical dysplasia extends to endocervix and is involving the endocervical glands, HE × 120.

giving it a 'verrucous' appearance (Figure 2c). Parakeratosis was often found at sites adjacent to hyperkeratosis. Parakeratosis was seen in 67 (4.3%) of the 1556 cases examined (Figure 1). In the majority of cases the hyperkeratotic change involved the portio vaginalis but in some it extended to the squamo-columnar junction (Figure 2d). Some cases having Bowenoid appearance were difficult to grade. Isolated abnormal cells were found at all levels throughout the epithelium with sudden maturation at the granular layer. Such cases were graded as severe dysplasia (Figure 1).

A practical problem is how to grade the severity of the dysplasia. Initially, the lesions were graded from basement membrane to surface and from basement membrane to keratotic layer. Grading to the surface resulted in significant undergrading of severity. In some biopsies the keratin layer was as thick as the epithelium beneath it. Development of a granular layer is evidence of maturation and it can be argued that hyperkeratotic lesions should be graded as only severe dysplasia. However, in this series and other reported series (Burghardt 1972), cases with invasive disease were seen with the entire surface showing normal keratinization. Thus, proper grading of these lesions should be from basement membrane to granular layer. A lesion showing full thickness change to the granular layer would be graded as carcinoma *in situ*.

Severe hyperkeratotic dysplasia was often associated with typical *in situ* carcinoma in adjacent areas and these areas should be examined in order not to miss any significant disease. Today many biopsies are colposcopically directed. Biopsy of both the white lesions and tissue immediately adjacent to the lesion should yield the most significant diagnostic tissue as carcinoma *in situ* was often adjacent to foci of hyperkeratotic dysplasia.

III. CYTOLOGIC FEATURES

Thirty-seven of the 46 patients had cytologic examinations within the two months of the biopsy showing hyperkeratotic dysplasia. In 24 patients (65%), the cytologic and histologic diagnosis agreed. In 11 patients (30%), the cytologic diagnosis undiagnosed the severity of the lesion. In 8 patients with carcinoma the cytologic diagnosis was moderate or severe dysplasia. In three patients with severe dysplasia, the cytologic diagnosis was inflammatory. In two patients (5%), the cytologic diagnosis was more severe than seen on histology. In one patient with positive cytology, the histology was only moderate dysplasia and another patient had severe dysplasia on cytology but only mild dysplasia on histology (Table 2). None of the women in this series had prolapse, syphilis or other conditions known to predispose to hyperkeratotic dysplasia.

Hyperkeratotic lesions may be difficult to evaluate by Pap smears because of poor shedding of abnormal cells (Koss et al. 1963). Cytologic examination underdiagnosed 11 of the 37 patients (30%)

of a single grade prior to biopsy. A histologic carcinoma may have been interpreted as dysplasia on cytologic examination. In no case was the cytologic examination normal if the histologic diagnosis was moderate dysplasia or worse. Thus, while cytologic examination may underdiagnose this group of lesions, sufficient abnormal cells are shed to arouse suspicion and indicate the necessity of additional studies.

IV. COMMENT

Although grading of hyperkeratotic lesions remains controversial (Christopherson 1977) recognition of hyperkeratotic dysplasia is not new. Prior to the advent of cytology, such lesions were described and their significance debated (Schiller 1938). Names given to a cervix that had a keratotic surface and a granular layer with or without associated dysplasia, included: leukoplakia, leukokeratosis, leukohyperkeratosis cervical pachydermia and hornifying dysplasia. Such lesions were associated with syphilis, vitamin deficiency and uterine prolapse. There was controversy over whether they were premalignant or associated with malignancy (Baker 1949).

With the development of cervical cytology and the general acceptance of the definitions of the Committee on Histological Terminology for Lesions of the Uterine Cervix (Weid 1961) which defined carcinoma *in situ* as a full thickness epithelial change keratotic lesions, were described as a separate entity, namely, leukoplakia (Henderson and Buck 1961; Olson and Nichols 1961). This term is confusing because some use the term to mean a white patch or a clinical lesion, while others describe a histologic lesion. The significance of such lesions is not clear. The keratinized surface may be

Table 2. Comparison of histological and cytological diagnosis in keratinizing dysplasia.

Diagnosis		Number
Histology and cytology agree		24 (65%)
Underdiagnosis by cytology		11 (30%)
Histology carcinoma/cytology dysplasia	8	
Histology severe dysplasia/cytology inflammation	3	
Overdiagnosis by cytology		2 (5%)
Histology moderate dysplasia/cytology positive	1	
Histology mild dysplasia/cytology severe dysplasia	1	
Total		37 (100%)

a result of metaplastic process associated with dysplasia or carcinoma in up to 10% of cases (Brown et al. 1973). The term leukoplakia is more commonly known as having no place in histopathology.

Since this series of hyperkeratotic dysplasia was obtained by reviewing biopsies diagnosed as dysplasia or carcinoma *in situ* all cases had dysplasias or worse. To see if there were instances of hyperkeratosis of the cervix without dysplastic changes, 500 cervical biopsies without dysplasia were reviewed and none with hyperkeratosis were found. The reason that hyperkeratosis without dysplasia is uncommon today may be that the major associated condition – prolonged uterine prolapse – is rare.

A number of related lesions were excluded from this study. Surface keratinization without a granular layer was seen only a few times in this review and was not associated with underlying dysplasia. Parakeratosis was seen in 67 biopsies (4.3%) and was often found adjacent to areas of hyperkeratotic dysplasia. This suggests that hyperkeratotic and parakeratotic dysplasia may be variants of the same process. Individual cell keratinization was not considered in this study because it is part of the standard classification of cervical dysplasia. A similar incidence rate was found in both nonkeratotic and hyperkeratotic dysplasia.

Hyperkeratotic dysplasia is significant because it is a lesion that does not readily fit into the standard classification of cervical dysplasia. There are at best two postulates that could explain this process. First, hyperkeratotic dysplasia could be just another expression of cervical dysplasia. There were cases where hyperkeratotic, parakeratotic and individual cell keratinization were all seen in the same case of cervical dysplasia. This lesion thus, would represent one end of the spectrum of cervical dysplasia.

This select group of hyperkeratotic lesions, comprising 3% of lesions of the cervix may in fact *de novo* from the ectocervix and not from the endocervical reserve cells. The origin of these primary ectocervical tumors would be analogous to primary squamous cell carcinomas of the vagina. Support of this postulate is found in electron microscopy studies (Williams et al. 1973) on nonkeratinizing *in situ* lesions of the cervix, where microvilli are seen on the surface of the *in situ* carcinoma similar to the surface of squamous metaplasia. These cells with microvilli originate from the reserve cells of the cervix. Since keratinized surfaces do not have microvilli this lesion may be of ectocervical origin in that ectocervical cells are known to have the capacity to produce a keratinized surface.

V. CONCLUDING REMARKS

Hyperkeratotic dysplasia of the cervix, defined as cervical dysplasia with a granular layer and a keratotic surface was noted in 3% of biopsies of cervical dysplasia in a 20 year span. The majority of patients were less than 50 years of age (38 of 46) and had severe dysplasia or carcinoma (36 of 46). Cervical cytologic examination underdiagnosed the severity of the lesion in 11 of 37 (30%) patients. To avoid underdiagnosis, hyperkeratotic cervical dysplasia should be graded from the basement membrane to the granular layer.

REFERENCES

Baker EM: Leucoplakia of the cervix uteri. Am J Obstet Gynecol 57: 575, 1949.
Brown D Jr, Kaufman RH, Gardner HL: Leukoplakia of the cervix. Am J Obstet Gynecol 116: 214, 1973.
Burghardt E: Early histological diagnosis of cervical cancer. Philadelphia: W.B. Saunders, 1973, 228.
Christopherson WM: Dysplasia, carcinoma *in situ* and microinvasive carcinoma of uterine cervix. Human Pathology 8: 489, 1977.
Henderson PH Jr, Buck CE: Cervical leukoplakia. Am J Obstet Gynecol 82: 887, 1961.
Koss LG, Steward FW, Foote FW, Jordan MJ, Bader GM, Day E: Some histological aspects of behavior of epidermoid carcinoma *in situ* and related lesions of the uterine cervix. Cancer 16: 1160, 1963.
Lambert B, Woodruff JD: Spindle cell atypia of the cervix. Cancer 16: 1141, 1963.
Olson AW, Nichols EE: Leukoplasia of the cervix – the mosaic and papillary pattern. Am J Obstet Gynecol 82: 895, 1961.
Richart RM: Cervical intraepithelial neoplasia. *In:* Sommers CC (ed): Pathology Annual. New York: Apleton – Century-Crofts, p 301, 1973.
Schiller W: Leucoplakia, leucokeratosis and carcinoma of the cervix. Am J Obstet Gynecol 35: 17, 1938.
Weid GL: Proceedings of the First International Congress on Exfoliative Cytology 1st ed. Philadelphia: J.B. Lippincott, 1961.
Williams AE, Jordan JA, Allen JM, Murphy JF: The surface ultrastructure of normal and metaplastic cervical epithelial and of carcinoma *in situ*. Cancer Res 33: 504, 1973.

13. MUCOEPIDERMOID CARCINOMA OF THE CERVIX

H.P. DINGES and J. ZEITLHOFER

The term mucoepidermoid tumor refers to growths that are composed of epidermoid cells and contain variable amounts of mucin (Stewart et al. 1945). While these two characteristics are consistently present, other features may be quite variable. In the major and minor salivary glands, mucoepidermoid tumors occur in a relatively favorable and a highly unfavorable form (Stewart et al. 1945; Koblin and Koch 1974). By contrast, mucoepidermoid carcinomas localizing in other regions of the body are almost invariably malignant.

Mucoepidermoid carcinomas also occur in the uterine cervix. In squamous cell carcinomas, sporadic mucin production is present throughout. In 7% of cases, mucin production is so pronounced that the diagnosis mucoepidermoid carcinoma appears to be well justified (Hellweg 1957). Mucin-containing epidermoid carcinomas of the cerix require a better distinction and definition of the different mucin containing growth in this area. This chapter deals with the re-evaluation of histological sections of 147 invasive cervical carcinomas: stages Ia to III.

I. METHODOLOGY

Special staining techniques were employed for re-evaluation of prominent mucin production on H & E stained routine sections. Sections were stained with PAS and with combined alcian blue + PAS (Runge et al. 1956). PAS- staining was preceded by diastase exposure in selected cases for specific visualization of mucin substances.

II. MORPHOLOGICAL CHARACTERISTICS

Alcian blue + PAS stained MEC sections showed 8 cases to be MECs, i.e. 5.4% of the 147 cases re-examined. This percentage is somewhat lower than that reported by Hellweg (1957) (7%), even if the few adenocarcinomas included are disregarded.

II.A. General description and definition

MECs have a basic epidermoid structure. Due to the variable mucin distribution and composition of the basic epidermoid structure, patterns are extremely variegated. Ordinary cervical squamous cell carcinomas and cases compatible with MEC due to their abundant mucin content, show considerable overlap. There are no specific indications which define the amount of mucin required for the diagnosis of cervical MEC.

II.A.1. Classifying cervical growths as MECs

Tumor masses are compatible with the diagnosis of MEC, if at least one third of the tumor tissue examined contains epidermoid and mucinous structures in more or less identical quantities (Dinges et al. 1977).

It is almost impossible to differentiate MECs from ordinary squamous cell carcinomas by macroscopic evidence. Threading of mucin at the cut surface is the most useful sign, but may be absent in some MECs.

II.B. Histological characteristics

II.B.1. Low power magnification

When viewing alcian blue + PAS stained MEC sections at low power, strongly violet staining

Hafez, E.S.E., Smith, J.P. (eds.), Carcinoma of the Cervix: Biology and Diagnosis. ISBN-13: 978-94-009-7487-6
© 1982, Martinus Nijhoff Publishers, The Hague/Boston/London.

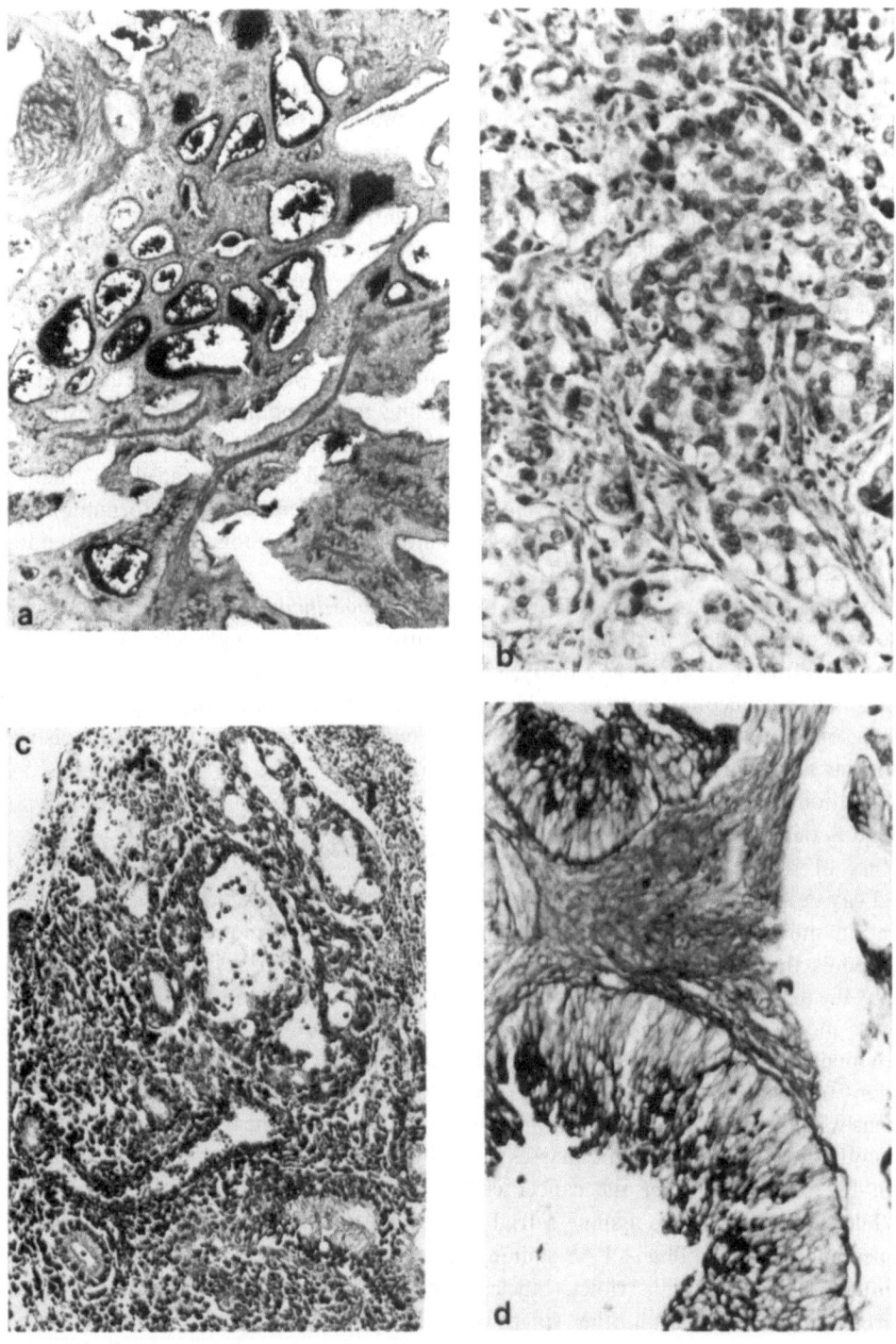

Figure 1. (*a*) MEC of the lacunar type. Note mucin pools. Fixation and preparation of specimen cause variable filling of pool (Alcian blue + PAS, × 100). (*b*) MEC of the monocellular type. Note ballooning single cells within epidermoid cancer cell masses (H & E, × 100). (*c*) Cervical biopsy specimen with evidence of *in situ* MEC. Top, cervical glands filled with dysplastic alveolar epithelium. The highly dysplastic epithelium shows characteristic bipotentiality with differentiation to squamous and glandular components. Bottom, normal cervical glands (H & E, × 100). (*d*) *In situ* MEC. Extent of mucin production is best shown by specific mucin stains (Alcain blue + PAS, × 100).

mucin is present in single ballooning cells and in larger cavities (Figure 1a). Most patterns show both monocellular mucin and mucin pools. Monocellular mucin clearly predominates, while larger mucin pools are absent (Figure 1b). The basic epidermoid structure equally shows considerable variability. Epithelial strands mostly formed by undifferentiated elements resembling basal and parabasal cells are found side' by side with more highly differentiated epithelial formations reminiscent of intermediate cells. In some areas, there is evidence of keratinization. Differentiation proceeds from the base towards the center of the strands.

II.B.2. High power magnification

Small and large mucin droplets are present in numerous cells. As the mucin droplets increase in size and coalesce, the nucleus becomes flatter and the cells distend to signet ring shapes (Figure 1b). Within the mucin vacuoles, acid mucopolysaccharides may be diffusely arranged and fluffy, but more often form homogeneous tightly-packed complexes. Mucin sometimes separates from the chromotropic cuticular seam of the vacuoles by a mucin-free ring (fixation artefact?), thus producing a pattern which is faintly reminiscent of a target.

Coalescence of single cells results in extensive mucin-filled cavities. These are produced by bursting of adjacent mucin cells which ultimately die. The mucin pools thus formed are sometimes recognizable by the naked eye. Towards the periphery of the pools, monocellular mucin production is seen, which maintains the process. Necrotic cell debris, mucin-streaked necrotic material and pure homogeneously packed mucin may be continuous with one another. Mucin and necrotic masses are localized in the central areas of the cancer cell strands. While the necrotic areas assume a friable reddish appearance on alcian blue + PAS staining, the pure mucin stains uniformly violet. Nuclear debris, necrotic single cells and all other stages of necrobiosis are suspended in the strongly staining mucin of the intermediate forms.

The stroma of the tumor masses is variable. At the tumor margins, the fibrous structure of the pre-existing tissue is loosened by edema with accumulation of neutral and acid mucopolysaccharides. Considerable lymphocytic and plasmocytic infiltration is seen in the tumor periphery, and sporadically foreign body giant cells are present. In the monocellular mucin type of MEC, the stroma tends to be less densely packed with fewer fibers and shows high vascularity.

II.B.3. Mucin types of MEC

In the MECs of the cervix, two distinctive mucin distribution patterns are seen. While there is considerable overlap, the two extremes present the following features:

a. Lacunar mucin type. Extracellular mucin forming mucin pools are characteristic of this type (Figure 1a). Mucin masses contain necrotic single cells and cell debris. Intracellular mucin is confined to the peripheral epithelial formations and empties into the mucin pools, thus being maintained.

b. Monocellular mucin type. Mucin is distributed intracellularly in single cells. A central mucin droplet is often optically separated from the cell periphery by an empty ring ('target' cells) (Figure 1b). Necroses are scant, and the stroma is well vascularized.

II.C. Histochemical characteristics

One of the advantages offered by the alcian blue + PAS technique is the differential staining of mucopolysaccharides and glycogen. At higher magnification, bright purple staining and finely and coarsely granular material is present. This is compatible with glycogen, as it disappears on exposure to diastase. At times, both glycogen and mucin are seen in one and the same cell – a sign of dysenzymia. In addition, purple material may abruptly show within the deep blue to violet staining mucin pools. Generally, acid mucopolysaccharides predominate. As the basic epidermoid tissue becomes more differentiated, the glycogen content gradually increases. Since glycogen is leached out on fixation of the material in aqueous formol solutions, its true content cannot be determined reliably.

III. IN SITU MUCOEPIDERMOID CARCINOMA

A special type of MEC was based on the cervical specimen obtained by curettage from a 29-year old female, who underwent conization and both cervical and endometrial curettage at different times.

III.A. Histology

The cervical scrapings contain polypoid structures both of normal and dysplastic cervical mucosa. In the preformed glandular spaces of the dysplastic mucosal portions, an atypical characteristically bipotential epithelium is present: dysplastic squamous structures predominate, but are continuous with glandular epithelium showing evidence of alveolar spaces and monocellular mucin (Figure 1c). The droplet-shaped mucin masses condense towards the gland lumen (Figure 1d). Epithelial dysplasia has progressed to the point of being compatible with *in situ* carcinoma. The preformed cavities, filled with dysplastic epithelium, border on a completely intact basement membrane. The conization specimen of this female shows no abnormality other than an extensive recent erosion at the squamocolumnar junction. In areas a dysplastic squamous lining is present. The endometrium contains few glands suggesting anti-ovulatory therapy.

III.B. Similarities to histological changes seen after anti-ovulatory therapy

The histological appearance of *in situ* MECs is strikingly similar to changes of the cervical mucosa that are seen under anti-ovulatory therapy and during pregnancy (Werner and Dinges 1976). This pattern is known as 'cribriform polypoid hyperplasia' (Joschko and Neuser 1975), and constitutes the intermediate developmental step lying half-way between benign 'cribriform polypoid hyperplasia' and malignant MEC (Dallenbach-Hellweg et al. 1971).

IV. GENERAL CHARACTERISTICS OF CERVICAL MUCOEPIDERMOID CARCINOMA

IV.A. Origin

MECs may originate from the small subcolumnar reserve cells that are bipotential and may differentiate both squamous and columnar epithelium (Hell-

weg 1957). All gland-forming and potentially metaplastic epithelia may constitute the matrix of mucoepidermoid carcinomas.

IV.B. Clinical data

The most prominent clinical symptom reported by patients with invasive MEC is extra-cyclical bleeding, which is either continuous or intermittent in nature or occurs on contact and has been present from several weeks to some months.

IV.C. Diagnosis and differential diagnosis

Diagnosis is usually based on exploratory excision or conization. The cytological diagnosis of MEC by smears is very difficult and needs great experience; however, malignancy can be easily diagnosed cytologically. Cervical MECs should primarily be differentiated from adenosquamous carcinoma and adenocancroid. The three types of carcinoma to be considered in the differential diagnosis have both squamous and glandular elements and may produce mucin. Special histochemical methods for visualizing mucin (PAS, alcian blue) are indispensable for determining the extent of mucin production.

The relative predominance of the three differentiation products constitutes the essential differential diagnostic criterion. Table 1 roughly illustrates the quantitative differences between the three cancer types. The extent of mucin production may be quite variable in carcinomas with predominantly glandular differentiation.

Table 1. Criteria for differentiating cervical carcinomas with squamous and glandular components.

	Squamous differentiation	Glandular differentiation	Mucin content
Squamous cell carcinoma	+ + +	+/−	+/−
Mucoepidermoid carcinoma	+ + +	+	+ + +
Adenosquamous carcinoma	+ +	+ +	+ +
Adenocancroid	+	+ + +	+ +
Adenocarcinoma	−	+ + +	+ +

+ low
+ + intermediate
+ + + high

Table 2. Annual incidence of invasive cervical carcinomas (all types) from 1970 through 1975 (annual mean, 24.5 cases).

Year	No. of cases	Mean age	Mucoepidermoid carcinoma
1970	31	5	1
1971	27	51	0
1972	28	51	1
1973	14	53	1
1974	27	45	3
1975	20	48	2
Total	147	50	8

IV.D. Prognosis

There is no clear-cut difference between MECs and other cervical carcinomas. Five females with stage 0 (MEC *in situ*) to Ib (mucoepidermoid carcinoma), followed up for periods of 6 months to 4 years, showed no evidence of local disease. One patient who had undergone surgery for stage IIa + b carcinoma died three years after surgery and showed multiple distant metastases on autopsy. Three women were lost to follow-up.

In the past few years, MECs have become more frequent and mucin production of squamous carcinomas has been more pronounced: while only 3 in 100 invasive cervical carcinomas were MECs from 1970 through 1973, the ratio was 3:27 and 2:20 in 1974 and 1975, respectively (Table 2).

IV.E. Treatment

Treatment of MECs is basically the same as other invasive cervical carcinomas. It consists of Wertheim's operation with bilateral lymphadenectomy in patients with clinically established invasive carcinoma. Females with far advanced cancer may undergo postoperative Co^{60} irradiation or other (adjuvant) therapies. It is still unclear whether MECs are radiosensitive.

V. CONCLUDING REMARKS

Two types of MEC can be distinguished: a lacunar mucin type and a monocellular mucin type. There is, however, considerable overlap. Squamous cell carcinoma can be distinguished from MEC on the basis of a defined mucin content. The cervical mucosa under progesterone-based anti-ovulatory therapy shows morphological similarities with MECs. MECs can be differentiated from adenosquamous carcinoma and adenocancroid due to the relative predominance of squamous and adenomatous structures.

ACKNOWLEDGEMENT

This study was supported by The Vienna Municipal Science Foundation (Wissenschaftlicher Fonds der Bundeshauptstadt Wien).

REFERENCES

Dallenbach-Hellweg G, Herting W, Momber F, Thorn V: Portioveränderungen unter Ovulationshemmern. *In* Seifert G (ed): Verhandlungen der Deutschen Gesellschaft für Pathologie. 55. Tagung. Jena: G. Fischer, pp 682–689, 1971.

Dinges HP, Werner R, Waidecker F: Über Mukoepidermoidkarzinome der Cervix uteri. Zbl Gynäk 99: 936, 1977.

Hellweg G: Über Schleimbildung in Plattenepithelcarcinomen. insbesondere an der Portio uteri (Mucoepidermoidcarcinome). Z Krebsforsch 61: 688, 1957.

Hellweg G: Über mukoepidermoidale Karzinome des Uterus. Geburtsh Frauenheilkd 10: 963, 1957.

Joschko K, Neuser D: 'Siebartige polypoide Zervixdrüsenhyperplasie' nach oralen Kontrazeptiva. Zbl Gynäk 97:15, 1975.

Koblin I, Koch H: On the nature of mucoepidermoid tumors of major and minor salivary glands. J maxillo-fac Surg 2: 19, 1974.

Runge H, Ebner H, Lidenschmidt W: Vorzüge der kombinierten Alcianblau-Perjodsäure-Schiff-Reaktion für die gynäkologische Histopathologie. Dt med Wschr 38: 1525, 1956.

Stewart FW, Foote FW, Becker WF: Muco-epidermoid tumors of salivary glands. Ann Surg 122: 820, 1945.

14. MORPHOMETRIC ANALYSIS OF BASAL CELL-STROMA INTERFACE IN NORMAL AND ABNORMAL CERVICAL EPITHELIUM

L.B. Twiggs, T. Okagaki and Barbara A. Clark

In the investigation of carcinogenesis and its product neoplasia, limits to the information derived from histopathological studies are evident. Interpretation of morphological alterations in neoplasia often have a subjective character which creates disagreements between investigators. A search for specific parameters which parallel and predict tissue behavior continues. Examples of such study include tissue culture methods, specific histochemical reactions, and electron microscopic observation. Descriptive morphology is the backbone of the histopathologic study. To give such descriptions quantitative character, a relatively new discipline has arisen. This discipline, morphometry, seeks to increase the scope of descriptive morphology by measuring recurring ordered structures. With these measurements, combined with mathematical conceptualization, models can be constructed which allow extrapolation from two dimensional to three dimensional space, hence the term sterology is also used. Sterology is a set of equations, namely, geometric-statistically derived, which have as their goal the attainment of quantifying information about three dimensional structures from two dimensional images. Such techniques have been used previously in the physical sciences, mainly geology and metallurgy, to estimate the specific contents of recurring mixtures (Weibel and Elias 1967).

In cervical epithelium, the interaction between the epithelium and its supporting stroma plays an important, but ill-understood, modulating role in epithelial differentiation and carcinogenesis. The interface between the basal cells and the stroma has recurring out-pouchings of the basal lamina designated as pseudopodia. The term pseudopodia is apparently a misnomer, since this structure has nothing to do with the locomotion of the basal cells of the epithelium. 'Basal processes' may be a better descriptive term. Appreciating that the pseudopodia is a convenient reference point and realizing that these recurring organelles are easily defined in electron microscopy, an application of a morphometric model to quantify these anatomical structures is possible. Such considerations combined with previous knowledge about the variability of this interface in preinvasive and invasive disease of the cervical epithelium make study of this anatomical area potentially useful (Ashworth et al. 1961; Hackemann et al. 1968).

Specifically, in cervical epithelium, this boundary, the basal lamina, is approximately 300 angstroms in width and is irregular in outline with protruding basal processes (pseudopodia). These pseudopodia frequently contain hemi-desmosomes with tonofilaments. The semi-quantitative loss of pseudopodia in CIN has been described (Shingleton et al. 1968).

Conventional transmission electron microscopy fails to demonstrate the exact size and number of pseudopodia per basal cell since the total basal cell surface cannot be depicted in a two-dimensional representation in the tissue sectioned. To estimate the number of pseudopodia per basal cell, a method to detach the basal cells from stroma with intact pseudopodia to avail themselves to a scanning electron microscope has not been forthcoming. Instead, a mathematical model is constructed from the observations by transmission electron microscopy (Okagaki et al. 1981).

I. MATHEMATICAL MODELS

In the construction of a mathematical model, two assumptions must be made. First, the basal cell is

Hafez, E.S.E., Smith, J.P. (eds.), Carcinoma of the Cervix: Biology and Diagnosis. ISBN-13: 978-94-009-7487-6

considered a solid cylinder standing on the plane of the basal lamina and secondly, the neck portion of the pseudopodia is also a smaller cylinder (Figure 1). In conventional transmission electron microscopy, the sectioned plane is nearly vertical to the basal lamina and intersects the bases of the cylindrical cell and its pseudopodia. The heights of the cylinders representing the basal cells and the pseudopodia are irrelevant to the measurement of the cross-sectional area of the basal cell base and the number of pseudopodia per basal cell. We estimate from transmission electron micrographs, the radii and the diameters of the cylinders representing a basal cell and pseudopodium, and then calculate the number of pseudopodia per basal cell.

Firstly, a theoretical model, consisting of multiple sections through a single cell was constructed (multiple section-single cell model). The application of the multiple section-single cell method of morphometry is a formidable task. In serial sections of a specimen, identical cells and the identical pseudopodia in different sectioned planes must be identified. This is impractical. From the model another more practical model was derived which was based on the

observations in a single section plane through a sufficiently large number of basal cells and, therefore, is designated the single section-multiple cell model. This extrapolation stands on the acceptable assumption that the tissue is homogeneous (mathematically, the measured values of a cell feature are dense and continuous) (Okagaki et al. 1981).

II. APPLICATION OF MORPHOMETRIC MODELS

Human uterine cervical tissues were obtained in the vicinity of the squamo-columnar junction by colposcopically directed biopsies. Tissues were then immediately fixed in McDowell's solution and prepared (Okagaki et al. 1981).

The electron microphotographs of the epithelial stroma interface were taken at the approximate magnification of 5,000 fold and then printed on $8'' \times 10''$ Kodak photographic paper. The final magnifications of the prints were calculated from the original magnification of the electron micrographs and enlarging factors of the prints. The lengths of the intersects of the section planes of the base of the basal cells ($\overline{L}_i$) and the lengths of the intersects of the section plane with the basal pseudopodia ($\overline{l}_{ik}$) were measured with a ruler, and the number of pseudopodia ($\bar{n}_i$) were counted as shown in Figure 2. The suffix i indicates the sequential number of the cell, and suffix k indicates the sequential number of pseudopodia. The values of $\overline{L}_i$, and $\overline{l}_{ik}$ were converted to original sizes, dividing the observed sizes on prints by the magnification factor. $\overline{L}$, the mean of L_i, and $\Delta\overline{L}$, the standard errors were computed. $\overline{l}^*$, the mean of $\overline{l}_{ik}$ was also calculated.

The theoretical derivation of the single section-multiple cell model shows that the $\overline{R}$, the mean radius of the cell; $\overline{D}$, the mean diameter of the cell; $\overline{A}$, the base area of the cell; $\overline{r}$, the mean radius of the pseudopodia; $\overline{d}$, the mean diameter of the pseudopodia; and $\bar{a}$, the mean base area of the pseudopodia were calculated from $\overline{L}$ and $\overline{l}^*$ as follows (Okagaki et al. 1981):

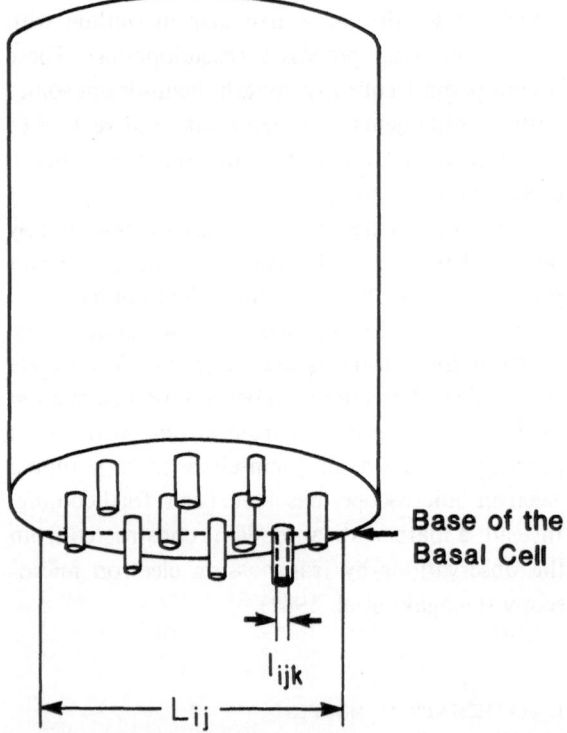

Figure 1. Schematic representation of base of basal cell with dotted line representing section plane. Measured values L_{ij} and l_{ijk} are depicted.

$$\overline{R} = \frac{2}{\pi} \overline{L}, \tag{1}$$

$$\overline{D} = \frac{4}{\pi} \overline{L}, \tag{2}$$

$$\overline{A} = \frac{4}{\pi}\,\overline{L}^2, \qquad (3)$$

$$\overline{r} = \frac{2}{\pi}\,\overline{1}^*, \qquad (4)$$

$$\overline{d} = \frac{4}{\pi}\,\overline{1}^*, \qquad (5)$$

and

$$\overline{a} = \frac{4}{\pi}\,\overline{1}^{*2}. \qquad (6)$$

Their standard errors, $\Delta\overline{R}$, $\Delta\overline{D}$, $\Delta\overline{A}$, $\Delta\overline{r}$, $\Delta\overline{d}$ and $\Delta\overline{a}$ were calculated as follows:

$$\Delta\overline{R} = \frac{2}{\pi}\,\Delta\overline{L}, \qquad (7)$$

$$\Delta\overline{D} = \frac{4}{\pi}\,\Delta\overline{L}, \qquad (8)$$

$$\Delta\overline{A} = \frac{8}{\pi}\,\overline{L}\cdot\Delta\overline{L}, \qquad (9)$$

$$\Delta\overline{r} = \frac{2}{\pi}\,\Delta\overline{1}^*, \qquad (10)$$

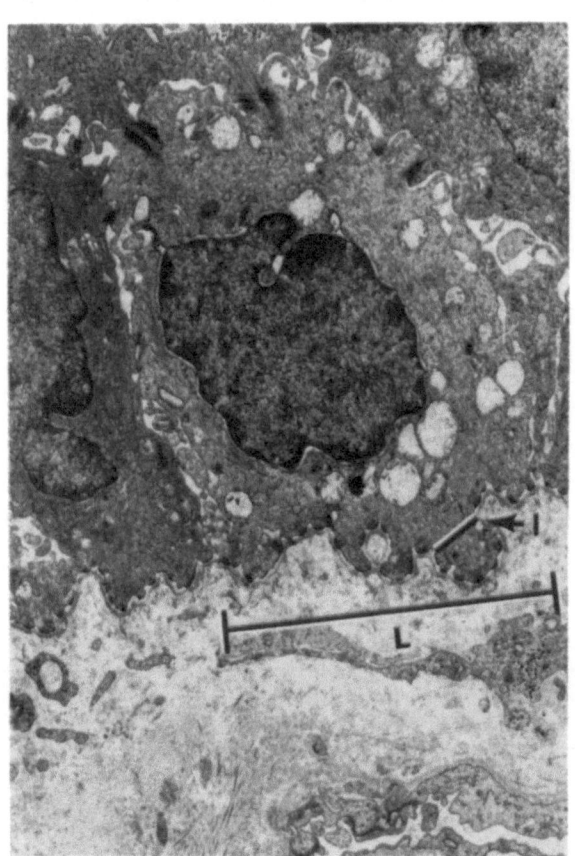

Figure 2. Actual measurement of electron photomicrograph showing length of intersect (*L*) of basal cell base and length of intersect (*l*) of pseudopodia.

$$\Delta\overline{d} = \frac{4}{\pi}\,\Delta\overline{1}^*, \qquad (11)$$

and

$$\Delta\overline{a} = \frac{8}{\pi}\,\Delta\overline{1}^*\cdot\Delta\overline{1}^*. \qquad (12)$$

The number of pseudopodia of the ith cell was calculated using the equation

$$\overline{N}_i = \frac{\overline{n}_i\cdot\overline{L}_i}{\overline{l}_i} \qquad (13)$$

where

$$\overline{l}_i = \frac{1}{\overline{n}_i}\sum\overline{l}_{ik}.$$

Likewise, $\overline{F}_i$, the ratio of the total area occupied by the pseudopodia to the base area of the basal cell (the ith cell) was calculated using the equation

$$\overline{F}_i = \frac{\sum_k^{\overline{n}_i}\overline{l}_{ik}}{\overline{L}_i} = \frac{\overline{n}_i\cdot\overline{l}_i}{\overline{L}_i}. \qquad (14)$$

$\overline{N}$ and $\overline{F}$, the mean values of N_i and F_i, are then calculated by

$$\overline{N} = \frac{1}{M}\sum_i^M\overline{N}_i, \qquad (15)$$

and

$$\overline{F} = \frac{1}{M}\sum_i^M\overline{F}_i. \qquad (16)$$

Further, $\Delta\overline{N}$ and $\Delta\overline{F}$, the standard errors, were calculated by

$$\Delta\overline{N} = \frac{1}{M}\sqrt{\sum_i^M\overline{N}_i{}^2 - MN^2}, \qquad (17)$$

and

$$\Delta\overline{F} = \frac{1}{M}\sqrt{\sum_i^M\overline{F}_i{}^2 - MF^2}. \qquad (18)$$

It should be noted that $\overline{N}$ and $\overline{F}$, thus calculated, converges to the expectancies $\hat{N}_i$ and $\hat{F}_i$ (true values) in terms of i.

Actual computation was performed using Digital Equipment Corporation PDP 8 F computer. The observations were made on three cases each of normal cervical epithelium and lesions consisting of reactive atypia (synonymous to healing erosion or basal cell hyperactivity), mild dysplasia, moderate dysplasia, severe dysplasia and carcinoma *in situ*. The number of the basal cells observed in each group was approximately fifty.

Table 1. Calculated values of radius ($\overline{R}$), diameter ($\overline{D}$), base area ($\overline{A}$) of the basal cell; radius ($\bar{r}$), diameter ($\overline{d}$), area ($\bar{a}$) of the pseudopodia, the number of pseudopodia per cell ($\overline{N}$) and the ratio of total base areas of pseudopodia to base area of basal cell ($\overline{F}$) in normal cervical epithelium. Standard errors are shown in parentheses. The calculations were made using Eqs. 3–18.

$\overline{L}$:　4.239 μm ± 0.182 (S.E.)
$\overline{l}^*$:　0.453 μm ± 0.018 (S.E.)
$\bar{n}$:　3.214 μm ± 0.176 (S.E.)

Basal cell			Pseudopodium			Number of pseudopodia per cell	Ratio of areas
radius ($\overline{R}$)	diameter ($\overline{D}$)	area ($\overline{A}$)	radius ($\bar{r}$)	diameter ($\overline{d}$)	area ($\bar{a}$)		
2.70 μm (±0.116)	5.40 μm (±0.232)	22.9 μm² (±1.97)	0.289 μm (±0.012)	0.577 μm (±9.023)	0.262 μm² (±0.021)	34.31 (±2.92)	0.338 (±0.018)

III. RESULTS

Using the mathematical models derived previously, the calculated values of the radius, $\overline{R}$, diameter, $\overline{D}$, base area, $\overline{A}$, of the basal cell and the similar qualities of the pseudopodia along with the estimation of the number of pseudopodia $\overline{N}$ and the ratio of the total base area of the pseudopodia to the base area of the basal cell $\overline{F}$ in the normal cervical epithelium are shown in Table 1. Using these as controls, the similar values were obtained on the cervical epithelium of the various grades of histological abnormality, ranging from reactive atypia, mild dysplasia through all grades of cervical intraepithelial neoplasia. The measured values of $\overline{L}$ are depicted in Table 2 for these histological categories. The calculations were then performed. The diameter of the basal cell, the area of the basal cell base, and similar quantities in the pseudopodia are depicted in Table 3. Reactive atypia and CIS had cells with the largest diameter and, therefore, the largest

base area. This variability was also reflected in the diameter of the pseudopodia and the area of the pseudopodia in these lesions.

The mean number of pseudopodia correlated in each histopathologic category and *p* values between classes and between normals computed by the students *t*-test are shown in Table 4. The numbers of pseudopodia per basal cell in reactive atypia and in mild dysplasia were essentially equal and there was no statistical significant difference. There were statistically significant differences between each successive grade of cervical intraepithelial neoplasia between each class and against normal after moderate dysplasia. Looking at the ratio of the area of the pseudopodia to the area of the basal cell base in each histological category, a similar statistically significant change was seen in the intraepithelial changes between classes and against normal (Table 5). There was a statistically significant difference in $\overline{F}$ in reactive atypia and mild dysplasia. This was a reflection of the increasing size of the reactive

Table 2. Measured values of section planes ($\overline{L}$), ($\overline{l}$) through basal cell base correlated with histopathologic diagnosis.

Histologic diagnosis	Normal	Reactive atypia	Mild dysplasia	Moderate dysplasia	Severe dysplasia	C.I.S.
Intersect basal cell base ($\overline{L}$) (μm) SE	4.239 ± 0.182	6.310 0.431	4.294 0.307	4.847 0.258	3.923 0.332	5.792 0.362
Intersect pseudopodia ($\overline{l}$) (μm) SE	0.453 ± 0.018	0.663 0.0418	0.497 0.040	0.495 0.040	0.251 0.063	0.633 0.076

Table 3. Calculated values of diameter and area of basal cell base and pseudopodia relative to histopathologic diagnosis.

Histologic diagnosis	Normal	Reactive atypia	Mild dysplasia	Moderate dysplasia	Severe dysplasia	C.I.S.
diameter of cell ($\bar{D}$) μm $\pm$SE	5.398 $\pm$ 0.232	8.034 $\pm$ 0.549	5.468 0.391	6.171 0.389	4.995 0.432	7.374 0.461
Area of cell ($\bar{A}$) sq μm $\pm$SE	22.882 $\pm$ 1.965	50.6905 $\pm$ 6.923	23.481 3.354	29.910 03.185	19.597 3.320	42.717 5.343
Diameter pseudo-podia ($\bar{d}$) μm $\pm$SE	0.577 $\pm$ 0.023	0.790 $\pm$ 0.039	0.630 0.036	0.590 0.044	0.690 0.074	0.763 0.076
Area of pseudo-podia ($\bar{a}$) sq μm $\pm$SE	0.262 $\pm$ 0.021	0.491 $\pm$ 0.047	0.311 0.036	0.274 0.041	0.374 0.080	0.458 0.091

atypia cells, presumably due to edema, with no relative increase in the number of pseudopodia.

IV. SIGNIFICANCE

Previous electron microscopic studies of cells originating in cervical intraepithelial neoplasia have demonstrated progressive decreases in intercellular cytoplasmic glycogen and desmosomes (Ashworth et al. 1961). The density of gap junction in epithelial solid tumors has been shown to be reciprocal to cellular differentiation and may hold some clues as to carcinogenesis (McNutt et al. 1969). These alterations in the epithelium have been combined with progressive increases in microvilli, free and bound ribosomes, and mitochondria (Shingleton et al. 1968). Recently, intercellular desmosomes in patients with cervical intraepithelial neoplasia were studied and a decreasing number per unit membrane in CIN III versus normal epithelium was noted (Lawrence et al. 1980). Using a morphometrically derived model investigating the differences in the basal cell stromal interface, further data describing the quantitative differences in well-recognized classes of preinvasive cervical neoplasia was generated.

While direct two-dimensional visualization of the stroma-epithelium interface with the electron microscope has demonstrated qualitative differences (Ashworth et al. 1961; Hackemann et al. 1968; Shingleton et al. 1968), we resorted to an indirect sterological method to quantitate the number of pseudopodia per basal cell in the squamous epi-

Table 4. The mean number of pseudopodia correlated to the histologic diagnosis. *p* value computed by students *t*-test.

Histologic diagnosis	Normal	Reactive atypia	Mild dysplasia	Moderate dysplasia	Severe dysplasia	C.I.S.
Mean No. of pseudopodia per cell ($\bar{N}$) $\pm$S.E.	34.312 $\pm$3.01	23.622 $\pm$4.391	26.983 $\pm$4.125	13.256 $\pm$2.285	7.527 $\pm$3.088	4.439 $\pm$1.373
p between classes	$0.01 < 0.025$	$p > 0.25$	$0.001 < p < 0.005$	$0.05 < p < 0.1$	$0.1 < p < 0.25$	
p against normal	$p < 0.001$	$p < 0.001$	$p < 0.001$	$p < 0.001$	$p < 0.001$	

thelium in the uterine cervix. Noting that cell to cell interactions are better studied in tissue culture systems, the basal cell stroma interface was looked at in detail with this morphometric model. With this single section-multiple cell model, decreasing numbers of pseudopodia per basal cell with statistical significance was seen in successive grades of cervical intraepithelial neoplasia (Twiggs et al. 1981). Considering the basal cell pseudopodia as a morphologic representation of differentiation, the loss of these structures may be considered a representation of the dedifferentiation in cellular structure which is seen in preinvasive cervical neoplasia. Loss of anatomical markers was seen in animal models when specific epithelia were treated with promoter substances (Raick 1973). Similarly, in specific tissue culture systems in the course of promoter use, inhibition of cellular differentiation with specific biochemical alterations was noted (Diamond et al. 1978). Moreover, the density of gap junctions in epithelial cell tumors was reciprocal to cellular differentiation (McNutt et al. 1969). Thusly, the loss of basal cell pseudopodia with advancing grades of CIN may be considered an analogous phenomenon. Conceptually, then, the loss of this anatomic apparatus may be considered dedifferentiation.

In contrast, it is possible with the loss of this parameter, basal cell pseudopodia, while correlating well to the well-adopted histological categories of CIN may be only a preparatory step in the onset of cell division (Twiggs et al. 1981). It was possible that reduction in pseudopodia we observed reflected a relative increase in cells in the proliferative phase of the mitotic cycle in CIN. That is, as cells enter G_0 and S phases of the cell cycle, a specific decrease in pseudopodia might have occurred. The increasing length of S phase relative to the G_0 in CIN has been elucidated with microspectrophotometric studies (Okagaki and Izuo 1978). However, contrary to this idea, in viewing our electron microscopic specimens, we did not observe a cell population in the higher grades of CIN possessing large numbers of pseudopodia which are cells presumably in G_0 or resting phase, comparable to that seen in normal controls (Twiggs et al. 1981). Certainly this may be due to a small sample population, but a more tenable explanation is that the loss of basal cell pseudopodia is an aspect of dedifferentiation which is commonly seen in neoplastic cells.

Certainly, the adherence of the basal cell to the stroma results from interfolding of the basal lamina and its pseudopodia. However, the basal cell pseudopodia may act as receptor organelles and may modulate stimuli from the stroma controlling the proliferation of these cells. Certainly, it has been demonstrated that tissue stroma may enhance cellular differentiation by regulating the cell growth (Cunha 1976). Moreover, supportive tissue stroma may modulate cellular differentiation and malignant transformation by regulating the replication of cells. The exact role stromal tissue plays in carcinogenesis is ill-understood at present, but epidermal growth factors have been implicated as an intermediary in stromal epithelial interactions (Marks 1976). In tissue culture models, membrane, proteins, and their intercellular connections are intimately related to controlled cell division (Jazwinski et al. 1978). Consequently, the loss of the basal cell pseudopodia may reflect an alteration in

Table 5. The ratio of area of pseudopodia to the area of the basal cell base. *p* value computed by students *t*-test.

Histologic diagnosis	Normal	Reactive atypia	Mild dysplasia	Moderate dysplasia	Severe dysplasia	C.I.S.
Ratio of areas of pseudopodia and base ±S.E.	0.338 ± 0.018	0.188 ± 0.026	0.266 ± 0.021	0.083 ± 0.012	0.064 ± 0.018	0.040 ± 0.010
p between classes	$p < 0.001$	$0.1 < p < 0.25$	$p < 0.001$	$0.1 < p < 0.025$	$0.1 < p < 0.25$	
p against normal		$p < 0.001$	$p < 0.001$	$p < 0.001$	$p < 0.001$	$p < 0.001$

cytoplasmic membrane receptors, which are necessary for control of replication. The intrinsic character of neoplastic cells is the loss of control of cell division. The loss of these structures in preinvasive cervical neoplasia may be an indirect representation of the loss of interaction and, therefore, loss of control cell division.

In its infancy, this technique holds promise as an adjuvant to histopathological study as abnormalities seen in the basal cell stromal interface may be quantitated. Obviously, the technique is time consuming and cannot be applied in a routine fashion to cervical biopsies. However, its application as a research tool in demonstrating where the tissues have undergone dedifferentiation may be possible. Vitamin A derivatives have been shown to cause reversion of cellular dedifferentiation (Elias et al. 1980). The measurement of pseudopodia from a large area of cervical intraepithelial neoplasia prior to the application of these derivatives, then measurement after an application, may give further evidence that not only do these derivatives cause cellular differentiation, but specific anatomical markers can be correlated to such reversal of dedifferentiation.

A proper application of this technique may differentiate between dysplastic lesions developing in areas of metaplasia as in DES exposed patients from dysplasia arising in the transformation zone in normal patients. Following correlation with clinical behavior such structural differences may allow refined predictors of neoplastic potential. The intercellular desmosomes are different in number comparing intraepithelial changes in DES exposed women and intraepithelial changes that develop in nonexposed individuals (Lawrence et al. 1980). Possibly, the demonstration of normal numbers of pseudopodia in patients histologically recognized dysplasia who are DES exposed may allow a more conservative management in these patients.

The multiple cell-single section morphometrically derived model was applied to normal cervical epithelium and abnormal cervical epithelium to ascertain its correlation to standard histopathological criteria. As noted, there was a statistically significant progressive decrease in pseudopodia in each successive grade of intraepithelial change. Speculation that the modification of the basal cell stroma interface might be an essential factor of epithelial carcinogenesis was presented.

ACKNOWLEDGEMENTS

Acknowledgements are made to Joan Wuertz Fredson and Jean A. Engbring for preparing the electron microphotographs and to Julie D. Wand for typing the manuscript.

REFERENCES

Ashworth CT, Stembridge VA, Luibel FJ: A study of Basement Membranes of Normal Epithelium, Carcinoma *in Situ*, and Invasive Carcinoma of Uterine Cervix, Utilizing Electron Microscopy and Histochemical Methods. Acta Cytol 5: 369–383, 1961.

Cunha GR: Stromal Induction and specification of morphogenesis and cytodifferentiation of the epithelia of the Mullerian ducts and urogenital sinus during development of the uterus and vagina in mice. J Exp Zool 196: 361–370, 1976.

Diamond L, O'Brien T, Rovena G: Tumor promotors inhibit terminal cell differentiation in culture. *In* Slaga TJ, Sivak A, Boutwel RK, (eds.): Carcinogenesis. Vol. , Mechanisms of Tumor Promotion and Carcinogenesis. New York: Raven Press, 1978, p 335.

Elias PM, Grayson S, Caldwell TM, McNutt NS: Gap junction proliferation in retinoic acid-treated human basal cell carcinoma. Lab Invest 42: 469–475, 1980.

Hackemann M, Grubb C, Hill K R: The ultrastructure of normal squamous epithelium of the human cervix uteri. Ultrast Res 22: 443–457, 1968.

Jazwinski SM, McLain DA, D'Eustachio P, Edelman OM: Surface signals and cellular recognition of growth. *In*: Slaga TJ, Sivak A, Boutwell RK (eds.): Carcinogenesis. Vol 2, Mechanisms of Tumor Promotion and Carcinogenesis. New York: Raven Press, 1978, pp 343–359.

Lawrence WD, Shingleton GH, Soong S: Ultrastructure and morphometric study of diethylstilbestrol associated lesions diagnosed as cervical intraepithelial neoplasia, III. Cancer Research 40: 1558–67, 1980.

Marks F: Epidermal growth control mechanisms, hyperplasia and tumor romotion in the skin. Cancer Res 36: 2636–2643, 1976.

McNutt NS, Weinstein RS: Carcinoma of the cervix: Deficiency of nexus intracellular junction. Science 165: 597–599, 1969.

Okagaki T, Clark BA, Twiggs LB: Measurement of number and cross sectional area of basal cell pseudopodia: A new morphometric method. Journal of Cell Biology 91: 629–636, 1981.

Okagaki T, Iuzo M: Correction of modal DNA values obtained by microspectrophotometry and test for their shifts. J Nat Cancer Instit 60: 1251–1258, 1978.

Raick AN: Ultrastructural, histological, biochemical alterations produced by 12-0-Tetradecanoylphorbol-13-acetate in mouse epidermis and their relevance to skin tumor pomotion. Cancer Res 33: 1096–1103, 1973.

Shingleton HM, Richart RM, Wiener J, Spiro D: Human cervical intraepithelial neoplasia: Fine structure of dysplasia and carcinoma *in situ*. Cancer Res 28: 695–706, 1968.

Twiggs LB, Okagaki T, Clark BA: Basal cell pseudopodia in cervical intraepithelial neoplasia; progressive reduction of number with severity: A morphometric quantification. Am J Ob-Gyn 139: 640–644, 1981.

Weibel ER, Elias H (eds): Proceedings of the Symposium on Quantitative Methods in Morphology. New York: Springer-Verlag, 1967, pp 7–10.

15. SEM OF NEOPLASIA OF THE CERVICAL EPITHELIUM

J.A. Jordan and J.M. Allen

Examination of the normal and abnormal epithelium of the human uterine cervix by Scanning Electron Microscopy (SEM) has revealed characteristic surface ultrastructural appearances. The different types of epithelium examined include stratified squamous, columnar, metaplastic squamous and cervical intraepithelial neoplasia (CIN), these appearances have been previously reported (Jordan and Williams 1971; Williams et al. 1971; Ferenczy and Richart 1973; Williams et al. 1973).

On the basis of histological and colposcopic criteria, cervical neoplasia has three recognized stages of development: CIN I, II and III. Similar stages are also identifiable on SEM examination (Jordan et al. 1975). In this chapter, the SEM appearance of CIN I, II and III will be described and compared with the appearance of normal epithelium.

I. PREPARATION OF SPECIMENS

The specimens are of human cervical epithelium obtained by wedge or punch biopsy taken under

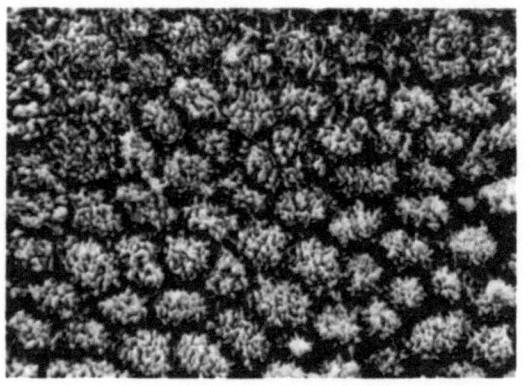

Figure 1. Columnar epithelium with only the tips of the cells visible, × 500.

colposcopic direction using the saline technique of colposcopy (Koller 1963; Kolstad and Stafl 1972). All specimens were washed in saline, fixed critical point dried and coated with gold (Boyde and Wood 1969), prior to SEM examination. In order to confirm the SEM identification of the epithelium examined, each specimen was subsequently processed for conventional light microscopy (Ayres et al. 1971).

II. NORMAL CERVICAL EPITHELIUM

II.A. Columnar epithelium

Columnar epithelium consists of closely packed, elongated cells, of which only the luminal end is normally visible on SEM examination. The diameter of each cell is approximately 4 μm and the arrangement of those cells is frequently described as having a 'cobblestone' appearance (Figure 1). Two types of columnar cells are seen: secretory (nonciliated) and ciliated. The surface of the secretory cells consists of microvilli of up to 2 μm in length and 0.2 μm in width. Secretory cells produce mucus and the ciliated cells interspersed with them (Figure 2) are responsible for the movement of the mucus.

II.B. Stratified squamous epithelium

Stratified squamous epithelium consists of numerous layers of cells at various stages of maturation. On SEM examination, only the mature superficial layer of cells is visible. This layer is made up to large, flattened, overlapping, polygonal cells of up to 40 μm in size. On examination at higher magnifications, the cell boundaries are prominent and the surface ultrastructure consists of branching and

Hafez, E.S.E., Smith, J.P. (eds.), Carcinoma of the Cervix: Biology and Diagnosis. ISBN-13: 978-94-009-7487-6
© 1982, Martinus Nijhoff Publishers, The Hague/Boston/London.

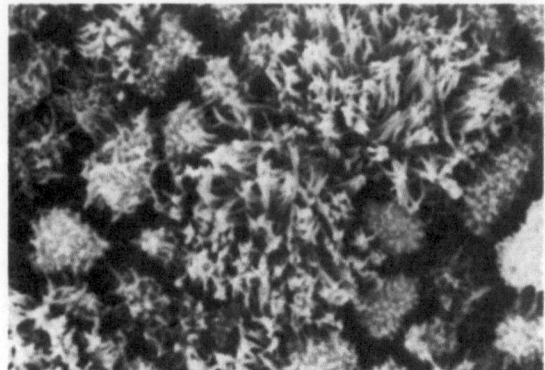

Figure 2. Ciliated cells surrounded by secretory cells, × 5,000.

anastomizing microridges which are approximately 0.15 μm in width and up to 10 μm in length with 0.25 μm spaces between them (Figure 3). These microridges increase the area of contact between the cells and interdigitate, thus contributing to a resistance to sideways movement of the cells.

II.C. *Metaplastic squamous epithelium*

Metaplasia is the physiological process whereby columnar epithelium is transformed to stratified squamous epithelium; the colposcopic recognition of metaplasia and its relationship to the development of CIN are well accepted. On SEM examination, the earliest visible stage of the metaplastic process is seen as the presence of larger cuboidal-type metaplastic cells at the tips of columnar villi

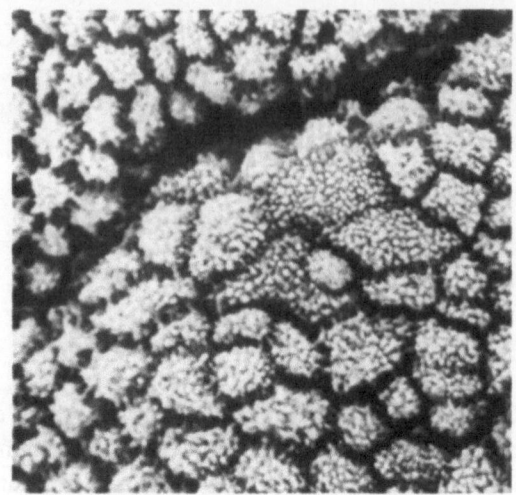

Figure 4. The earliest visible stage of metaplasia with the presence of cuboidal-type cells at the tip of a columnar villus, × 1,000.

(Figure 4). As metaplasia proceeds, the number of metaplastic cells increases and become flattened with prominent intercellular junctions, and a surface ultrastructure consisting of microvilli (Figure 5). The columnar villi subsequently fuse, resulting in the appearance of islands of metaplastic cells surrounded by columnar cells. Eventually, the columnar epithelium is completely replaced by flattened, polygonal cells which still retain a microvillous ultrastructure (Figure 6). The metaplastic process is complete at the stage where mature stratified squamous epithelium is evident at the site where there was once columnar epithelium.

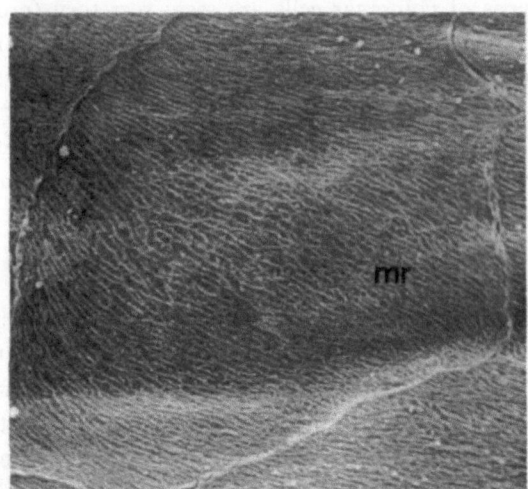

Figure 3. A normal superficial squamous cell. Cell boundary (b), microridges (mr), × 2,000.

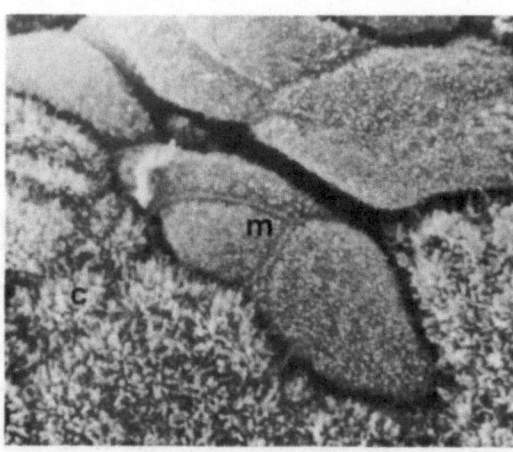

Figure 5. Metaplastic cells (m) surrounded by columnar cells (c), × 2,000.

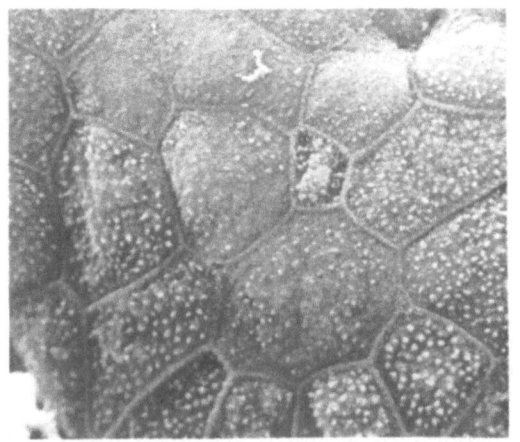

Figure 6. Flattened, polygonal metaplastic cells in the later stages of metaplasia, × 2,000.

III. NEOPLASTIC CERVICAL EPITHELIUM

III.A. CIN I

At the earliest pre-invasive stage of neoplasia, the superficial layer of cells when viewed at low magnification has a disorganized appearance compared with that of normal squamous epithelium. The constituent cells are smaller (approximately 20 μm), more rounded and the cell junctions less prominent than normal superficial squamous cells (Figure 7). The surface ultrastructure consists of microvilli which are short (less than 1 μm in length and 0.15 μm wide) and closely packed.

III.B. CIN II

At this stage, the degree of disorganization of the epithelium is more marked (Figure 8). The cells are small (15–20 μm) and rounded, and do not overlap; their cell junctions are not evident. Their surface ultrastructure consists of numerous microvilli with similar dimensions to those described for CIN I cells.

III.C. CIN III

At low magnification, the lack of organization of the superficial layer of cells is very marked. The constituent cells are generally rounded and variable in size (10–15 μm), with no distinguishable cell boundaries. In some cases, the cells form more bizarre shapes. As in CIN I and II, the surface ultrastructure of these cells is microvillous.

IV. CONCLUDING REMARKS

The SEM examination of human cervical squamous epithelium and its constituent cells in the various observable stages of the neoplastic process, demonstrates a gradual alteration of the normal appearance of the epithelium. Furthermore, these stages of abnormality have characteristic appearances which are distinguishable from those of benign conditions, especially metaplasia. At low magnifications, a comparison between normal and neoplastic squamous epithelium shows a dramatic

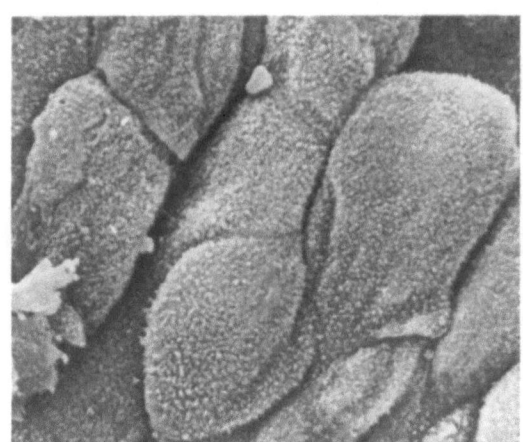

Figure 7. Detail of an area of CIN I with smaller, more rounded cells, × 2,000.

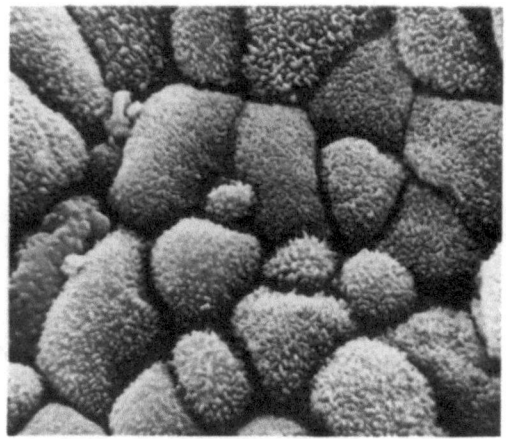

Figure 8. Detail of cells from CIN II, with surface microvilli, × 20,000.

90

alteration in epithelial organization due to the change in size, shape and surface ultrastructure of the constituent cells.

The presence of microvilli observed on certain types of cells, including secretory columnar, metaplastic and neoplastic squamous cells, would appear to be a reflection of the degree of activity within the cells. The rounded shape of the neoplastic cells, in addition to the presence of microvilli, also contributes to a reduction in cell to cell adhesion, thereby increasing cell exfoliation.

REFERENCES

Ayres A, Allen JM, Williams AE: A method for obtaining conventional histological sections from specimens after examination by scanning electron microscopy. Journal of Microscopy 93: 247, 1971.

Boyde A, Wood C: Preparation of animal tissue for surface scanning electron microscopy. Journal of Microscopy 19: 221, 1969.

Coppleson M, Reid B: Pre-clinical carcinoma of the cervix uteri. London: Pergamon Press, 1967.

Ferenczy A, Richart RM: Scanning electron microscopy of the cervical transformation zone. American Journal of Obstetrics and Gynaecology 115: 151, 1973.

Jordan JA, Williams AE: Scanning electron microscopy in the study of cervical neoplasia. Journal of Obstetrics and Gynaecology. British Commonwealth 78: 940, 1971.

Jordan JA, Murphy JF, Allen JM, Williams AE: The neoplastic cervix. In Hafez ESE (ed): Scanning Electron Microscopic Atlas of Mammalian Reproduction. Tokyo: Igaku Shoin Ltd, 21: 250, 1975.

Koller O: The Vascular Patterns of the Uterine Cervix. London: Scandinavian University Books, Pall Mall, Vol 16, 1963.

Kolstad P, Stafl A: Atlas of Colposcopy. London: Scandinavian University Books, Pall Mall, 1972.

Williams AE, Jordan JA, Rimmer D, Ratcliffe NA: Scanning Electron Microscopy of the normal cervix and of carcinoma in situ. In the Early Diagnosis of Cancer of the Cervix. Hull, England: University of Hull, 1971.

Williams AE, Jordan JA, Allen JM, Murphy JF: The surface ultrastructure of normal and metaplastic cervical epithelium and of carcinoma in situ. Cancer Res 33: 504, 1973.

16. SURFACE ULTRASTRUCTURE OF THE UTERINE CERVIX AND EARLY DETECTION OF IRREVERSIBLE NEOPLASIA

P. Kenemans, J.H.M. Davina, R.W. de Haan, P.H.T. van der Zanden, G.P. Vooys and A.M. Stadhouders

I. CELL SURFACE ORGANIZATION IN MALIGNANCY

The plasma membrane-cell surface complex is of crucial significance for the social behavior of cells within cell populations (Nicolson 1977; Poste 1977; Nicolson et al. 1977). Alterations in cell surface organization may account for cellular misbehavior. This asocial behavior is termed malignancy when it meets two criteria: loss of growth control (resulting in excessive proliferation) and loss of positional control (resulting in invasion and metastasis).

Transformed and malignant cells are characterized by specific modifications of their cell surface organization (Nicolson and Poste 1976a, b; Poste and Weiss 1976; Nicolson et al. 1977; Hynes 1979). Invasion and metastasis are very complex phenomena. Both can be broken down into several steps, each of which must involve a number of specific properties. Due to the difference between these two phenomena, and thus between the required cellular properties, the cellular surface organization in metastasis may differ from that in pure invasion, while both are different from that in normal cells. Therefore, the cellular phenotype is of potentially great diagnostic significance. Recognition of the cellular surface organization pattern may not only allow (early) diagnosis (discrimination between normal and (pre-) malignant cells) but also pretreatment staging (discrimination between the ability to metastasize or not).

Altered cell surface organization is reflected in detectable changes in cell surface properties which may be structural or functional in nature. In the latter, attention is given to alterations in molecular composition (cell surface proteins, glycoproteins and mucopolysaccharides) and therefore, in specific (e.g., hormone) or non-specific (e.g., lectin) receptor sites. The involvement of membrane enzymes is also studied. Finally, and most promising, the antigenic composition of the neoplastic cell surface is an object of intensive investigations. The study of these functional aspects requires mostly highly sophisticated methods, including some laborious and meticulous labeling methods.

II. MORPHOLOGY OF CELL SURFACE IN MALIGNANCY

The morphology of the cell surface can be studied with several methods. Transmission Electron Microscopy (TEM) reveals, next to cell surface features in cross section, important membrane-associated cytoskeletal components and functional complexes. The latter (i.e., desmosomes, tight junctions and gap junctions), are membrane areas specialized in cell to cell contact, which can also be studied effectively with the freeze-fracture technique. In neoplasia, significant changes can be seen (e.g., Gilula 1975; Weinstein et al. 1976).

Scanning Electron Microscopy (SEM) provides a rather simple and appropriate method for the study of relatively large areas of cell surface at high magnification. Due to its high depth of field and large range of magnification, it allows local changes in microstructure to be related to the overall spatial organization of the area of interest. SEM ultrastructural features as microridges, microvilli, filopodia, blebs, ruffles and other lamellipodia can be defined on *in vitro* transformed cells (e.g., Vesely and Boyde 1973) and on *in vivo* malignant cells (e.g., Murphy et al. 1973; Domagala and Woyke 1975).

SEM therefore, offers a most powerful approach to diagnostic cytopathology, especially if any of the ultrastructural cell surface parameters could be

Hafez, E.S.E., Smith, J.P. (eds.), Carcinoma of the Cervix: Biology and Diagnosis. ISBN-13: 978-94-009-7487-6
© 1982, Martinus Nijhoff Publishers, The Hague/Boston/London.

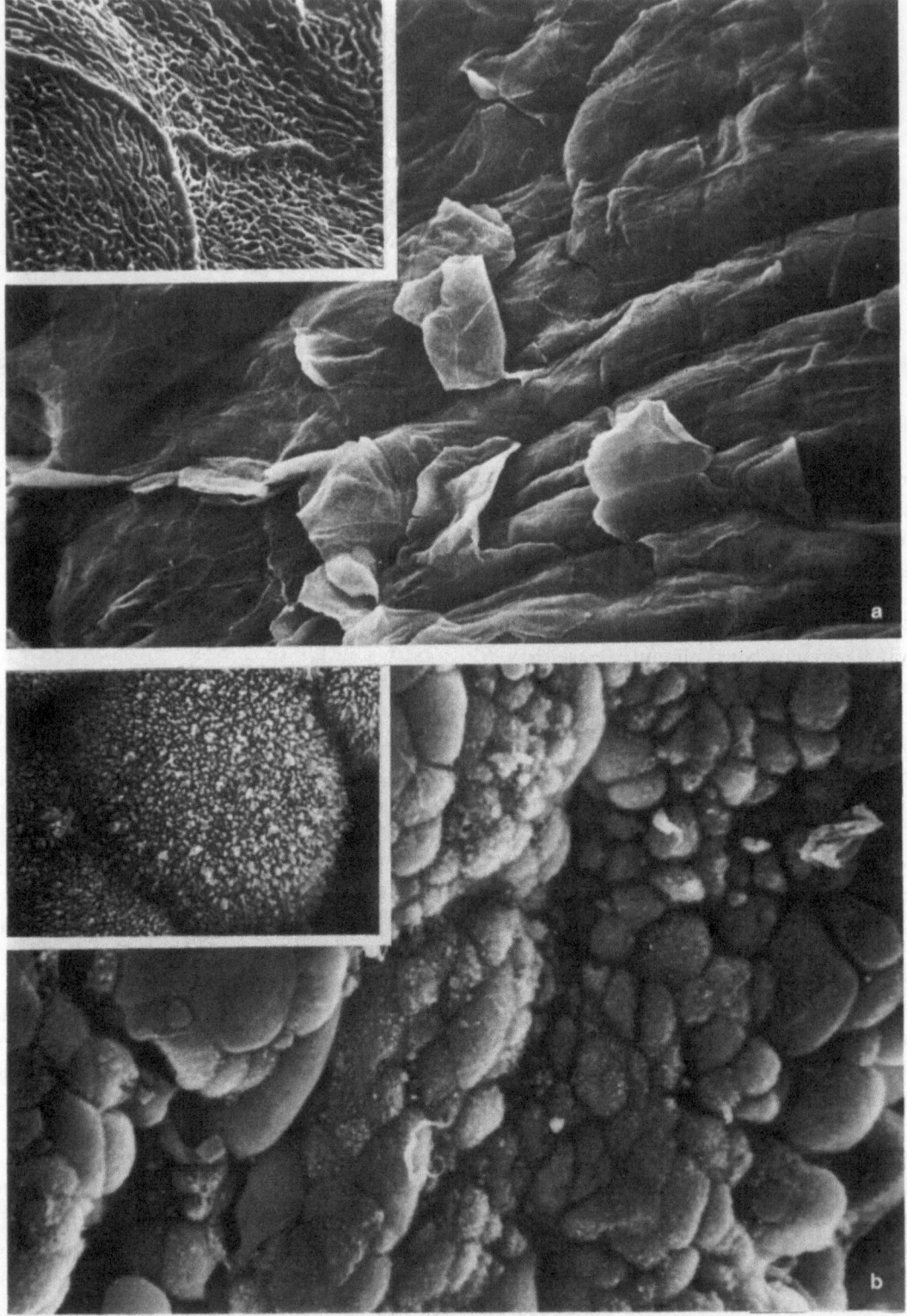

Figure 1. Scanning Electron Microscopy (SEM) showing tissue organization, and cell surface micromorphology (inset) at the free, luminal side of the ectocervical epithelium of the human uterine cervix. SEM of normal cervical squamous epithelium (a) reveals a superficial layer consisting of exfoliating flat, polygonal cells ($\times$ 320). *Inset*: Cell surface ultrastructure of the free, luminal side of the superficial cells showing microridges and linear bars ($\times$ 5,000). SEM of carcinoma *in situ* of the cervix (b) reveals areas with disorganization of the superficial layer which consists of rounded cells of irregular shape and size ($\times$ 640). *Inset*: Cell surface ultrastructure of the free, luminal side of these dome-shaped cells, showing abundant microvilli ($\times$ 5,000).

considered as an early marker of irreversible neoplastic transformation (Allen et al. 1976; Wilbanks 1976).

III. THE SURFACE ULTRASTRUCTURE OF THE
ECTOCERVICAL EPITHELIUM

Transmission electron microscopy (TEM) and Freeze-etch studies (McNutt and Weinstein 1969; McNutt et al. 1971; Shingleton and Wilbanks 1974) have shown that differences in surface architecture exist between normal and abnormal ectocervical cells. There is an increased number of microvilli on the surface of neoplastic cells together with a decreased number of desmosomes, which may explain the decrease in cohesiveness of malignant cells.

The nonkeratinizing, squamous stratified epithelium of the human ectocervix generally comprises some 20–25 cell layers in total. In relation to the question of diagnostic cytopathology, the uppermost layer is especially important. SEM studies show that in the normal uterine cervix, the superficial layer consists of large, flattened and polygonal cells, that show a continuous tendency to exfoliate (Figure 1a). Higher magnification reveals a typical microarchitecture of the free cell surfaces, directed to the lumen of the vagina; viz., a system of longitudinal elevations of the plasma membrane, the so-called microridges. Moreover, the cell surface displays next to the terminal bars, which line the edges of the cells, linear bars protruding from the surface (Figure 1a, inset). Essentially, the same cell surface characteristics are found on exfoliated cells in cervical smear preparations (Figure 2a).

In carcinoma in situ (CIS), the upper layer of the ectocervix shows a totally different structural organization. The smaller, rounded cells do show a rich variability in shape and size (Figure 1b), while their free surfaces are covered with abundant microvilli (Figure 1b, inset).

The above mentioned characteristics of normal and abnormal cervical epithelia have been demonstrated unequivocally by numerous SEM studies of both single, exfoliated cells (Murphy et al. 1973; Llanes et al. 1973; Ferenczy and Richart 1974; Murphy et al. 1975a, b; Allen et al. 1976) and of biopsies of the uterine cervix (Murphy et al. 1974;

Williams et al. 1975; Jordan et al. 1975; Jordan 1976a, b; Rubio and Kranz 1976; Sherman 1977; Ferenczy and Gelfand 1979). These unanimous reports have also provoked a tendency to reverse the relationship by hypothesizing that cell surface microridges indicate normality, while cell surface microvilli imply abnormality.

While studying individual exfoliated cells by a correlative LM/SEM method, it was shown that SEM could, on the basis of surface morphology, separate a population of cells into subsets. These subsets, when viewed by LM, appeared identical (Murphy et al. 1973; Murphy et al. 1975). A microvillous surface pattern of exfoliated cervical cells reflects the malignant potential of these cells (Allen et al. 1976). Irreversible neoplastic transformation could be established if a microvillous pattern on mature squamous cells (excluding microvilli on immature cells, e.g. parabasal and metaplastic cells) exists in that subgroup of CIN cells that show a progression towards malignancy. The SEM method of diagnostic cytology would, in this case, overrule the highly sophisticated Papanicolaou LM method, which is limited in terms of optimum patient management since it allows neither prognostication of individual lesions (Patten 1978), nor tumor staging.

IV. THE DIAGNOSTIC NON-SIGNIFICANCE
OF MICRORIDGES AND MICROVILLI
ON ECTOCERVICAL CELLS

In order to assess the feasibility of ultrastructural cell surface features as microvilli and microridges, to be used as early markers of irreversible neoplastic transformation, both exfoliated cells as well as biopsies were studied (Kenemans et al. 1980; Davina et al. 1980).

Using a technique in which LM and SEM were applied consecutively to the same cells, LM normal superficial and (mature) intermediate cells could show globular microvilli on their surface instead of the expected microridges (Figures 2b, 3f, 4c and 4f). In LM normal material, these microvilli most probably do *not* reflect a malignant potential, but merely serve to identify the cell sides that contain microvilli at those sides of the flat cells which were originally directed to the basement membrane (the 'basal'

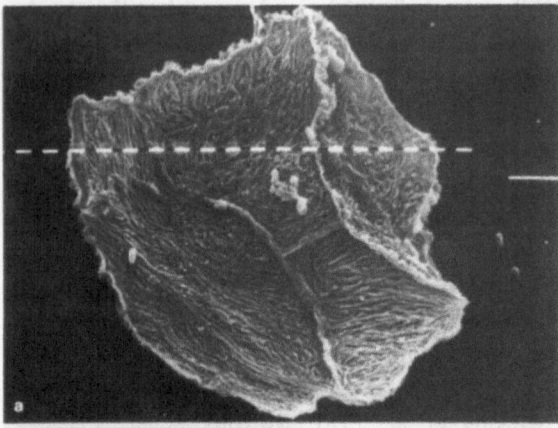
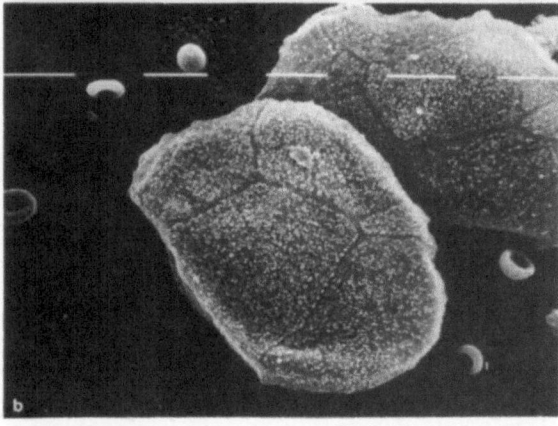

Figure 2. SEM of exfoliated superficial ectocervical cells, illustrating the 'luminal' cell side/'basal' cell side difference found in the squamous epithelium of the human cervix.

The 'luminal' cell side (a), i.e., the sides of the flat cells which were orginally directed to the vaginal lumen, have a typical surface pattern with microridges, and linear bars protruding from the surface (bar = 1 μm). The 'basal' cell sides (b), i.e., the cell sides which were originally directed to the basement membrane, show globular microvilli and surface grooves (bar = 10 μm).

sides) while the other side of the cells (the 'luminal' side) display the well-known microridge pattern.

Thus, a simple new working hypothesis was formulated, stating that normal superficial and intermediate ectocervical cells display different cell surface patterns on both sides (Kenemans et al. 1981). The 'luminal' cell side is characterized by microridges (and 'linear bars', Figures 2a, 3c), while the 'basal' cell side is characterized by (globular) microvilli (and 'grooves' (Figures 2b, 3f), which correspond to the linear bars).

The 'basal side/luminal side difference hypothesis' was obtained by using the following methodological approaches: (A) LM/SEM study parallel on sedimented cells; (B) LM/SEM study consecutively on folded cells; (C) SEM study of adjoining cell surfaces in tissue.

IV.A. LM/SEM parallel on sedimental cells (Kenemans et al. 1980)

Cervical cells obtained from 7 patients with a routine-cytological and colposcopically normal cervix, were studied parallel with LM and SEM, using 100 cells from each population every time. Where the LM method revealed that the population contained some 96% normal superficial and intermediate cells, with the SEM-method (Figure 2) an almost equal incidence of cell surfaces with microvilli (49%) and of surfaces with microridges (44%) was found. With random sedimentation, half of the cells may lie upside down, thus revealing the basal side (a situation which may be different from that in normal smears). There is a great variety of cell surface characteristics (Figure 3), including several types of microvilli and microridges, which may be related to such factors as degree of maturity and hormonal stimuli.

IV.B. LM/SEM consecutively on folded cells (Kenemans et al. 1980)

This technique permits both preservation of ultrastructure as well as identification of LM classified cells. Folded LM normal exfoliated cells allow both sides of the cell to be studied when examined by SEM. Frequently, a microridge pattern was found on one cell side and a microvillous one on the other side of the *same* flat cell (Figure 5).

IV.C. SEM study of adjoining cell surface in tissue (Davina et al. 1980)

Using a fracturing technique, and later a more refined stripping technique, it was possible to study 'complementary' surfaces of adjacent cells. After pressing double adhesive tape against the tissue surface of fixed and properly processed biopsies, a layer of epithelial cells was stripped off. Both the sheet of cells on the tape and the remaining biopsies were processed further and studied in the SEM. The basal side of a particular cell can then be compared with the luminal side of the underlying cell. Stripping can be repeated approximately ten times,

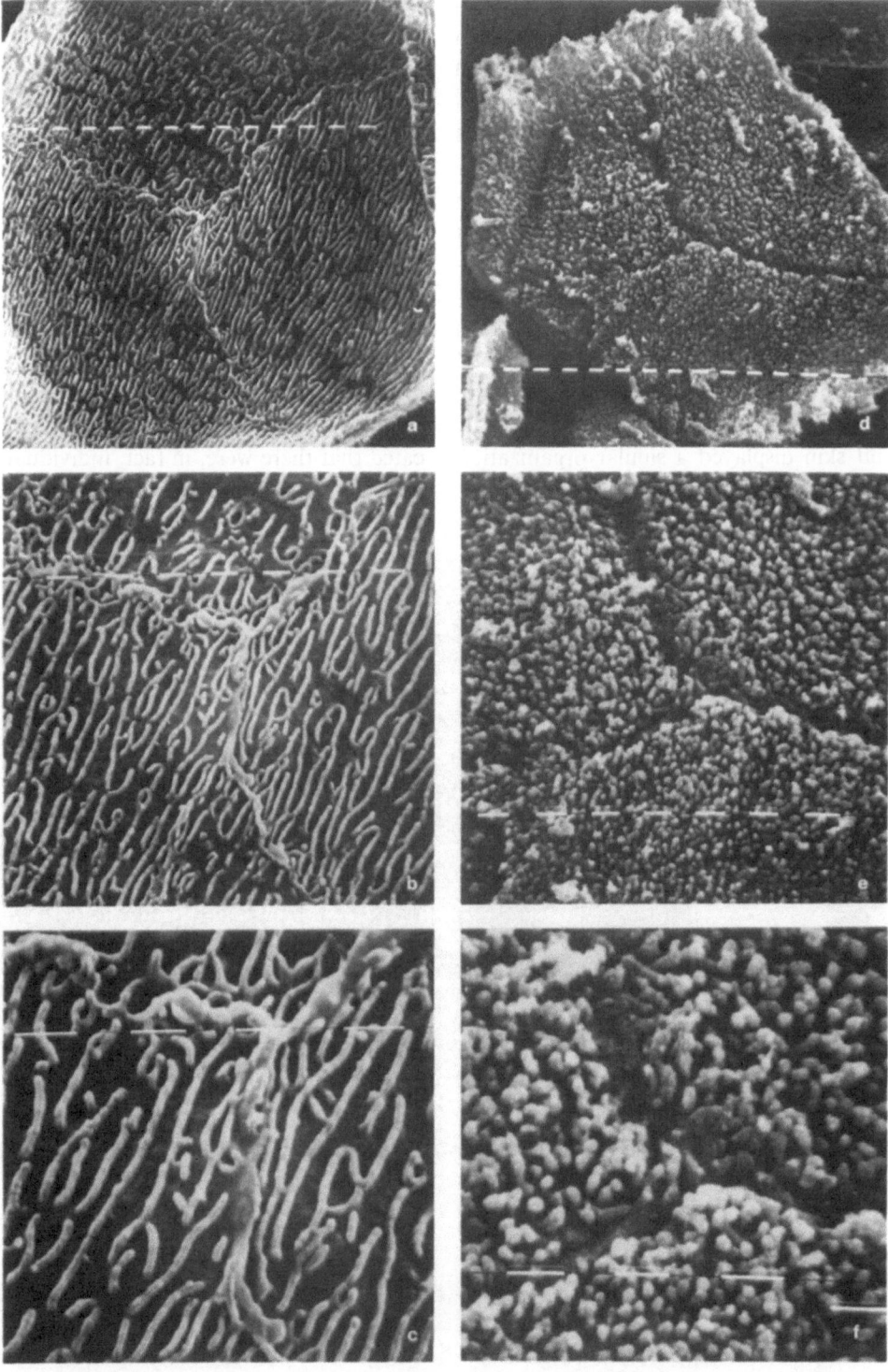

Figure 3. Different ultrastructural cell surface characteristics of two normal exfoliated cervical cells as revealed by SEM with different magnifications (bar = 1 μm). Surface microstructure of the 'luminal' cell side (a, b, c) shows a microridge pattern with protruding linear bars, while the surface microstructure of the other cell shows a 'basal' cell side pattern (d, e, f) with microvilli and linear grooves.

96

when the cleavage plane then occurs in the cyto-plasm and not intercellularly. This may be due to the altered cell surface organization in more basal layers. Stripping of the ectocervix has been pre-viously reported (e.g., Murphy et al. 1973) but was always performed *in situ* without comparing lu-minal and basal sides of the adjoining cells.

Results of the stripping technique indicate that neighboring cell surfaces appear to be complemen-tary to one another (Figure 6), with villi-like struc-tures on one side (the basal side of the upper cell) and microridge patterns on the other (the luminal side of the underlying cell). By using fracture methods, the squamous epithelium cells of both the vagina, and skin displayed a similar organization (Kenemans et al. 1980).

V. CONCLUDING REMARKS

It has become evident that all types of stratified squamous epithelia emerge from one basic struc-tural plan. This structural plan is characterized by a luminal cell side, covered with microridges and a basal cell side, covered with microvilli. These lu-minal microridges intermesh with the basal micro-villi of the adjacent cell, just as the basal microvilli intermesh with the luminal microridges.

Until now, reports could not be found which define these separate characteristics. However, one study (Rubio 1976) described the vaginal epithe-lium in the rat after estrogen treatment, and indi-cated that there were, in fact, individual character-istics between the luminal cell side and the basal cell side.

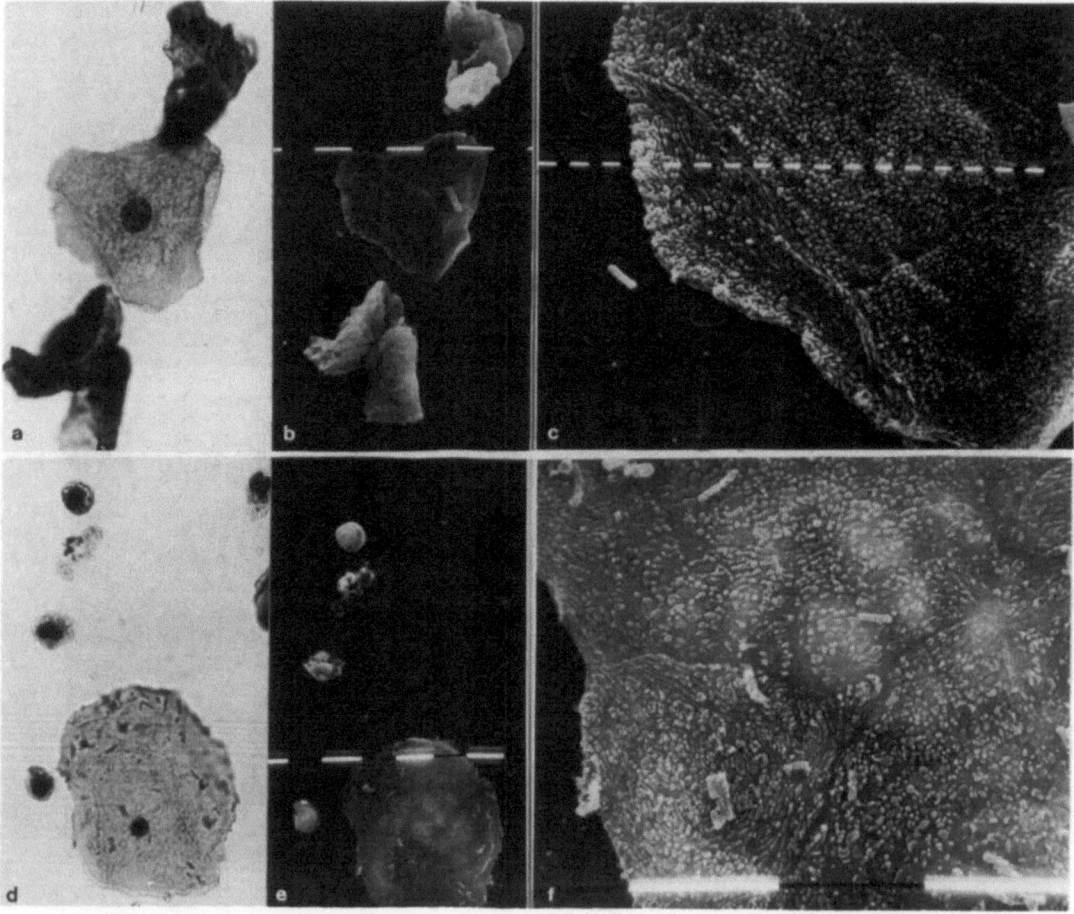

Figure 4. Consecutive observations on the same ectocervical cell by LM and SEM. The technique permits both identification in SEM of LM classified cells, as well as preservation of ultrastructure. An intermediate squamous cell observed in LM (a) and low-magnification SEM (b, bar = 10 μm). The high-magnification view reveals globular microvilli, and grooves (c, bar = 1 μm). A superficial squamous cell observed in LM (d) and low-magnification SEM (e, bar = 10 μm). The higher magnification micrograph demonstrates globular microvilli, and grooves (f, bar = 10 μm).

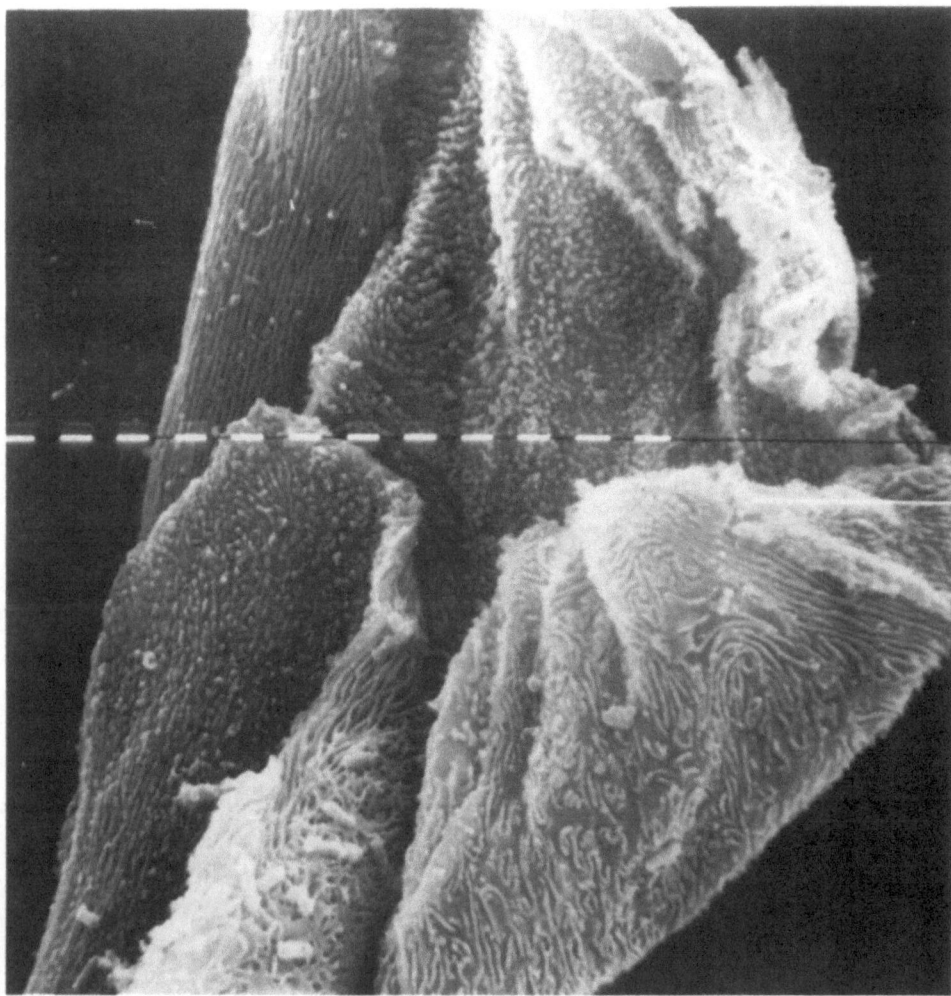

Figure 5. A SEM observation on two folded exfoliated normal ectocervical cells, allowing both sides of the cell to be studied. The surface difference between the 'basal' cell side and the 'luminal' cell side of each cell is evident, each cell showing microvilli on one side and microridges on the other (bar = 1 μm).

98

Because all normal squamous epithelial cells exhibit such definite structures, the microvilli cannot be used as early indicators of irreversible neoplastic transformation of the human ectocervical epithelium.

ACKNOWLEDGEMENTS

The authors wish to thank Miss G.E.M. Lamers for technical assistance and Mr. G.W. Klickermann for photographic work. The work presented was supported by a grant from the Dutch Cancer Society (KWF – NUKC – SMM 79–7).

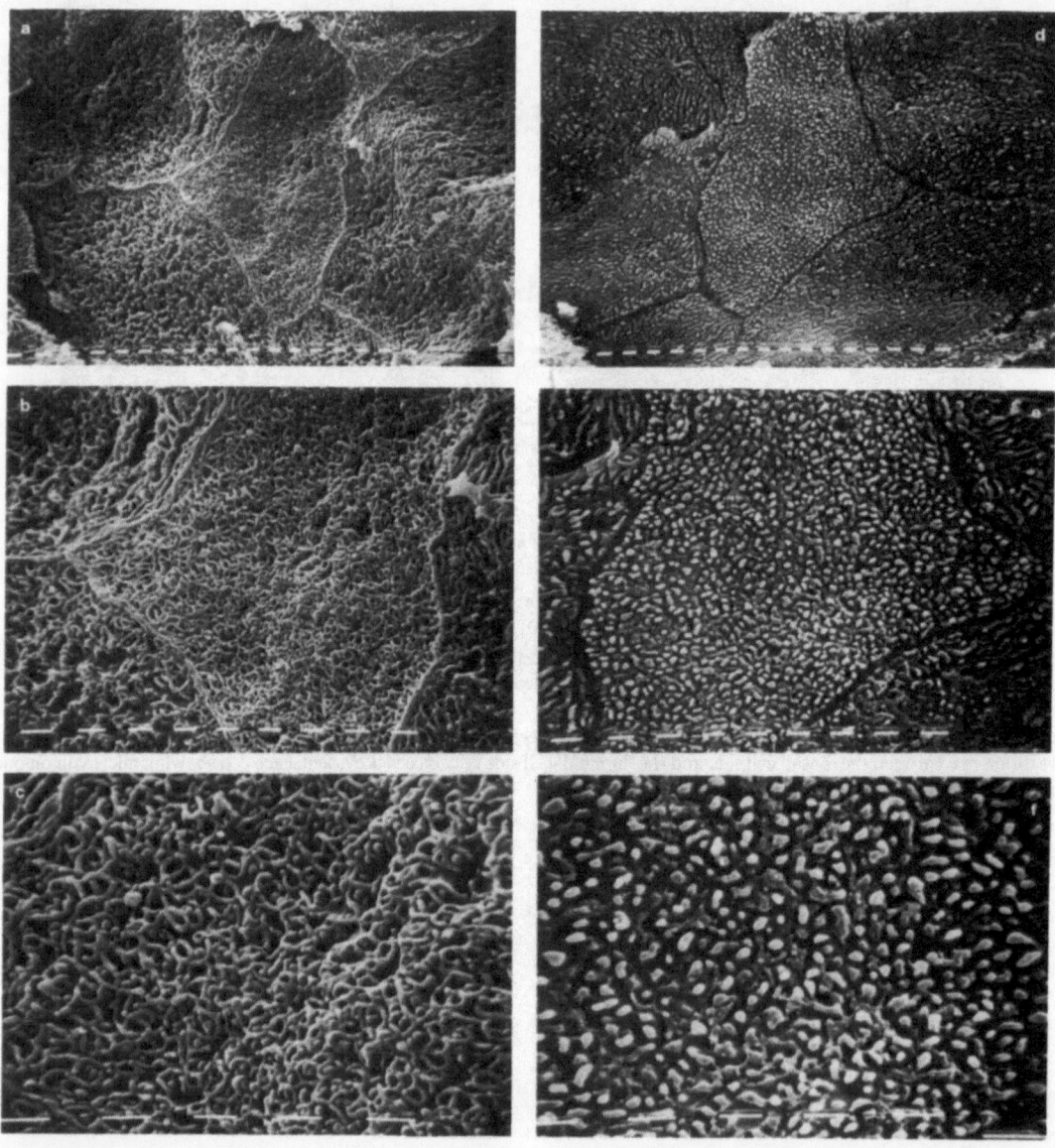

Figure 6. Adjoining cell surfaces of normal ectocervical cells within the tissue are observable in SEM after intercellular cleavage of the stratified tissue using a special stripping technique. After pressing adhesive tape against the tissue surface of biopsies a layer of cells is stripped off, and the surfaces of both the sheet of cells and that of the remaining biopsy are studied in SEM (bar = 1 μm). Cells which have been adjacent show 'complementary' surfaces after stripping (compare a with d, b with e, and c with f). Cell surfaces which were directed to the original lumen of the *tractus genitalis* ('luminal' cell surfaces) situated on the remaining biopsy (a) show with higher magnifications (b, c) a microridge pattern (and protruding bars), while the cell surfaces which were originally directed to the basement membrane ('basal' cell surfaces) situated on the tape (d), show at higher magnification (e, f) microvilli (with grooves, which correspond to the bars).

REFERENCES

Allen JM, Murphy JF, Jordan JA, Williams AE: The use of scanning electron microscopy in cervical cytology: results from the examination of 218 patients. Scanning Electron Microscopy/1976 (Part IV). Proceedings of the Workshop on SEM in Reproductive Biology. Chicago: IIT Research Institute, 315, 1976.

Davina JHM, Stadhouders AM, Kenemans P, van Haelst UJGM: A stripping technique for scanning electron microscopical study of adjoining cell surfaces in stratified squamous epithelium of the uterine ectocervix. BEDO 13: 253, 1980.

Domagala W, Woyke S: Transmission and scanning electron microscopic studies of cells in effusions. Acta Cytol 19: 214, 1975.

Ferenczy A, Gelfand MM: The cytodynamics of normal and neoplastic cervical epithelium. Obstet Gynecol Surv 34: 808, 1979.

Ferenczy A, Richart RM: Normal exfoliative cytology. *In* Ferenczy A, Richart RM (eds): Female Reproductive System: Dynamics of Scan and Transmission electron microscopy. New York: John Wiley & Sons, 1974, p 78.

Gilula NB: Junctional membranes in normal and neoplastic tissues. *In*: Cellular Membranes and Tumor Cell Behavior. 28th Annual Symp on Fundamental Cancer Research. Baltimore: Williams & Wilkins, 1975, p 219.

Hynes RO: Tumorigenicity, Transformation and Cell Surfaces. *In* Hynes RO (ed): Surfaces of Normal and Malignant Cells. New York: John Wiley & Sons, 1979, p 1.

Jordan JA, Murphy JF, Allen JM, Williams AE: The neoplastic Cervix. *In* Hafez ESE (ed): Atlas of Mammalian Reproduction. Stuttgart: Georg Thieme Verlag, 1975, p. 250.

Jordan JA: Scanning electron microscopy of the physiological epithelium. *In* Jordan JA and Singer A (eds): The Cervix. London: Saunders, 1976, p 44.

Jordan JA: Scanning electron microscopy of the cervical neoplasia. *In* Jordan JA and Singer A (eds): The Cervix. London: Saunders, 1976, p 372.

Kenemans P, Zanden v d PHT, Stolk JG, Vooys GP, Stadhouders AM: Cell Surface Ultrastructure in Neoplasia of the Uterine Cervix. *In* Letnansky K (ed): Biology of the Cancer Cell. Amstelveen: Kugler Publications, 1980, p 307.

Kenemans P, Davina JHM, Haan de RW, Zanden v d PHT, Stolk JG, Stadhouders AM: Cell surface morphology in epithelial malignancy and its precursor lesions. *In* Johari O (ed): Scanning Electron Microscopy, part III, 1981, p 23.

Llanes AT, Farre CB, Ferenczy A, Richart RM: Scanning electron microscopy of normal exfoliated squamous cervical cells. Acta Cytol 17: 507, 1973.

McNutt NS, Hershberg RA, Weinstein RS: Further observations on the occurrence of nexuses in benign and malignant human cervical epithelium. J Cell Biol 51: 805, 1971.

McNutt NS, Weinstein RS: Carcinoma of the cervix – deficiency of nexus intercellular junctions. Science 165: 597, 1969.

Murphy JF, Allen JM, Jordan JA, Williams AE: Examination of exfoliated cervical cells by the scanning electron microscope. Scanning Electron Microscopy. Proceedings of the Workshop on Scanning Electron Microscopy in Pathology, IITRI. Chicago: 605, 1973.

Murphy JF, Jordan JA, Allen JM, Williams AE: Correlation of Scanning Electron Microscopy, Colposcopy and Histology in 50 patients presenting with abnormal cervical cytology. J Obstet Gynaecol Br Commonw 81: 236, 1974.

Murphy JF, Allen JM, Jordan JA, Williams AE: Scanning electron microscopy of normal and abnormal exfoliated cervical squamous cells. Brit J Obstet Cynaecol 82: 44, 1975a.

Murphy JF, Allen JM, Jordan JA, Williams AE: Exfoliated cervical cells (man). *In* Hafez ESE (ed): Atlas of Mammalian Reproduction. Stuttgart: Georg Thieme Verlag, 1975b, p 242.

Nicolson GL: Cell surface and Blood-Borne Tumor Metastasis. *In* Day SB, Myers WPL, Stansly P, Garattini G, (eds): Cancer Invasion and Metastasis. Biologic Mechanisms and Therapy. Progress in Cancer Research and Therapy, Vol 5. New York: Raven Press, 1977, p 163.

Nicolson GL, Poste G: The Cancer Cell: Dynamic Aspects and Modifications in Cell-Surface Organization. I. New Engl J Med 295: 197, 1976a.

Nicolson GL, Poste G: The Cancer Cell: Dynamic Aspects and Modifications in Cell-Surface Organization. II. New Engl J Med 295: 253, 1976b.

Nicolson GL, Birdwell CR, Brunson KW, Robbins JC, Beattie G, Fidler IJ: Cell interactions in the metastatic process: Some cell surface properties associated with successful blood-borne tumor spread. *In* Burgers MM and Lash J (eds): Cell and Tissue Interactions. New York: Raven Press, 1977, p. 225.

Patten SF: Diagnostic Cytology of the Uterine Cervix. Baltimore: The Williams & Wilkins Comp., 1978.

Poste G: Cell surface and Metastasis. *In* Day SB, Myers WPL, Stansly P, Garattini S, (eds): Cancer Invasion and Metastasis. Biologic Mechanisms and Therapy. Progress in Cancer Research and Therapy, Vol 5. New York: Raven Press, 1977, p 19.

Poste G, Weiss L: Some considerations on cell surface alterations in Malignancy. *In* Weiss L (ed): Fundamental Aspects of Metastasis. Amsterdam: North-Holland, 1976, p 25.

Rubio CA: The exfoliating cervico-vaginal surface. Anat Rec 185: 359, 1976.

Rubio CA, Kranz I: The exfoliating cervical epithelial surface in dysplasia, carcinoma *in situ* and invasive squamous carcinoma. Acta Cytol 20: 144, 1976.

Sherman AI: Comparison of cancer cell surfaces of the lower reproductive tract by scanning electron microscopy. Am J Obstet Gynecol 129: 893, 1977.

Shingleton HM, Wilbanks GD: Fine Structure of Human Cervical Intraepithelial Neoplasia *in Vivo* and *in Vitro*. Cancer 33: 981, 1974.

Vesely P, Boyde A: The significance of SEM evaluation of the cell surface for tumor cell biology. IITRI/SEM 1973: 690, 1973.

Weinstein RS, Selles WD, Young IT: Quantitative analyses of membrane topography in normal and malignant epithelium. Proc Sixth Europ Congr on electron Microscopy, Jerusalem, 1976: 104, 1976.

Wilbanks GD: *In Vivo* and *in Vitro* 'Markers' of Human Cervical Intraepithelial Neoplasia. Cancer Res 36: 2485, 1976.

Williams AE, Jordan JA, Murphy JF, Allen JM: The cervix uteri. *In* Hafez ESE (ed): Atlas of Mammalian Reproduction. Stuttgart: Georg Thieme Verlag, 1975, p 223.

17. HISTOCHEMISTRY OF ALKALINE PHOSPHATASE IN CERVICAL NEOPLASIA

S. Nozawa, H. Oota, K. Arai, S. Izumi, F. Tsutsui and S. Kurihara

I. HISTOCHEMICAL ISOENZYME PATTERNS OF ALKALINE PHOSPHATASE

Alkaline phosphatase (ALP) is a substance thought to participate in active transport. Formerly it was thought that only diseases of the bone, liver or bileduct result in a rise of serum ALP. However, owing to improved methods for the analysis of isoenzymes, e.g., electrophoresis and various inhibition tests, it is now possible to identify ALP isoenzymes originating not only in the bone or liver, but also in the small intestine or placenta.

Methodology of the histochemical heat stability and L-P sensitivity tests was reported (Nozawa et al. 1980) and results of these morphological investigations were in close agreement with results derived by biochemical heat stability and L-P inhibition tests. These two histochemical tests were employed in the classification of ALP isoenzymes.

In this chapter, ALP enzymes are classified histochemically into type I, II and III, using heat stability and L-P inhibition tests concomitantly.

The type I isoenzyme, which shows marked heat stability and L-P sensitivity, resembles the Regan isoenzyme which is heterotopically produced by some cancers (Fishman et al. 1968). The histochemical properties of this isoenzyme are identical to those of the ALP in placental cells observed under the same conditions.

Type II isoenzyme, which is heat sensitive and L-P sensitive, resembles the intestinal ALP isoenzyme. It shows the identical histochemical properties as intestinal ALP when viewed under the same conditions.

Type III isoenzyme, which is heat sensitive and slightly L-P sensitive, has the same characteristics as ALP in liver or bone and the same properties as the ALP of these organs when observed under the same conditions.

II. REGAN ISOENZYME

Diagnosis of cancer is primarily based on morphological methods which determine atypia as a result of increased nucleic DNA in cancer cells. However, abnormalities in phenotypic expression due to transformed genes have been noted and the results of investigations on various types of enzymes are gradually being used in diagnosing cancer.

Fishman et al. (1968) reported a heat-stable, L-phenylalanine (L-P) sensitive ALP isoenzyme – the Regan isoenzyme – in the serum, exudate and tumor tissue of a pulmonary cancer patient, which could not be biochemically or immunologically distinguished from placental ALP. This placenta-like ALP was a protein produced ectopically in tumors (Nakayama et al. 1970; Kellen et al. 1976) and is now being used as a carcino-placental antigen (Fishman 1973) in supplementing the diagnosis of malignant tumors.

The Regan isoenzyme was originally thought to derive only from tumor cells (Stolbach et al. 1969; Usategui-Gomez et al. 1974; Nathanson and Fishman 1977), however, it was recently found in non-cancer patients (Malkin et al. 1979).

The identification of morphologically normal cells that produce heat-stable ALP was difficult when biochemical methods were employed. Using enzyme histochemical methods, the existence of a Regan-like (heat-stable, L-P sensitive) ALP isoenzyme was documented in cells derived from the Müllerian duct, e.g. reserve and columnar cells (Figures 1a, 1b, 4) of the uterine cervix and cells from the luminal surface of the endometrial lining epithelium (Nozawa et al. 1975, 1980, 1981; Izumi 1977). Any of these cells may represent a tissue source of the Regan-like substance in non-cancer and non-pregnant patients, a suggestion supported biochemically.

Hafez, E.S.E., Smith, J.P. (eds.), Carcinoma of the Cervix: Biology and Diagnosis. ISBN-13: 978-94-009-7487-6

During the course of carcinogenesis of the uterine cervix, reserve cells may undergo a malignant change.

Via the stages of dysplasia and carcinoma *in situ*, progression to invasive cancer may occur. Therefore, enzyme histochemical methods were used to study the changes in the ALP isoenzymes of reserve cells during the course of carcinogenesis.

III. HISTOCHEMICAL STUDIES OF ALKALINE PHOSPHATASE

III.A. Non-specific ALP activity

III.A.1. Light microscopic study

The materials consisted of samples from 4 atypical reserve cell hyperplasia, 42 dysplasia, 53 cancer *in situ* and 88 invasive cancer patients (Table 1). Tissues were fixed for 9 hr at 4°C in Baker's 10% formol calcium (Baker 1946), washed overnight at 4°C in Holt's gum sucrose (Holt 1959), then 6 μm thick serial section were cut with a cryostat and mounted on glass slides. The modified method of Burstone (1958) was used as ALP staining. The substrate was naphthol AS-BI phosphate (1.1 mM), the azo dye was fast-red-violet LB salt (0.75%), and the buffer consisted of 0.05 M propandiol (pH 9.8). The pH of the incubation medium was 9.3–9.5; incubation was for 15 min at room temperature. Nuclear staining was done by the Azur-A-Schiff method.

ALP activity in various kinds of uterine cervical epithelial cells was visualized light-microscopically primarily along the plasma membrane, as a red

Table 1. Non-specific ALP activity.

	No. of total cases	Non-specific ALP
Atypical reserve cell hyperplasia	4	100%
Dysplasia	42	29%
Cancer *in situ*	53	34%
Invasive cancer	88	34%
Toal	187	34%

From: Nozowa et al., 1981.

homogeneous precipitate of the azo dye pigment. Sections which, in a circumscribed area, exhibited any non-specific ALP activity in the plasma membranes were designated as ALP-positive. The section was designated as ALP-negative only if there was no ALP activity. ALP-positivity was classified into four grades ranging from $\pm$ to 3+. The enzyme activity in the capillary endothelial cells of the same section was used as the standard of comparison.

Of 187 cases, 34% were positive for non-specific ALP activity (Table 1). Invasive cancers with ALP positive regions were either of the undifferentiated or the intermediate type (Figures 2a, 3a); there was no ALP activity in regions which revealed a tendency towards differentiation to squamous epithelium. Although weak ALP activity was occasionally noted in the surface keratinized layer of squamous epithelia, this type of ALP activity was disregarded in this chapter.

III.A.2. Electron microscopic study

For electron-microscopic histochemical investigations of ALP, 28 samples were divided into two parts; one part was used for study by light microscopy, the other for electron microscopy. The latter group included 10 dysplasia, 6 cancer *in situ* and 12 invasive cancer cases. Fresh tissues were cut into $0.5 \times 0.5 \times 5$ mm rectangles and pre-fixed by the double fixation method. They were first paraformaldehyde (4.5%) fixed for 4 hr at 4°C followed by 1 hr 2.5% glutaraldehyde fixation at 4°C. The tissues were then washed overnight at 4°C in 0.05 M tris-maleate buffer (pH 7.4), 40 μ sections were cut with a tissue sectioner and incubated for 30 min at room temperature according to the method of Mayahara et al. (1967), in 40 ml of a medium consisting of 7.6 ml 0.1 M Na, β-glycerophosphate (350 mg/10 ml), 6.4 ml 0.2 M tris-HC1 buffer (pH 7.5), 10 ml 0.015 M MgSo$_4$. 7H$_2$O, and 16 ml 0.5 M lead citrate (pH 10.0–11.5). The sections were dehydrated in a graded series of alcohol, embedded in epoxy-resin and thick and thin sections were double-stained with uranyl acetate and lead citrate.

Electron microscopic inspection revealed that epithelial cells manifested no ALP activity when they were well differentiated, as evidenced by the presence of many tonofilaments and desmosomes. However, when the cells were poorly differentiated,

Table 2. Criteria of heat stability and L-phenylalanine sensitivity.

		Category 1	Category 2	Category 3	Category 4
Heat stability[a]	Non-specific ALP	(+) (++) (+++)	(+++)	(++) (+++)	(+) (++) (+++)
		↓	↓	↓ ↓	↓ ↓ ↓
	ALP after heat inactivation	(−)	(+)	(+) (++)	(+) (++) (+++)
L-P sensitivity[a]	ALP after D-P inhibition	(+) (++) (+++)	(±) (+)	(+) (++) (+++)	(++) (+++)
		↓ ↓ ↓	↓ ↓	↓ ↓ ↓	↓ ↓
	ALP after L-P inhibition	(+) (++) (+++)	(−) (±)	(−) (+) (++)	(−)(±)(−)(±)(+)

[a] Category 1 – none; Category 2 – slight; Category 3 – moderate; Category 4 – marked.
From: Nozawa et al. 1980; reproduced with permission of the publisher: Chapman & Hall Ltd.

as evidenced by the presence of fewer tonofilaments and desmosomes (Figures 5, 6), ALP activity was occasionally recognized as black dots, primarily on plasma membranes.

III.B. Heat-stability test

The heat stability test was performed on serial sections which were derived from 48 lesions manifesting non-specific ALP activity. Heat-stability test was performed with or without heat-inactivation at 65°C for 30 min in a 0.005 M MgCl$_2$ solution (Jensen et al. 1968).

With respect to heat stability, 4 categories were established by comparing the intensity of ALP-staining between sections that had, or had not, been heat-inactivated (Table 2). Category 1 sections were heat-sensitive and showed no ALP-activity after heat-inactivation. Category 2 (slightly heat-stable) was applied when there was a considerable difference between the heat-inactivated and inactivated sections. If there was little or no difference between the sections, they were categorized as heat-stability 3 (moderate) and 4 (marked), respectively. Only 4 of 48 (8.3%) sections (2 each deriving from dysplasia and invasive cancer cases) were markedly heat-stable (Category 4); the other 44 sections manifested no heat stability (Table 3, Figures 2b, 3b).

Table 3. Type of ALP determined by heat stability and L-phenylalanine sensitivity.

Lesions \ Alkaline phosphatase	No. of serial section cases	Heat stability none	slight	moderate	marked	L-P sensitivity none	slight	moderate	marked	No. of cases	Type of ALP
Atypical reserve cell hyperplasia	4	X					X			4	III
Dysplasia	7				X				X	1	I
					X		X			1	?
		X							X	1	II
		X						X		1	?
		X					X			3	III
Carcinoma *in situ*	12	X							X	1	II
		X					X			11	III
Invasive carcinoma	25				X				X	2	I
		X							X	2	II
		X						X		3	?
		X					X			18	III
Total	48	44	0	0	4	0	37	4	7	48	

III.C. L-phenylalanine inhibition test

The serial sections of 48 cases which had been examined for heat-stable ALP activity were examined by the L-P inhibition test. For the L-P inhibition test, the method described by Watanabe and Fishman (1964) was used. ALP staining was performed after 15 min incubation at room temperature in a medium containing 0.03 M L-P. For the control, the incubation medium contained 0.03 M D-phenylalanine, which is stereo-specific for L-P.

The tissues were then dehydrated in a graded series of alcohol. Regarding L-P sensitivity, four categories were established (Table 2); the higher the assigned number, the greater the L-P sensitivity. Sections were classified according to the difference in ALP-staining after incubation in the presence of L-phenylalanine or D-phenylalanine. All sections were L-P sensitive; 37 were assigned to Category 2 (Figures 2c, 2d, 3c, 3d), 7 to Category 4 and 4 to Category 3 (Table 3).

IV. ALP ISOENZYME PATTERNS IN CERVICAL NEOPLASIA

The 48 cases that were examined for non-specific ALP activity, heat stability of ALP and sensitivity to L-P, were classified according to the ALP isoenzyme type. The type I ALP isoenzyme manifested both marked heat stability and L-P sensitivity, and was similar to the ALP isoenzyme produced heterotopically in some cancers, although it was also found in the placenta and reserve cells of non-cancer patients. The type II isoenzyme is heat-sensitive and markedly L-P sensitive and resembles the ALP of the small intestine. The type III isoenzyme is heat-sensitive and slightly L-P sensitive and resembles the ALP of the liver, bone, and endothelial cells of blood vessel.

While 43 of 48 cases could be categorized under one of these 3 types, five could not (Table 3). Of these five cases, one had dysplasia with marked heat stability and slight L-P sensitivity, one was of dysplasia and three were of invasive cancer which were heat-sensitive and moderately L-P sensitive. These five cases were unclassifiable according to this system, probably due to limitations inherent in the present enzyme-histochemical methods.

V. 'ENZYME DEVIATION' DURING CARCINOGENESIS

The heat-stable, L-P sensitive ALP (type I) is similar to the Regan isoenzyme found in the plasma membrane of reserve cells (Nozawa et al. 1975, 1980, 1981; Izumi 1977), which are thought to be the origin of most uterine cancers. However, the present study revealed non-specific ALP activity in 4 cases of atypical reserve cell hyperplasia and all of these ALPs were classified as type III. The isoenzymes in these cases were entirely different from those existing in normal cells. Normal reserve cells, by a process of malignant transformation, have resulted in the manifestation of atypical reserve cell hyperplasia, which contain a different type of isoenzyme from that present in normal reserve cells. Furthermore, while 'enzyme deviation' already exists at this stage, it goes undetected by conventional morphological methods.

The type I isoenzyme was detected in only one dysplasia and two invasive cancer cases, suggesting that reserve cells continued to maintain the same type I isoenzyme even after malignant transformation. The other classifiable lesions (4 cases of dysplasia, 12 of cancer in situ (Figures 2a–2d), 20 of invasive cancer (Figures 3a–3d)) had type II or III ALP; which may represent an alteration in the phenotypic expression of transformed genes.

When a malignant transformation occurred, various kinds of isoenzymes which are not found in normal reserve cells, appeared. Schapira et al. (1963) and Weinhaus (1970) have made a similar observation regarding the enzyme aldolase. In the course of hepatic carcinogenesis, a new isoenzyme appears. To explain the mechanism of such an alteration of isoenzymes ('enzyme deviation'), dedifferentiation and disdifferentiation have been proposed.

Advocates of the dedifferentiation hypothesis consider carcinogenesis to represent a shift to an undifferentiated stage. Isoenzymes may also be converted into a more undifferentiated, uniform pattern (Greenstein 1954). Since in hepatomas, the enzyme patterns are converted into those of embryonal liver cells, the hypothesis of dedifferentiation prevailed at one time. However, in a certain type of the Yoshida ascitic liver cancer, there appears an isoenzyme – the C type aldolase – which is not observed in embryonal liver cells. This

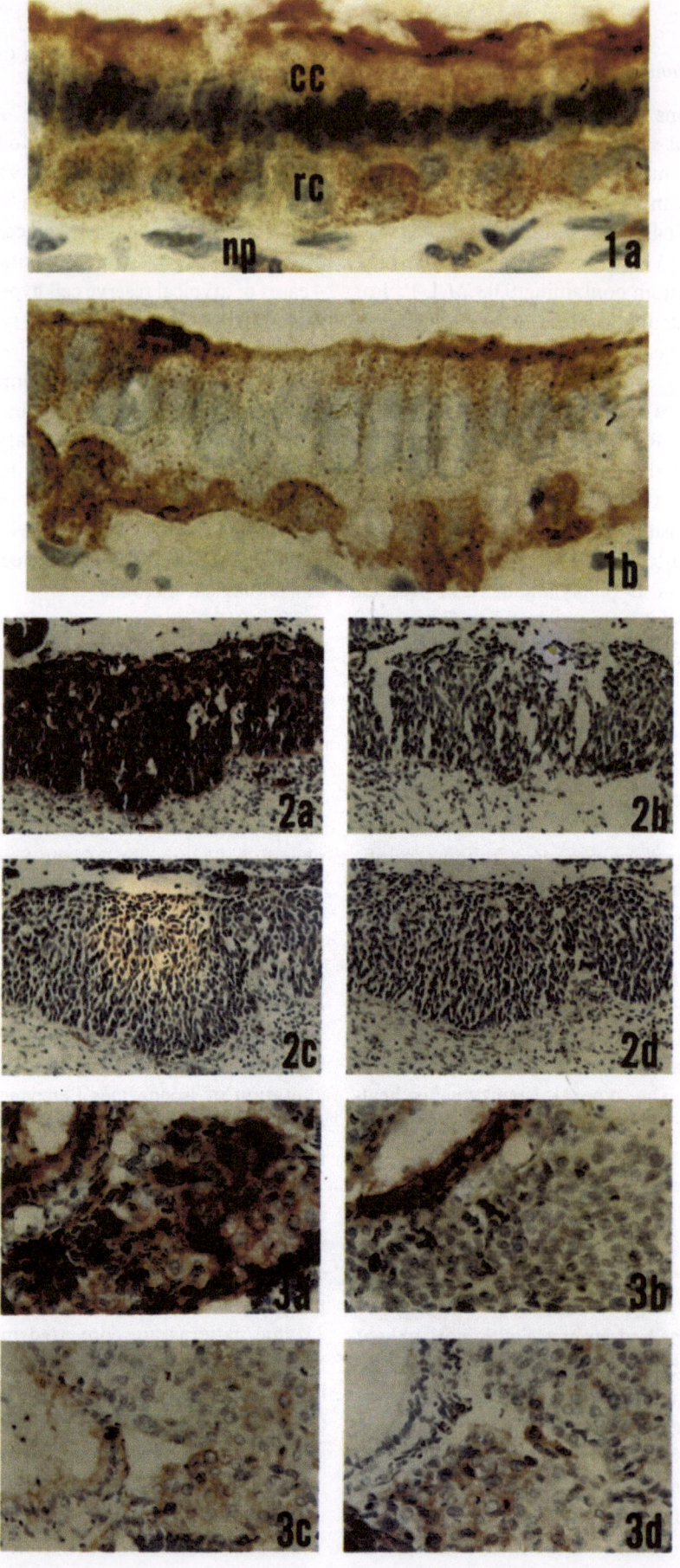

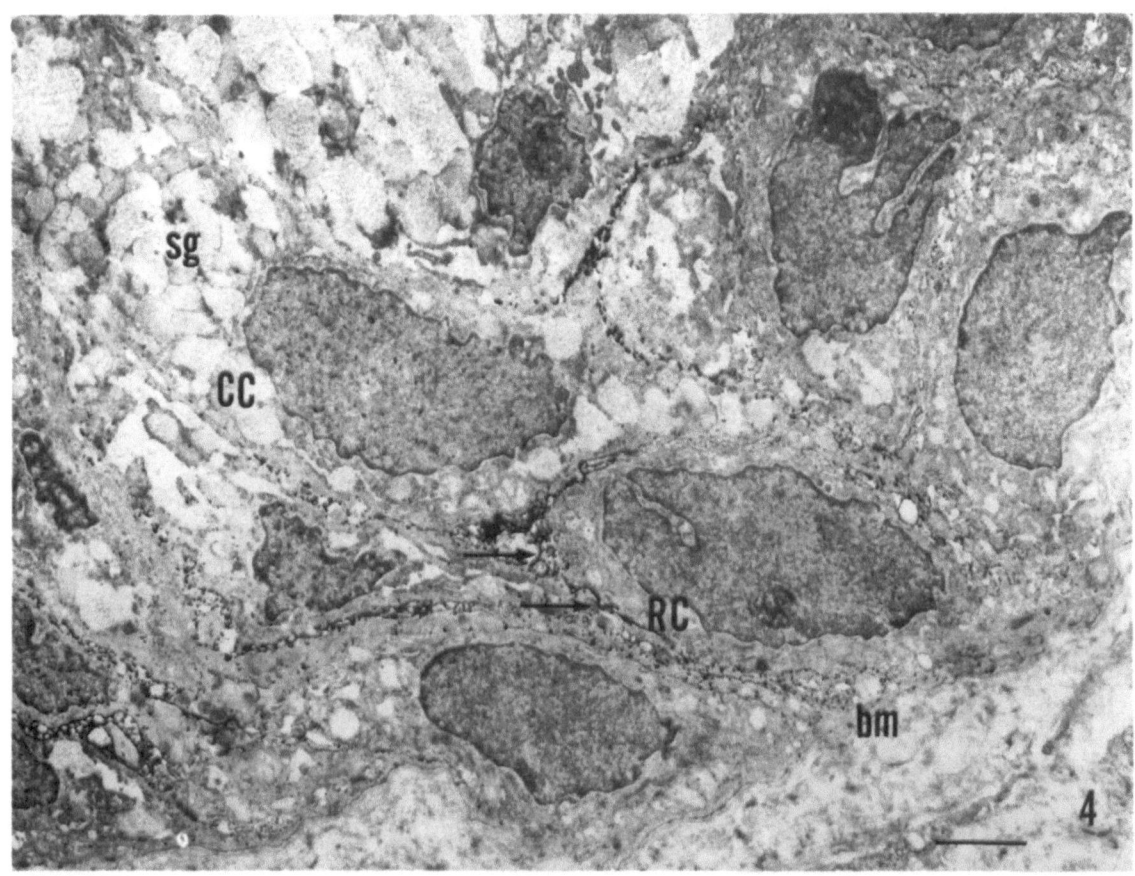

Figure 4. ALP localizations are observed at the lateral plasma membrane of reserve cells of uterine cervix; arrow – ALP activity; columnar cell (CC); secretory granule (sg); reserve cell (RC); basement membrane (bm).

Figure 1. (a) Red-colored precipitate in columnar cells (cc) and reserve cells (rc) of uterine cervix and neutrophils (np) shows ALP activity; (b) After heat inactivation, heat-stable ALP of columnar cells and reserve cells persisted, while ALP of neutrophils is heat-inactivated. The ALP in cervical columnar cells and reserve cells resembles placental ALP or the Regan isoenzyme produced heterotopically by tumors (*From:* Nozawa et al. 1980; reproduced with permission of the publisher: Chapman & Hall Ltd.).

Figure 2. (a) Red precipitate in cancer *in situ* shows ALP activity; (b) Heat-inactivation of ALP activity; (c) After D-phenylalanine inhibition test (control); (d) After L-phenylalanine inhibition test. A slight difference in inhibition is seen. ALP in this cancer *in situ* resembles liver or bone ALP (*From:* Nozawa et al. 1981; reproduced with permission of the publisher).

Figure 3 (a) Strong ALP activity is seen in both cancer cells and endocervical columnar cells; (b) After heat inactivation, heat-stable ALP activity in columnar cells persists, while ALP in cancer cells is heat-inactivated; (c) After D-phenylalanine inhibition test (control); (d) After L-phenylalanine inhibition test. A marked difference in inhibition is seen in ALP activity in columnar cells, while a slight difference in ALP of cancer cells is seen. ALP in columnar cells resembles Regan or placental or reserve cell ALP, while ALP in cancer cells resembles liver or bone ALP (Nozawa et al. 1981).

106

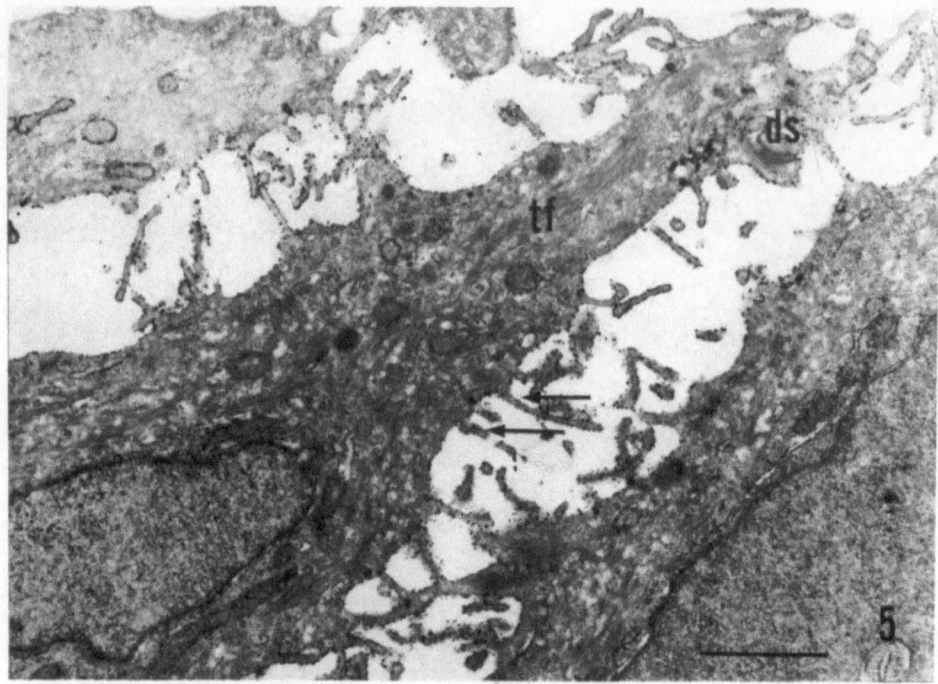

Figure 5. Localizations of ALP activity are seen as black dots at microvilli and plasma membranes of dysplastic cells; arrow – ALP activity; tonofilament (tf); desmosome (ds).

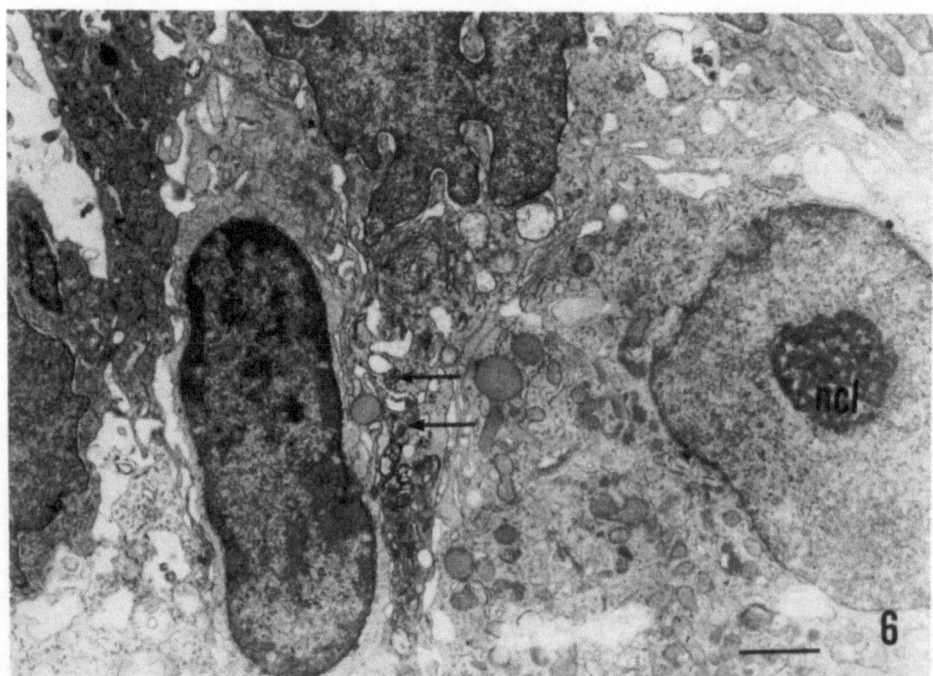

Figure 6. ALP localizations are observed at the plasma membrane of cancer cells; arrow – ALP activity; nucleolus (ncl).

phenomenon could not be explained solely by dedifferentiation, therefore, the disdifferentiation hypothesis has been proposed (Sugimura et al. 1972). Embryonic differentiation is stated as taking place according to a time schedule and is controlled by the switching on or off of genes in a sequential manner. The phenotypic expressions are also believed to be under specific control. However, in the case of cancer cells, because of a malfunction of the control system, various phenotypic expressions of genes, not normally found, are noted.

Instead of one kind of the Regan-like ALP isoenzyme in the reserve cells, various types of isoenzymes appear in precancerous lesions or cancer tissues. The enzyme deviation of the ALP in uterine cervical cancers, may be more appropriately interpreted as the result of disorder in the system controlling the phenotypic expression of genes, rather than by the dedifferentiation hypothesis, according to which various isoenzyme patterns are converted into a single pattern.

VI. CONCLUDING REMARKS

Histochemical studies on 187 patients with precancerous and cancerous lesions of the uterine cervix, were undertaken to ascertain the incidence of alkaline phosphatase (ALP) and the isoenzyme types. Of 187 cases, 64 (34.2%) manifested non-specific ALP activity, serial sections from 48 of these were subjected to heat stability and L-phenylalanine (L-P) inhibition tests. One mild dysplasia and 2 invasive cancer cases manifested an ALP isoenzyme similar to reserve cell ALP; based on its marked heat stability and L-P sensitivity, it was classified as type I ALP. One severe dysplasia, 1 cancer *in situ* and 2 invasive cancer cases revealed an ALP isoenzyme similar to small intestine ALP; based on its marked heat and L-P sensitivity, it was classified as type II. Four atypical reserve cell hyperplasia, 3 severe dysplasia, 11 cancer *in situ*, and 18 invasive cancer cases had an ALP isoenzyme similar to liver or bone ALP; based on its marked heat and slight L-P sensitivity, it was classified as type III.

During the course of carcinogenesis, the heat stability and L-P sensitivity of reserve cell ALP undergoes a change, and 'enzyme deviation' occurs.

REFERENCES

Baker JR: The histochemical recognition of lipine. Quart J Micr Sci 87: 441, 1946.

Burstone MS: Histochemical comparison of naphthol As-phosphates for the demonstration of phosphatases. J Nat Canc Inst 20: 601, 1958.

Fishman WH, Inglis NR, Stolbach LL, Krant MJ: A serum alkaline phosphatase isoenzyme of human neoplastic cell origin. Cancer Res 28: 150, 1968.

Fishman WH: Carcinoplacental isoenzyme antigens. *In* Weber G (ed): Advances in enzyme regulation, Vol XI. New York: Pergamon Press, 1973, pp 293–321.

Greenstein TP: Biochemistry of cancer, 2nd ed. New York: Academic Press, 1954.

Holt SJ: Factors governing the validity of staining methods for enzymes, and their bearing upon the Gomori acid phosphatase technique. Exp Cell Res Suppl VII, 1, 1959.

Izumi S: Histochemical characterization of reserve cell alkaline phosphatase – with a special reference to heat stability test and L-phenylalanine test. Acta Obst Gynec Jpn 29: 149, 1977.

Jensen H, Lynghye J, Davidsen S: Histochemical investigation of the thermostable alkaline phosphatase in the normal full-term placenta. Acta Obst Gynec Scandinav 47: 437, 1968.

Kellen JA, Bush RS, Malkin A: Placenta-like alkaline phosphatase in gynecological cancers. Cancer Res 36: 269, 1976.

Malkin A, Kellen JA, Caplan B: The presence of placenta-like alkaline phosphatase in normal human uterine cervix and endometrium. *In* Lehman FG (ed): Carcino-Embryonic Proteins, Vol II. Amsterdam: North Holland: Elsevier, 1979, pp 679–684.

Mayahara H, Hirano H, Saito T, Ogawa K: The new lead citrate method for the ultracytochemical demonstration of activity of non-specific alkaline phosphatase. (Orthophosphoric monoester phosphohydrolase). Histochemie 11: 88, 1967.

Nakayama T, Yoshida M, Kitamura M: L-leucine sensitive, heat-stable alkaline-phosphatase isoenzyme detected in a patient with pleuritis carcinomatosa. Clin Chem Acta 30: 546, 1970.

Nathanson L, Fishman WH: New observations on the Regan isoenzyme of alkaline phosphatase in cancer patients. Cancer 27: 1388, 1977.

Nozawa W, Izumi S, Ohta H, Shinozuka T, Tsutsui F, Kurihara S, Watanabe K: Histochemical studies on alkaline phosphatase in uterine cervical reserve cell, precancerous and cancerous lesions. *In* Shanmugaratnam K (ed): Proc 2nd Asian Cancer Conference. Singapore: Stanford College Press, 1975, pp 324–326.

Nozawa S, Ohta H, Izumi S, Hayashi S, Tsutsui F, Kurihara S: Watanabe K: Heat-stable alkaline phosphatase in normal female genital organ – With special reference to the histochemical heat-stability test and L-phenylalanine inhibition

108

test. Acta Histochem Cytochem 13: 521, 1980.

Nozawa S, Ohta H, Izumi S, Hayashi S, Tsutsui F, Kurihara S: Heat stable alkaline phosphatase in uterine cancer. Histochem J 13: 941, 1981.

Schapira F, Dreyfuss JC, Schapira G: Anomaly of aldolase in primary liver cancer. Nature 200: 995, 1963.

Stolbach LL, Krant MJ, Fishman WH: Ectopic production of an alkaline phosphatase isoenzyme in patients with cancer. Ann NY Acad Sci 166: 760, 1969.

Sugimura T, Matsushima T, Kawachi T, Kogure K, Tanaka N,

Miyake S, Hozumi M, Sato H: Disdifferentiation and Decarcinogenesis. Gann Monograph Cancer Res 13: 31, 1972.

Usategui-Gomez M, Yeager FM, Castro AF: Regan isoenzyme in normal human sera. Cancer Res 34: 2544, 1974.

Watanabe K, Fishman WH: Application of stereospecific inhibitor, L-phenylalanine to the enzymorphology of intestinal alkaline phosphatase. J Histochem Cytochem 12: 252, 1964.

Weinhaus S: Homologies in enzymes and metabolic pathways. *In* Whelam WJ, Schultz J (eds): Metabolic alternative in cancer. Amsterdam: North-Holland, 1970, pp 462.

18. MORPHOLOGY OF THE BASEMENT MEMBRANE IN CARCINOMA OF THE CERVIX

U.M. SPORNITZ and E.S.E. HAFEZ

Basement membranes are found wherever plasma membranes of parenchymal cells come into contact with connective tissue elements as seen by electron microscopy (Vracko 1974). Opinions about the existence of a basement membrane in cervical epithelium have previously been rather controversial (Ashworth et al. 1961). Ever since the basement membrane in this tissue had been demonstrated to exist, it has attracted considerable attention; particularly because of the unsettled question of the role which is played by the basement membrane in the transition of carcinoma *in situ* in to invasive carcinoma. The determination of the invasive status of cervical carcinoma depends, to a large extent, on the structural integrity of the basement membrane underlying the neoplastic epithelium (Coppleson 1976). Most investigators of cervical neoplasma have focused on the absence or presence of the basement membrane rather than on its morphology in different conditions such as dysplasia, carcinoma *in situ* and invasive carcinoma.

I. MORPHOLOGY AND FUNCTION OF BASEMENT MEMBRANES

Two main functions are generally attributed to the basement membrane which are not necessarily mutually exclusive: (1) basement membranes act as semipermeable filters (e.g. the renal glomerular basement membrane; Farquhar 1980); (2) basement membranes provide support for one cell type and/or serve as a boundary between different cell types (e.g. epithelial cells and connective tissue; Vracko 1974).

Much of the knowledge that has been accumulated in recent years about the function of basement membranes has been gathered from experimental studies with renal glomerular basement membranes, a model system particularly suitable to study the filter functions of basement membranes. With few exceptions (cf. Kefalides 1979) the other types of basement membranes are less well known. Basement membranes in most tissues, including cervical epithelium, are generally composed of three distinguished zones:

1. The *lamina densa* (or basement membrane proper), consists of tightly packed fibrils, about 30 to 40 Å in diameter, which are randomly oriented in an amorphous matrix. In the case of normal cervical epithelium, the lamina densa is a continuous sheath approximately 300 Å thick.

2. The lamina densa is separated from the basal epithelial cells by a lighter zone: the *lamina lucida* (sometimes called lamina rara). This name is used because it does not stain with electron stains. The lamina lucida is thought to contain electron lucent material responsible for the attachment of basement membranes to plasma membranes (Vracko 1974). This interpretation appears likely since the lamina densa always keeps the same distance from the plasma membrane. The lamina lucida must be composed of some substantial material rather than being an empty space, which is relevant when considering the penetration of invasive epithelium into the underlying stroma. In the case of normal cervical epithelium, the lamina lucida is about 300 Å thick, thus having the same dimension as the lamina densa.

3. The side of the lamina densa facing the stroma is characterized by so-called 'anchoring fibrils' about 100 Å in diameter, which are believed to connect the basement membrane to connective tissue fibrils of the stroma, namely collagen fibrils.

The chemical composition of basement membranes varies considerably in different species or even in different organs from the same species (cf. Kefalides 1979). Basement membranes are generally composed

Hafez, E.S.E., Smith, J.P. (eds.), Carcinoma of the Cervix: Biology and Diagnosis. ISBN-13: 978-94-009-7487-6
© 1982, Martinus Nijhoff Publishers, The Hague/Boston/London.

110

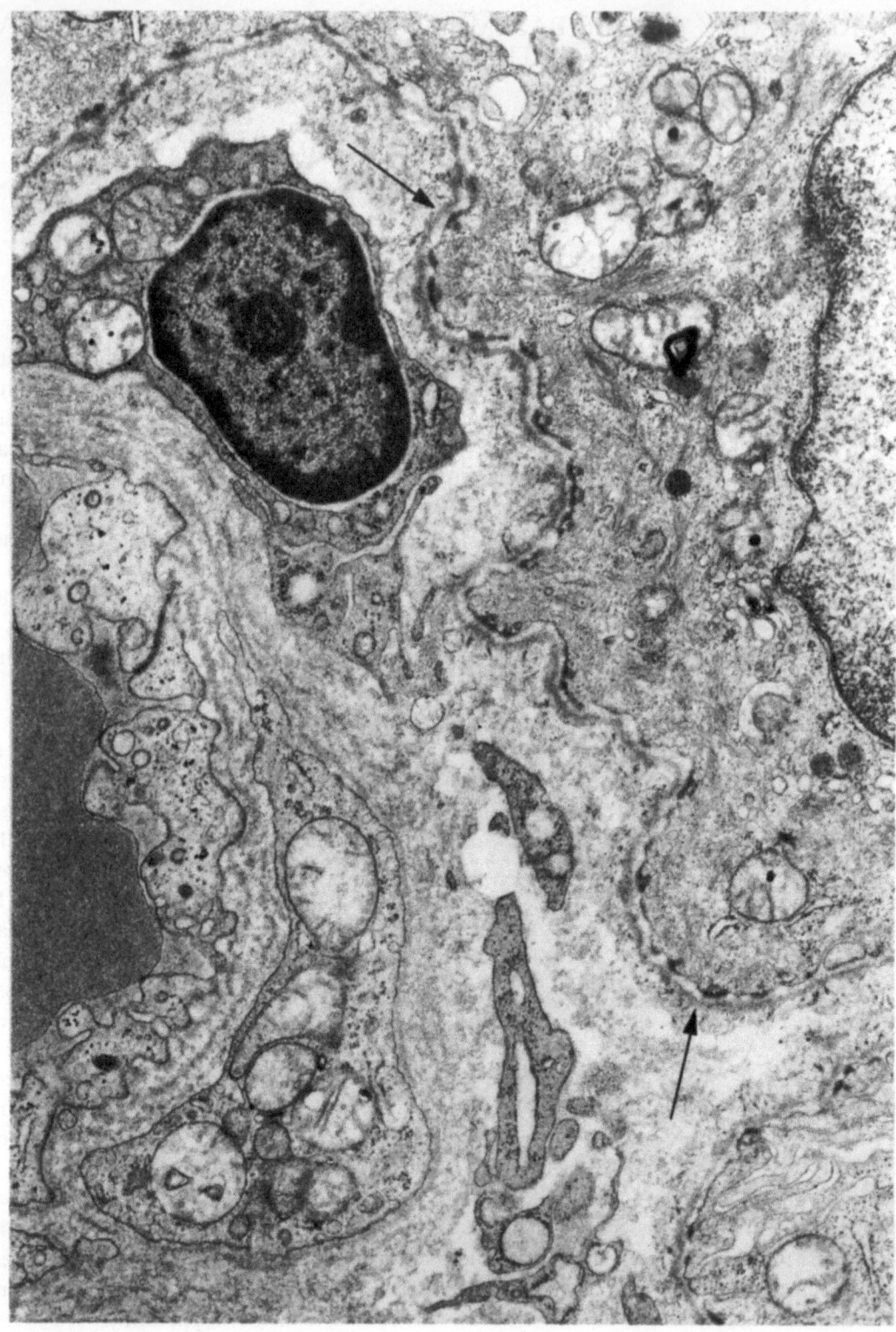

Figure 1. Electron micrograph of normal cervical epithelium. In the basal region several foot processes are present. The arrows point at the basement membrane, × 22,000.

of 90% protein, 8% carbohydrate and only 2% lipids (Vracko 1974). Because of this relatively low content in lipids, single fixation with osmiumtetroxide does not appear to be appropriate. Double fixation with glutaraldehyde followed by osmium-tetroxide is strongly recommended for basement membrane studies.

In squamous epithelia, such as epidermis and cervical epithelium, the basal layer of cells is attached to the basement membranes by means of hemidesmosomes. Hemidesmosomes are present at the basal plasma membrane and like 'full' desmosomes possess tonofilaments projecting from the desmosomes into the cytoplasm.

II. THE BASEMENT MEMBRANE OF NORMAL CERVICAL EPITHELIUM

In normal cervical epithelium the basement membrane has a constant thickness of 300 Å which varies only within narrow limits (290–310 Å). The basement membrane is separated from the plasma membrane of basal cells by a lamina lucida which is also about 300 Å thick. Undulations of the basement membrane are caused through foot processes of the basal cells. These are irregularly shaped projections at the basis of the cells. On the average section through a normal basal cell of cervical epithelium, about 4–6 such projections are present. Semiquantitative calculations indicate that the basal surface area is enlarged 2–3 times by these foot processes. The foot processes are always covered by a continuous layer of basement membrane. Only in very rare instances can a discontinuity of the basement membrane be found. However, this always seems to be due to mechanical stress during preparation rather than to naturally occurring imperfections of the basement membrane itself.

On the stromal side of the basement membrane, anchoring fibrils frequently occur. These fibrils seem to be continuous on the side of the basement membrane with the basement membrane filaments and on the side of the stroma with the collagen fibrils. Hence, the anchoring fibrils are probably reticular fibrils. Hemidesmosomes occur quite frequently in normal cervical epithelium. On the average, the distance between individual hemidesmosomes is approximately 0.5 μm. The lamina lucida underlying the hemidesmosomes is not only thinner (Figure 1), but also consists of a finely dispersed granular matrix. The cytoplasm of the basal cells immediately adjacent to the plasma membrane has essentially the same structural composition as the more central parts of the cytoplasm. A terminal web or network of cytoplasmic filaments is not present in normal cervical epithelium. The tonofilaments arising from the hemidesmosomes and projecting into the cytoplasm are not as pronounced as are the ones in the areas of the full desmosomes, which are responsible for the contact between epithelial cells. Sometimes tonofilaments are completely missing. Hemidesmosomes are not present in endocervical glandular epithelium, but may be present in columnar cells at the squamo-columnar junction (Figure 2).

III. BASEMENT MEMBRANE OF CERVICAL INTRAEPITHELIAL NEOPLASIA

Dysplasia may progress toward invasion without the intermediate stage of carcinoma *in situ*. In respective cases, dysplasia is assumed to be a true carcinoma *in situ* of special differentiation (Burghardt 1978). A gradual progressive change generally occurs from mild dysplasia to carcinoma *in situ*. This is particularly well reflected by changes in the basal plasma membrane and its associated structures like foot processes and the basal lamina.

With the development of cervical intraepithelial neoplasia from mild dysplasia to carcinoma *in situ*, a progressive loss of foot processes occurs. In normal cervical epithelium, the average number of foot processes per cell is approximately 35 which decreases to 13 in moderate dysplasia and finally reaches a low of 4 foot processes per cell in carcinoma *in situ* (Twiggs et al. 1980). Concomitantly occurring with the loss of foot processes, the basal lamina (or basement membrane), which generally adheres well to the basal plasma membrane, becomes much straighter and finally in carcinoma *in situ*, has almost totally lost its undulations (Figure 3). In earlier stages of this development, a relative increase in number of hemidesmosomes appears. This may be due to the life span of hemidesmosomes being longer than that of the basal lamina. Therefore, the reduction of the basal plasma membrane necessarily results in an increase in the

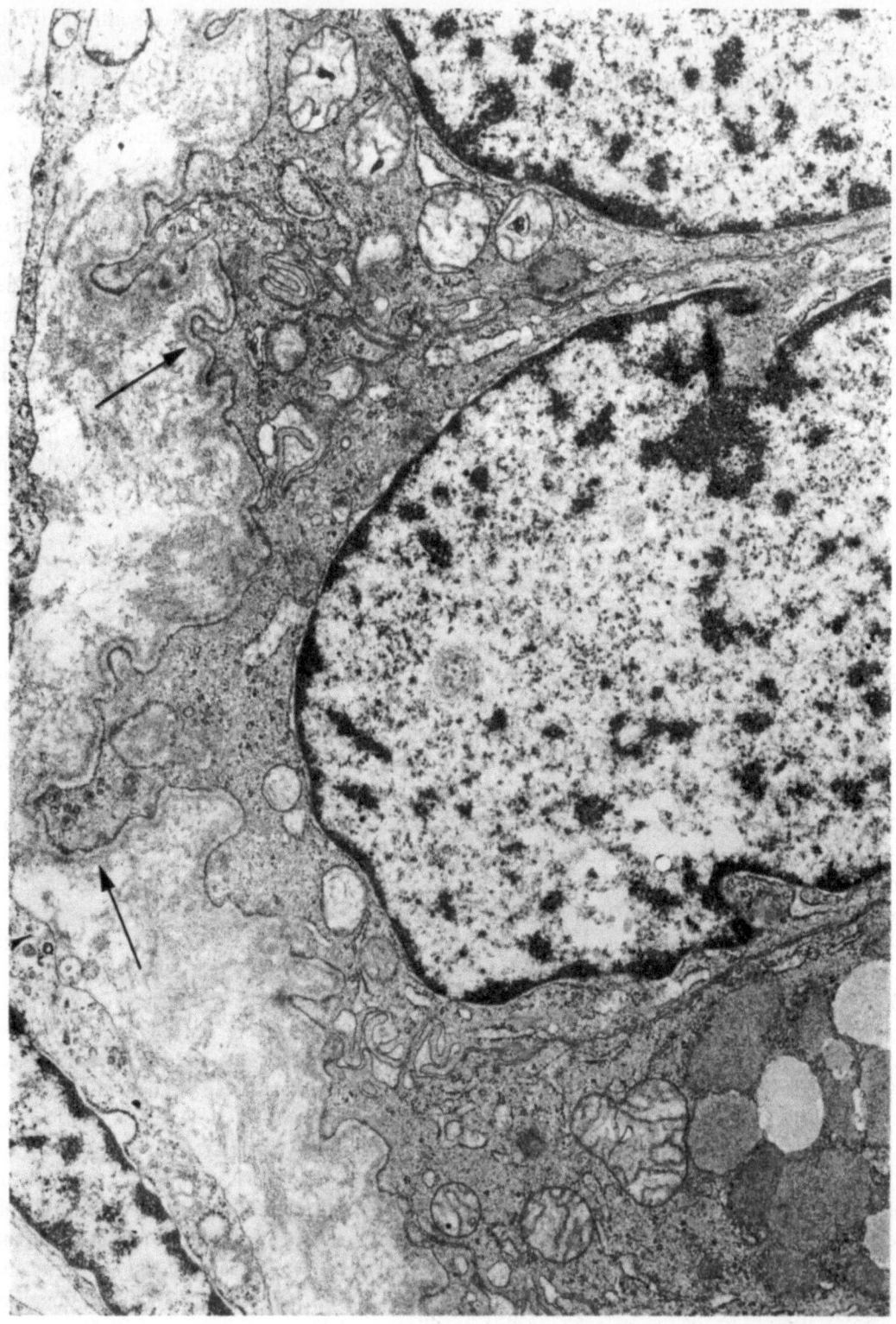

Figure 2. Basal region of normal endocervical glandular epithelium. In the lower third on the right-hand side several secretory granules are present (arrows: basement membrane), × 22,000.

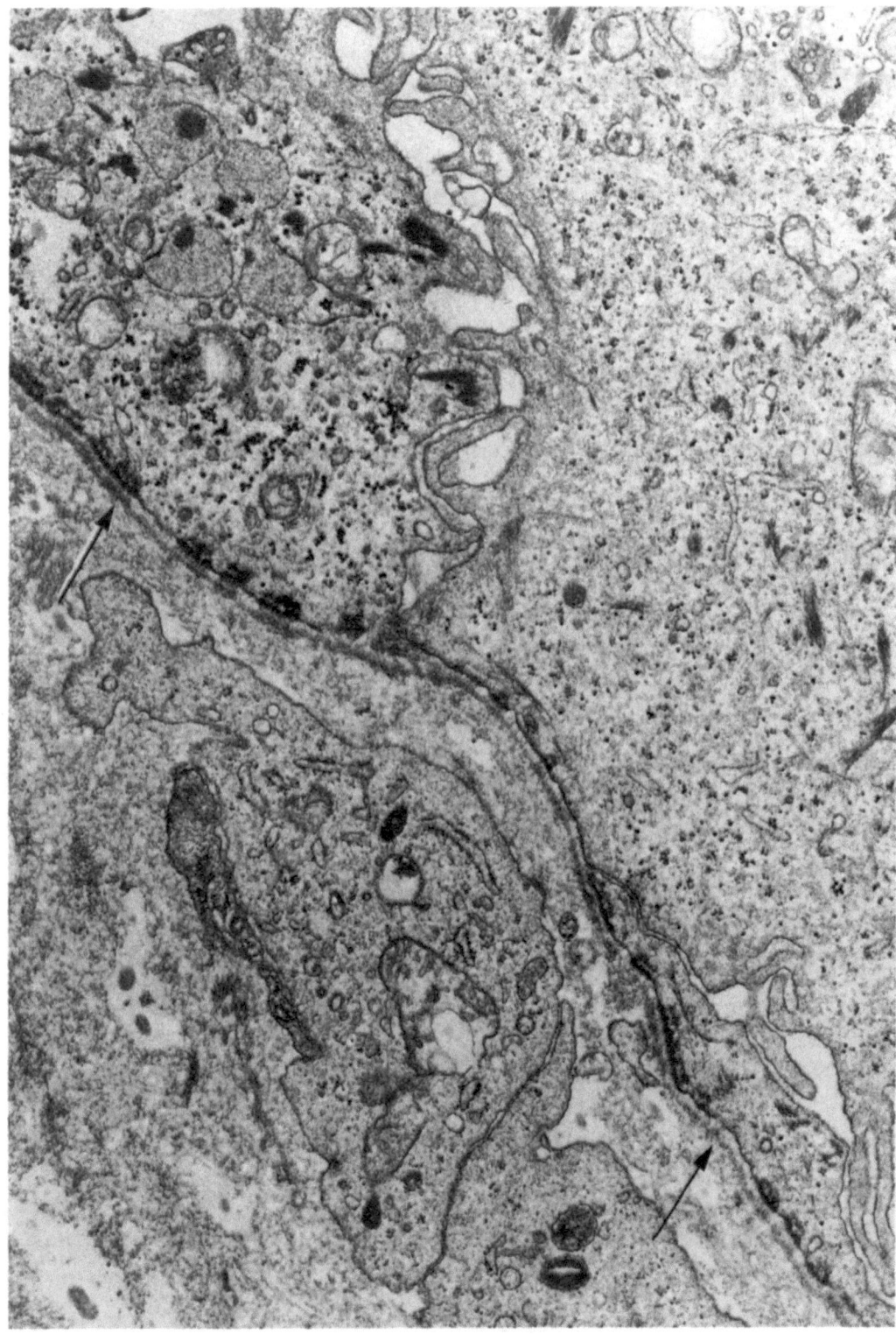

Figure 3. Cervical epithelium of carcinoma *in situ*. Note the straight basement membrane as compared to Figure 1. There are no foot processes present (arrows: basement membrane), × 22,000.

114

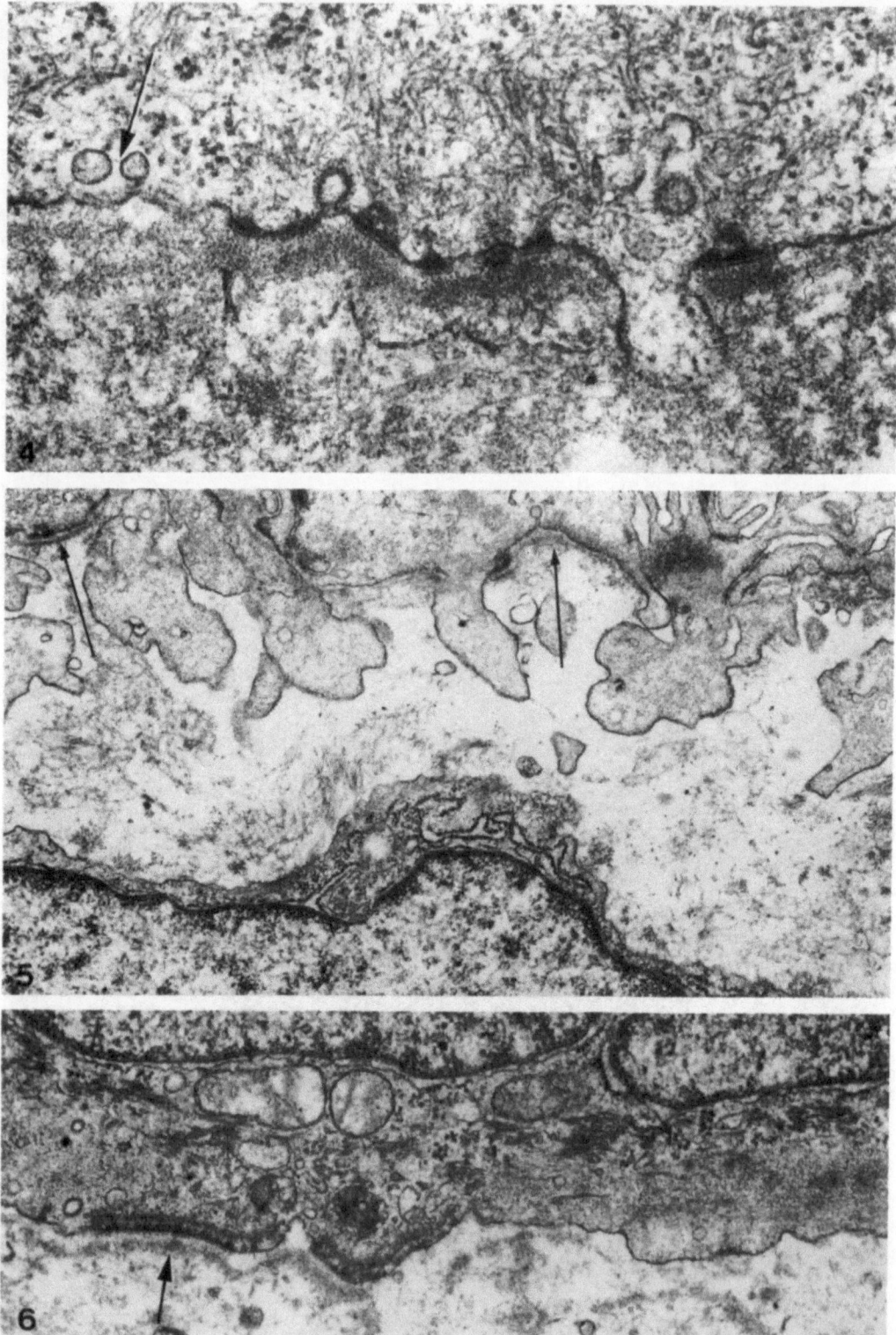

Figure 4. Microinvasive epithelium with penetrating foot process. Arrows point at cytoplasmic vesicles (probably exocytosis). Anchoring fibrils on the stromal side of the basement membrane are present, × 54,000.

Figure 5. Invasive carcinoma with numerous penetrating foot processes. The arrows point at remnants of basement membrane, × 18,000.

Figure 6. Electron micrograph of invasive carcinoma. Except for in the areas of the hemidesmosome (arrow) the basement membrane is absent. Note the microfibrillar web present on the right-hand side of the cell, × 30,000.

number of hemidesmosomes per unit length of plasma membrane. This increase is only of a temporary nature, since progressive development into the direction of carcinoma *in situ* finally results in a drastic reduction in number of hemidesmosomes. Another major difference between the basal lamina of normal and that of dysplastic epithelium is a decrease of the average thickness from a normal 300 Å to approximately 250 Å. The thickness of the lamina lucida remains unaltered. In carcinoma *in situ*, the number of anchoring fibrils adhering to the basement membrane also seems to be reduced.

IV. THE BASEMENT MEMBRANE OF MICROINVASIVE AND INVASIVE CARCINOMA

The transition between carcinoma *in situ* and microinvasion is marked through the reappearance of foot projections. The first reappearing foot processes measure only about 0.1 to 0.15 μm in diameter and have about one tenth of the diameter of the foot processes of normal cervical epithelium. In contrast to the latter (which are covered by a continuous basement membrane), the foot processes of microinvasive epithelium penetrate through the basement membrane into the underlying stroma. These penetrations always occur in the interspace between hemidesmosomes (Figure 4). In areas adjacent to the penetrating foot projections, cytoplasmic vesicles can frequently be observed in close opposition to the basal plasma membrane (Figure 4). The limiting membrane of these vesicles does not correspond with the basal plasma membrane in its morphology. There is a similarity to other cytoplasmic vesicular membranes, like those found in the vicinity of Golgi complexes. Therefore these vesicles reflect a process of exocytosis rather than pinocytotic uptake into the cells. Whereever these vesicles are present in the proximity of the basal plasma membrane, the basement membrane region underlying the plasma membrane seems to be altered morphologically. At the same time, the lamina densa has become narrower and the lamina lucida has become thicker.

In areas where the penetrating foot processes occur, the number of hemidesmosomes is drastically reduced and the anchoring fibrils have almost disappeared totally – particularly in later stages of invasion (Figure 5). Moreover the basal cytoplasm of the cells, which possess penetrating foot processes, show a thick network of microfilaments (terminal web) (Figure 6). Except for these microfilaments and a few vesicles, the foot processes and the basal peripheral cytoplasm do not contain any appreciable amount of cell organelles. Another very important feature of microinvasive cells is that the remaining basement membrane varies considerably in thickness ranging from 150 Å to 1200 Å. The penetrating processes seem to force their way through the basement membranes because the gaps in the basement membrane were only in the case of a clearly invasive epithelium found to be wider than the penetrating foot processes (Figure 7). The lamina densa – which usually maintains a distance of about 300 Å from the plasma membrane because of the material of the lamina lucida – sometimes comes into direct contact with the penetrating processes.

In clearly invasive carcinoma, the basement membrane is usually missing over large areas. The hemidesmosomes and anchoring fibrils disappear. The network of fibrils at the basal periphery of the cells is generally still present and in many cases, this zone of microfibrils even becomes wider (Figure 8). When a total loss of basement membranes exists, the hemidesmosomes apparently play a role in retaining the membrane for some time. The basement membrane of clearly invasive carcinoma remains in those places where hemidesmosomes have remained (Figure 6). With the degradation of hemidesmosomes, the basement membranes are also lost completely. In many cases, the microinvasive foot processes are covered by an amorphous ground substance, which however, does not form a lamina densa and lucida but comes into direct contact with plasma membrane of the penetrated process (Figure 9).

V. COMMENT

Although the basement membrane is involved in the process of invasion, it has obtained relatively little attention so far. Absence or presence of the basement membrane are mentioned in almost every paper dealing with ultrastructure of cervical lesions (Younes 1968; Shingleton and Lawrence 1976; Auersperg et al. 1973; Kocher et al. 1981). Because of conflicting reports regarding the structural integrity in differential cervical lesions, the reliability of the basement

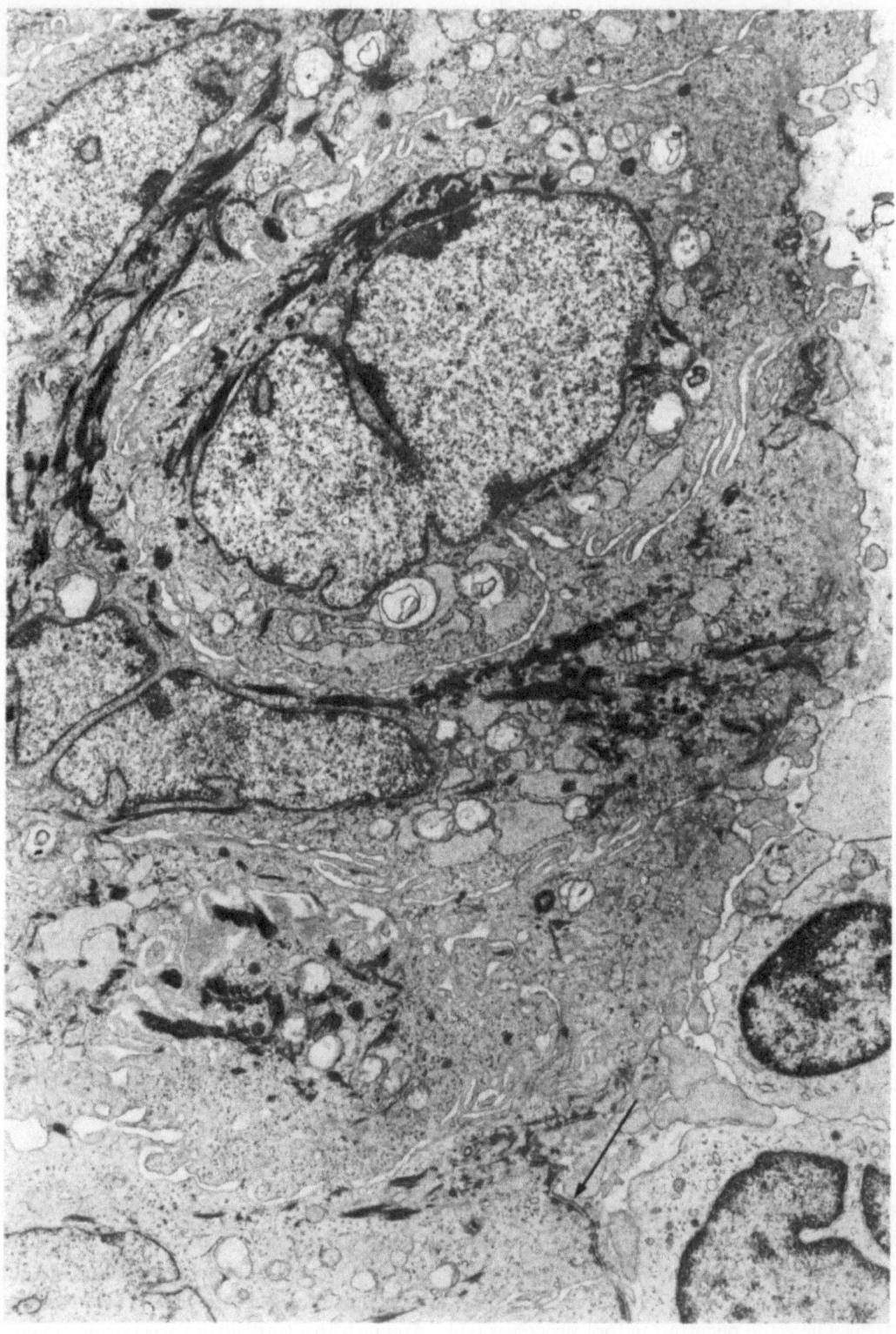

Figure 7. Electron micrograph of invasive carcinoma. Over the whole length of two cells the basement membrane is missing. The arrow points at the area where the basement membrane is still present, × 8,500.

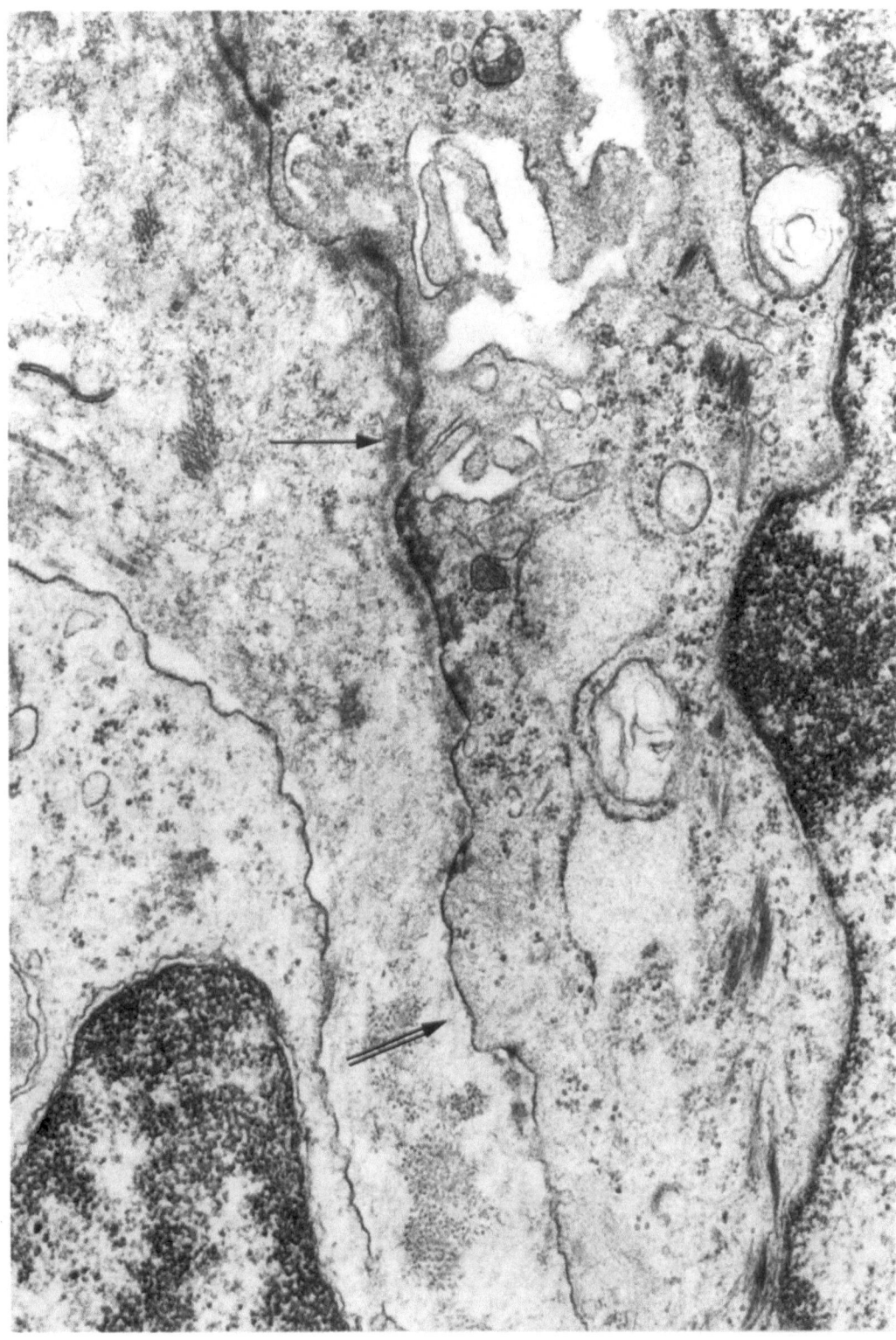

Figure 8. Basal region of an invasive cancer cell. The single arrow points at an area where the basement membrane is still present. The double arrow denotes the area where the basement membrane is missing, × 30,000.

118

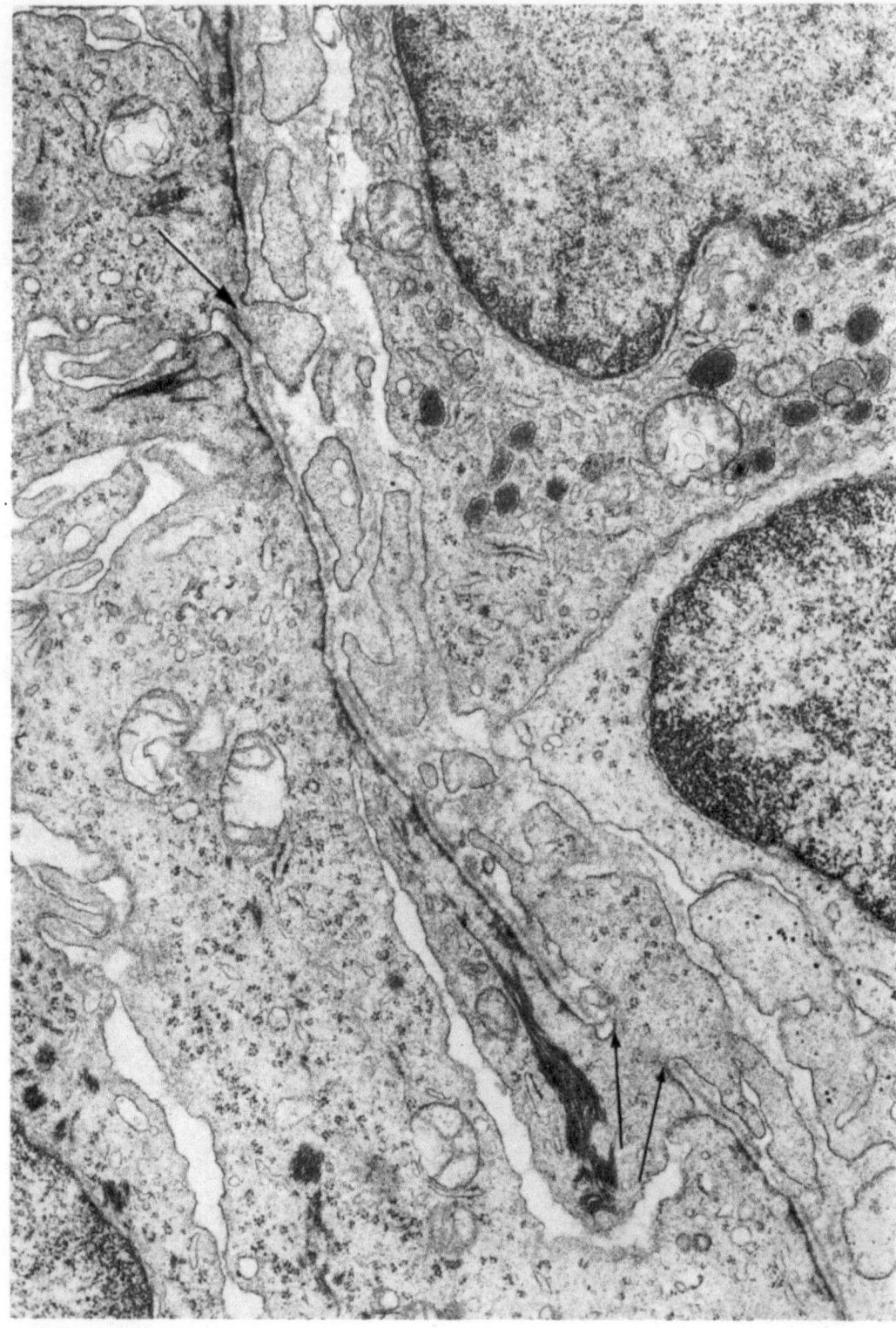

Figure 9. Two penetrating foot processes which have broken through the basement membrane (arrows). Note the amorphous ground substance covering the foot processes that have broken through, × 22,000.

membrane, as an indicator of the invasive status has been doubted (Luibel et al. 1960; Langley 1976; Coppleson 1976). The usual method of choice to investigate the integrity of the basement membrane is that of histology which uses specific stains applied to light microscopic sections. Because of the time involved in preparation and the difficulty in orienting the minute tissue blocks during preparation, electron microscopy is usually not used. The diagnostic value of light microscopy is somewhat limited when the determination of an invasive status of a lesion is most critical and important, i.e. at the borderline between carcinoma *in situ* and microinvasive carcinoma. Microinvasive foot processes cannot be detected by means of light microscopic sections. Because of the greater diagnostic reliability we suggest a routine fixing and embedding procedure for electron microscopy to be carried out. Whenever light microscopic sections fail to answer the question of an invasive status of a lesion, the electron microscopic block of the same cervix can then be sectioned and inspected.

Contrary to early belief (Ashworth et al. 1961), it has become clear now, that the epithelium synthesizes the material for the basement membrane upon which it rests. The stroma acts as an inductor, as shown in studies of the chick cornea (Hay and Dodson 1973), where the basement membrane is only formed in the presence of stroma acting as substrate. With the stroma being the inductor of basement membrane synthesis, the factor regulating the amount of synthesis must then be the relative size of the contact area with the stroma, i.e. the surface area of the basal plasma membrane. The time for a total basement membrane turnover lies between 100 and 150 days in the case of rat renal glomerular basement membrane (Price and Spiro 1977). If the same period is applicable to the cervical basement membrane, the intracellular synthesis of basement membrane constituent in the respective areas ceases in earlier stages of dysplasia. The reduction in number of the foot processes outbalances the loss of basement membrane over a long period of time. When the basal plasma membrane of dysplastic epithelium has finally been straightened out, (as is the case in carcinoma *in situ*) the situation becomes critical as the constant loss of basement membrane constituents is not replenished by newly synthesized material.

Reduced adhesion between microinvasive cells (as documented through the partial loss of desmosomes) (Kocher et al. 1981) is probably one of the factors responsible for the onset of invasion. Proteolytic activity which occurs in squamous cell carcinoma of the skin and is thought to participate in the process of invasion, probably also occurs in cervical carcinoma. The cytoplasmic vesicles particularly found during the early invasive stages in the vicinity of basement membrane irregularities (Figure 4) are probably the morphologic expression of this proteolytic activity. The gap formed in the basement membrane through this lysis enables the basal cells to penetrate with their foot processes into the underlying stroma. The active movement necessary in the initial steps of invasion is most likely carried out through the peripheral web of microfilaments which have been formed in the microinvasive cells (Figure 6). The fact that the contact of the penetrating foot process, with the underlying stroma, does not result in the synthesis of basement membrane in invasive cervical epithelium may be regarded as a reflection of the altered genetic make-up of these cells which led to the loss of basement membrane synthesis (Figure 10). Once the basement membrane, as a scaffold and a substrate for growth and orientation, has been destroyed, orderly cellular reconstitution does not occur (Vracko 1974).

More attention should be given to the ultrastructure of basement membranes and the basal region of cells in direct contact with the basement membranes since both may serve as a very valuable indicator of the invasive status of cervical lesions. Irregularities of the basement membrane, such as varying thickness and particularly discontinuities, can be taken as a sign of microinvasion either having already begun or just being at the point where it is about to start. The ultrastructural preservation of the tissue should be perfect and the mechanically induced rupture of the basement membrane can then be excluded.

ACKNOWLEDGEMENT

The authors wish to thank Mr. R. Betschart for his excellent technical assistance during preparation of electron microscopic specimen, Mr. G. Morson for drawing Figure 10 and Mr. H. Stöcklin for his assistance with the photography.

120

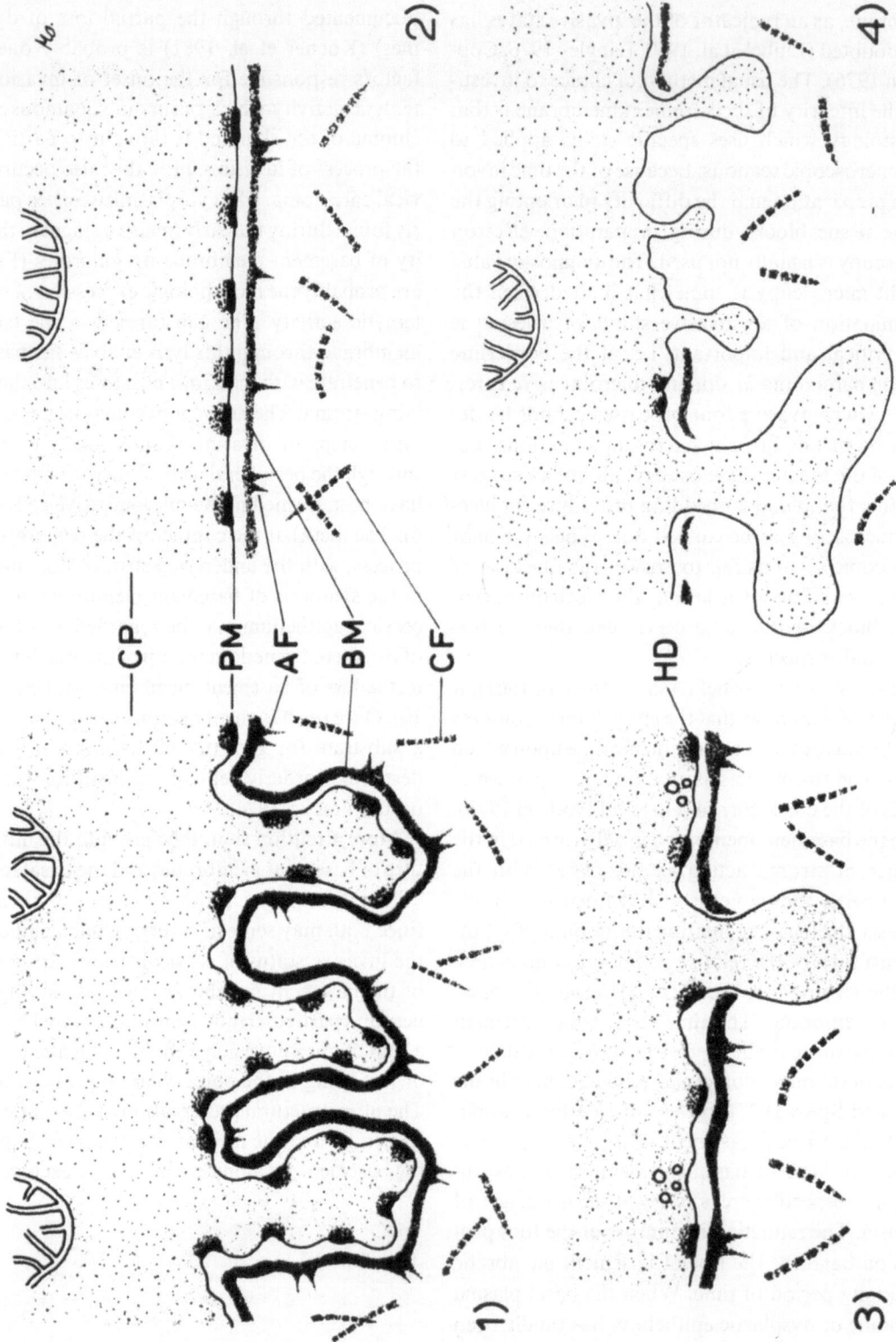

Figure 10. (1) Normal cervical epithelium; (2) Dysplastic epithelium; (3) Microinvasive epithelium; (4) Clearly invasive epithelium. CP = cytoplasm; PM = plasma membrane; AF = anchoring fibrils; BM = basement membrane; CF = collagen fibrils; HD = hemidesmosomes.

REFERENCES

Ashworth CT, Stembridge VA, Luibel FJ: A study of basement membranes of normal epithelium, carcinoma in situ and invasive carcinoma of uterine cervix utilizing electron microscopy and histochemical methods. Acta cytologica 5: 331, 1961.

Auersperg N, Erber H, Worth A: Histologic variation among poorly differentiated invasive carcinomas of human uterine cervix. J Natl Cancer Inst 51: 1461, 1973.

Burghardt E: Workshop session: Histological terminology. *In* Burghardt E, Holzer E, Jordan JA (eds): Cervical pathology and colposcopy. Stuttgart: G. Thieme Publishers, 1978.

Coppleson M: Management of preclinical carcinoma of the cervix. *In* Jordan JA, Singer A (eds): The Cervix. Philadelphia: Saunders Company Ltd, 1976, pp 453–474.

Farquhar M: Role of the basement membrane in glomerula filtration: Results obtained with electron-dense tracers. *In* Mausnbach AB, Olsen TS, Christensen EI (eds): Functional ultrastructure of the kidney. New York: Academic Press, 1980, pp 31–51.

Hay ED, Dodson JW: Secretion of collagen by corneal epithelium I. Morphology of collagenous products produced by isolated epithelia grown on frozen-killed lens. J Cell Biol 57: 190, 1973.

Kefalides NA, Alper R, Clark CC: Biochemistry and metabolism of basement membranes. Int Rev Cytol 61: 167, 1979.

Kocher O, Amaudruz M, Schindler AM, Gabbiani G: Desmosomes and gap junctions in precarcinomatous and carcinomatous conditions of squamous epithelia. J Submicr Cytol 13: 267, 1981.

Langley FA: The pathology of cervical neoplasia. *In* Jordan JA, Singer A (eds): The Cervix. Philadelphia: Saunders Company Ltd 1976, pp 345–363.

Luibel FJ, Sanders E, Ashworth CT: An electron microscopic study of carcinoma *in situ* and invasive carcinoma of the cervix uteri. Cancer Res 20: 357, 1960.

Price RG, Spiro RG: Studies on the metabolism of the renal glomerular basement membrane. J Biol Chem 23: 8597, 1977.

Shingleton HM, Lawrence DW: Transmission electron microscopy of cervical neoplasia. *In* Jordan JA, Singer E (eds): The Cervix. Philadelphia: Saunders Company Ltd, 1976, pp 363–371.

Twiggs LB, Okagaki T, Clark BA: Progressive loss of basal cell pseudopodia in cervical intraepithelial neoplasia. An example of inhibition of differentiation in vivo. Presented at the symposium: Carcinoma of the cervix. Charleston, SC, 1980.

Vracko R: Basal lamina scaffold: Anatomy and significance for maintenance of orderly tissue structure. Am J Pathology 77: 314, 1974.

Younes MS: Electron microscope observations on carcinoma *in situ* of the cervix. Obstetr Gynecol Survey 24: 768, 1968.

III. ETIOLOGY

19. ROLE OF SPERM BASIC PROTEINS AS CARCINOGENS IN CERVICAL CANCER

P.W. French, M. Coppleson, B.L. Reid and A. Singer

For much of the century of its existence cancer research has been concerned with a description of the extraordinary range of substances that are carcinogenic. In this description there is implicit the hope that a catalogue of carcinogens will some day somehow indicate the nature of the neoplastic process. A continuing and frustrating absence of a concept for the essential nature of neoplastic growth points up the failure of this approach and encourages the search for others. The idea is gaining ground that a physiological mechanism for the control of normal growth may be the site of action of all carcinogens. Rapid advances in cell biology are revealing mechanisms for normal growth control unsuspected even two decades ago, mechanisms which could be subverted by he action of the carcinogen. This report attempts to define such a mechanism operating in the presumptive cervical squamous epithelial cell. During its differentiation, it is proposed that actin and tubulin filaments of the surface mucoid coat are responsible for the formation of channels concerned with the entry of small ions and metabolites to the cell body. Strong polycations in the form of the sperm basic proteins present during the laying down of these channels in the embryonic cell compromise the structure of these channels so that they are no longer as responsive to controlling agents such as hormones or nerve trophic substances. The concept is treated more extensively elsewhere by Reid (1981).

I. ANTAGONISTS IN CERVICAL CANCER

I.A. The target cell

It was shown (Kaufmann and Ober 1959) that that portion of the cervical lining prone to develop cervical cancer had been at one stage covered by columnar cells. Such a portion was later covered with squamous epithelium and the transition then provided an entry point for the installation of the carcinogenic process. The study of these transitional stages was later made more opportune with the aid of the colposcope (Coppleson and Reid 1967). A survey of several thousand cervices by combined colposcope-microscope methods in women from foetal to senescent ages showed that the transitional process (termed metaplasia) although nearly always physiological occasionally succumbed to neoplasia. Biopsies of the tissues at the earliest phase of the transition disclosed a cell that was actively motile and often in a state of division (Reid and Coppleson 1978).

I.B. The carcinogen

Our earliest proposals concerned the role of virus. As parasites of the metaplastic cell of possible carcinogenic significance, a group of viruses known to be transmitted venereally was studied (Reid 1962). Later, the spermatozoon itself was studied because of similarities in the mechanism of its integration with host cell nucleic acid as had been proposed in viral oncogenesis. By a series of experiments it was shown DNA of gamete origin could come into intimate relation with host cell nuclear DNA (Coppleson and Reid 1967). It is to be noted that this intimacy, demonstrable in case of both virus and gamete, failed to lead to further concept and experiment on its role in carcinogenesis, a failure which persists to the present.

Hafez, E.S.E., Smith, J.P. (eds.), Carcinoma of the Cervix: Biology and Diagnosis. ISBN-13: 978-94-009-7487-6
© 1982, Martinus Nijhoff Publishers, The Hague/Boston/London.

II. THE SEARCH FOR NEWER CONCEPTS OF GROWTH CONTROL

The control of growth in microbes is an active field of possible relevance to the same topic in the cells of higher organisms. The idea that the cell wall may be directly concerned in microbial growth control is not new (Jacob et al. 1963). Cell biologists in the interim have tended to divert their interests from the nucleus toward the cell periphery. Such methods were applied to the periphery of presumptive squame cells (Reid and Coppleon 1978; Reid and Charlson 1979). Light microscope studies of living cells showed great motility of the periphery to be associated with similarly active nuclear movements. The cell periphery was thrown into ruffles and microspikes – the so-called microextensions – well known historically. The cytological basis of the microextension was a bundle of filaments up to one half micron in diameter. Their movement was shown in subsequent electron microscope study to produce varying states of disaggregation of the bundle into filaments which rapidly produced a network. The whole arrangement at the histological level could be recognized as the mucoid coat of the presumptive squamous cell whose main biochemical components were proteins, lipids and nucleic acids (Reid and Charlson 1979; Reid 1974). It was previously shown that the DNA of this coat was derived from the heterochromatin of the nuclear edge in the form of microtubule and microfilament bundles projected explosively toward the cell edge (Reid and Blackwell 1971).

Projection occurred over the surface of the cell; bundles then returned to the cell body where their place was taken by a second microextension suffering the same fate. Such a sequential exposure was viewed as the manifestation of a mechanism for the sequential exposure of the genome to the environment. The selection of that part of the genome best adapted to function in the area may occur. The instrument of this adaptation was seen as a continuing rearrangement of the filament component of the network of the surface mucoids as these filaments responded to energy flows present in their environment (Reid and Coppleson 1975). These rearrangements subtend channels in the mucoid coat along which flow ions and other metabolites. They thus provide the machinery for active transport in this differentiating embryonic cell. Proteins in this cell surface coat are the locus of action of many growth controllers such as steroid or peptide hormones whose final action is to regulate the entry of metabolites, metal ions, glucose, amino acids and so forth. In the presence of certain substances in the environment, development of the channels is proposedly compromised so that, for example, the active sites for hormone action are occluded or improperly exposed. The channel then transmits the metabolite but at a rate dependent solely on its ambient concentration, unrelated to the control pattern determined by the organism as a whole. Such agents are the carcinogens.

The problem then became the definition of a substance(s) in the sperm which could derange the orderly differentiation of the surface coat of the presumptive squamous epithelial cell in such a way.

The chief components of the surface mucoid are of overall polyanionic charge. They could therefore be electrostatically immobilized in their movement by polycationic substances. DNA is an example of one such polyanion in the surface coat (Reid and Charlson 1979) and the problem becomes the identification of substances which can bind to DNA. Such substances could attract DNA to the surface and there immobilize it. As assayed by electron microscopy in a suitable test system (Reid and Blackwell 1974) it was found that a variety of proteins was active in this regard and of these, the basic proteins, histones and protamines were most active. The human sperm head is a rich source of both basic proteins which are relatively easily extracted (French 1979) and purified. The proportion of basic proteins in the sperm head varies on an individual basis. There is another variation of importance: the DNA-binding capacity of the basic proteins varies with their basicity (Bode et al. 1977) a variation related to the amount of arginine in the amino acid analysis. The arginine content of the sperm histones is about 16% while that of the protamine is 40% (Puwaravutipanich and Panyim 1975) so that the latter could bind more avidly to the surface polyanions and in this way disrupt the surface filaments during cell differentiation more actively than the histones.

III. EXPERIMENTAL APPROACH

Observations were thus made on the response of cultured cervical cells to histones and protamines prepared from the sperm head and added to the culture fluid in which they were growing. In the experiment as undertaken, cinematography was used to study the changes produced in cell behavior after contact with the protein for several hours at a concentration of 25 μg/ml.

The main results were as follows:

1. The most striking effects were on the motility of the cell especially on that of its surface. The orderly ruffling and microspike pattern was disrupted by a marked retraction of the edge and the subsequent appearance of numerous spikes (Figures 1a and b). This was shown in electron micrographs to be associated with a disturbance of filament pattern in the outer layers of the cytoplasm, loss of the plasma membrane and release of surface debris to the culture medium.

2. The retraction of the cell edge left large bundles of microfilaments exposed on the surface. Some of these showed branching, irregular aggregation as well as prominent cross links.

3. For the same concentration of protein, protamines gave a more marked effect than histones.

4. These effects were reversible within the time period of study. Replacement with fresh medium without added protein was accompanied by a re-version to normal cell shape and behavior.

5. Use of higher concentration of protein e.g. 100 μg/ml produced cell death.

6. There was always considerable debris present amongst the surface filaments and being released to the culture medium. Some of this material was particulate, the particles being about 35 nm in diameter apparently budding from the surface of the filaments.

IV. DISCUSSION OF EXPERIMENTAL RESULTS

The surface of the normal cell beyond its plasma membrane exhibits morphological (Singer 1979), biochemical (Chen et al. 1978), behavioral (Vasiliev et al. 1978) and immunological (Willingham et al. 1974) evidence for the presence of microfibrillar and microtubular proteins just as does the cell cytoplasm. Such proteins proposedly participate in the formation of the transport channels on the surface (Reid 1981). Although the details of the formative process are presently unknown, there is evidence of great reciprocity in the interplay of these proteins at this time such that an abnormal persistence of actin filaments with or without attached myosin seems to derange the capacity of the tubulin filaments to form channels whose patency is controlled in turn by their content of appropriate hormone-binding proteins.

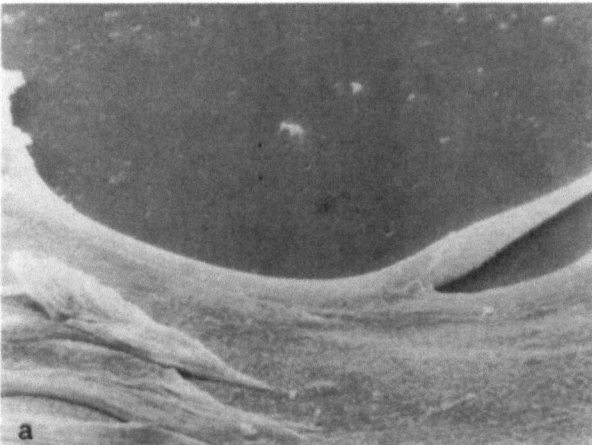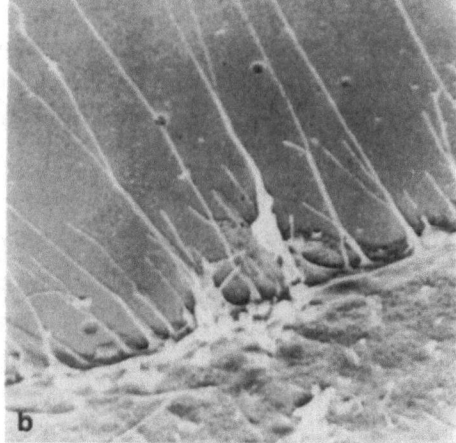

Figure 1. Scanning electron micrographs of cultured human cervical epithelial cells. (a) Before treatment with human sperm basic protein. Surface of an epithelial cell on the edge of the sheet showing smooth contours, × 4000; (b) After treatment with human sperm basic protein. Surface of affected cell showing large numbers of surface filaments some of them distorted, some branched, × 3600.

Other effects, well known to characterize the neoplastic state such as changes in the social behavior of cells, capacity for non-recognition by immune surveillance as well as failure to exhibit contact inhibition could be related to a derangement of the surface layers produced at the same time.

V. COLLABORATIVE EVIDENCE FROM OTHER DISCIPLINES

V.A. From epidemiology

Supportive evidence for the complicity of sperm basic proteins as carcinogens originates from an entirely unexpected direction. Cancer of the cervix is commonly described as a venereal disease by epidemiologists (Kessler 1976). Historically, the woman has been the subject of much concept and study on the nature of its origins and incidence. Attention was directed to the salient epidemiological features of the sexual partner of the affected woman (Singer 1973), features which were sufficiently striking as to enable the definition of a high risk male. One of the features of such a definition was his residence in the lower social classes (Singer et al. 1976). Semen samples from 200 males were collected and extracted basic proteins from their washed sperm characterized. The two types of protein already described were quantitated from densitometer traces of polyacrylamide gels and these values set against the social class of the donor as based on occupation or income (Reid et al. 1978). There was a significant correlation between the lower social classes and a higher relative content of protamine in the sperm basic protein complement. The broader biological implications of this finding have been discussed (Reid et al. 1979).

V.B. From chemical and viral carcinogenesis studies

Other known carcinogens exhibit the property of active cross-linkage of proteins and nucleic acids to which they are exposed. Examples include carcinogenic chemicals such as the coal tar derivatives (Fornace and Little 1979) and some oncogenic viruses by a mechanism presently under close scrutiny. The mechanism in the case of some of these viruses is important because it seems to involve altered physiological and not primarily neoplastic mechanisms which persist under conditions where the carcinogen is absent. It has been shown that the Rous sarcoma virus (Opperman et al. 1979) and mouse sarcoma virus (Sen and Todaro 1979) produce a manifold excess of a phosphoprotein in the cell surface at the instant of the transformation process. Such a mechanism would be worthy of investigation in the instance of the proposed herpes virus of cervical carcinogenesis. The phosphoproteins are important mediators of a wide range of physiological control mechanisms in cell function, control systems which are often concerned with cross-linking at surface membranes.

The effect of Rous sarcoma virus on the chick fibroblast cell edge some 12–24 hours after contact is remarkably similar at the morphological level to that produced by the concentration of sperm proteins used in these studies (Wang and Goldberg 1976). It remains to be seen whether such a morphological accompaniment of neoplastic transformation noted in these human cells is accompanied by other well-known features such as a capacity for unrestrained growth.

Collaborative chemical and viral carcinogenesis studies also disclose that many chemical carcinogens cause the liberation of oncogenic viruses from cells to which they are exhibited (Huebner and Todaro 1969). A miscellany of chemicals is involved and they all seem capable of raising the viscosity of the cell surface proteins on which they act. Sperm basic proteins would have such an action and further research is necessary to see if viral or proviral liberation accompanies their other striking effects on the differentiating squamous cell surface.

VI. CONCLUDING REMARKS

Studies of the structure and function of the cell surface of the eukaryote cell have progressed to a state where a mechanism for the control of growth can be defined. The proposed mechanism concerns the elaboration by the differentiating cell of a system of channels through its mucoid coat for the entry of metabolites. The instruments of this elaboration are the microfilaments and microtubules of the mucoid coat and the conduits which they subtend contain proteins, some of which are receptors for controllers such as the hormones. Carcinogens present in the environment at the time of differentiation compromise the formation of the conduits such that the controlling proteins either fail to be exposed or are inadequately exposed. Metabolites thus enter the cell in amounts related to their environmental concentration rather than to those determined by the organism. Sperm basic proteins, especially their protamine moiety, are active in disturbing surface and cytoplasmic microfilament organization in the growing cervical cell and it is proposed that this lesion, propagated via the DNA content of the filaments could form the basis of the neoplastic transformation. Because of an increased sperm protamine content, males in the lower social classes are viewed as more prone to initiate such changes in the target cell.

REFERENCES

Body JL, Willmetzer L, Opatz K: On the Competition between Protamines and Histones: Studies directed towards the Understanding of Spermatogenesis. Biochem 72: 393, 1977.

Chen LB, Murray A, Segal RA, Bushnell A, Walsh M: Studies on Intercellular LETS Glycoprotein Matrices. Cell 14: 377, 1978.

Coppleson M, Reid BL: Preclinical Carcinoma of the Cervix Uteri. London: Pergamon, 1967.

Fornace AJ, Little IB: DNA-Protein Cross Linking By Chemical Carcinogens in Mammalian Cells. Cancer Res 39: 704, 1979.

French P: Ethanol Extraction of Basic Proteins from Ejaculated Human Spermatozoa. Aust J Biol Sci 32: 443, 1979.

Huebner RJ, Todaro GJ: Oncogenesis of RNA tumour viruses and determinants of cancer. Proc Nat Acad Sci 64: 1087, 1969.

Jacob F, Brenner S, Cuzin F: On the Regulation of DNA Replication in Bacteria. Cold Spr Harb Symp Quant Biol 28: 329, 1963.

Kaufmann C, Ober KG: The Morphological Changes of the Cervix Uteri with Age and their significance in the Early Diagnosis of Carcinoma. In Wolstenholme GEW, O'Connor M (eds): CIBA Found Studies Cir 3. London: Churchill, 1959, p 61.

Kessler I: Human Cervical Cancer as a Venereal Disease. Cancer Res 36: 783, 1976.

Opperman H, Levinson AD, Varmus HE, Levintow L, Bishop JM: Uninfected Vertebrate Cells Contain a Protein that is closely related to the product of the avian sarcoma virus transforming gene (src). Proc Nat Acad Sci 76: 1804, 1979.

Puwaravutipanich T, Panyim S: The Nuclear Basic Proteins of Human Testes and Ejaculated Spermatozoa. Exp Cell Res 90: 153, 1975.

Reid BL: The Role of Virus in the Origin and Progression of Epithelial Anomalies of the Ectocervix. In Proc 1st Intern Congr Exfol Cytol Philadelphia: Lippincott, 1962.

Reid BL: Interaction of the Living Cell with its Environment; Speculation of the Function of the DNA content of Surface Mucoids. Biosystems 5: 207, 1974.

Reid BL: Carcinogenesis. In Coppleson M (ed): Gynecologic Oncology. London: Churchill Livingstone, 1981, p 36.

Reid BL, Blackwell PM: Nuclear Extensions of Cultured Cells: A Possible Mechanism of Cellular Differentiation in Informational Molecules in Biological Systems. In Ledoux LGH (ed). Amsterdam: North Holland, 1971, p 285.

Reid BL, Blackwell PM: Histone and Polyamine Acid-DNA Interactions at Molecular and Cellular Levels. 8th Intern Congr Electr Micros Canberra 2: 270, 1974.

Reid BL, Charlson AC: Cytoplasmic and Cell Surface Deoxyribonucleic Acids with Consideration of their Origin. Int Rev Cytol 60: 27, 1979.

Reid BL, Coppleson M: Natural History: Recent Advances. In Jordan J, Singer A (eds): The Cervix. London: Saunders, 1975, p 317.

Reid BL, Coppleson M: The Natural History of Cervical Cancer. In Macdonald RR (ed): Scientific Basis of Obstetrics and Gynaecology. Edinburgh: Churchill Livingstone, 1978, p 427.

Reid BL, Hagan B, Coppleson M: Heterogeneous Homo sapiens. Med J Aust 2: 377, 1979.

Reid BL, French PW, Singer A, Hagan BE, Coppleson M: Sperm Basic Proteins in Cervical Carcinogenesis: Correlation with Socio-economic Class. Lancet ii 60, 1978.

Singer A: The Male Factor in Cervical Cancer. Oxf Med Sch Gaz 25: 18, 1973.

Singer A, Reid BL, Coppleson M: A Hypothesis: The role of a high-risk male in the etiology of cervical carcinoma. Amer J Obstet Gynec 126: 110, 1976.

Singer IJ: The Fibronexus: a transmembrane association of fibronectin-containing fibres and bundles, Cell 16: 675, 1979.

Sen A, Todaro GJ: A murine sarcoma virus – associated protein kinase interaction with actin and microtubular protein. Cell 17: 347, 1979.

Vasiliev JM, Gelfand IM, Domnina LV, Ivanova LY, Komm SG, Olshevskaja LV: Effect of colcemid on the locomotory behaviour of fibroblasts. J Emb exp Morph 24: 625, 1970.

Wang E, Goldberg AR: Changes in Microfilament Organisation and Surface Topography upon Transformed Chick Fibroblasts with Rous Sarcoma Virus. Proc Nat Acad Sci 73: 4065, 1976.

Willingham MC, Ostland RE, Pastan I: Myosin is a component of the cell surface of cultured cells. Proc Nat Acad Sci 71: 4144, 1974.

20. EXPRESSION OF HERPES VIRUS ANTIGEN IN PREMALIGNANT AND MALIGNANT CERVIX

G.A. CABRAL, F. MARCIANO-CABRAL, D. FRY, H. TOMLIN, D. HALL and D. GOPLERUD

I. INTRODUCTION

I.A. Evidence linking herpes simplex virus to cervical neoplasia

I.A.1. Histological and epidemiological studies

There is considerable evidence which indicates a close relationship between herpes simplex virus type 2 (HSV-2) and cervical neoplasia. As early as 1966, it was suggested that the virus was associated with genital cancer following screening of Papanicolaou smears for both anaplastic and herpetic cytological markers (Naib et al. 1966, 1969, 1973). In this and later studies (Beilby 1968; Nowakovsky et al. 1968; An 1969; Naib et al. 1969, 1973; Ng et al. 1970; Wolinska and Melaned 1970; Jordan et al. 1972) increased incidence of cervical anaplasia was noted in women with cytologically identifiable genital herpes infections. Subsequent seroepidemiological studies have confirmed the associative relationship between HSV-2 and cervical cancer (Rawls et al. 1973; Kessler 1974; Nahmias et al. 1974; Anzai et al. 1975) and, in addition, have demonstrated that women with cervical dysplasia, carcinoma *in situ* (CIS), or invasive squamous cell carcinoma tend to have higher titers of neutralizing antibodies to HSV-2 than matched controls.

I.A.2. In vitro transformation studies

The oncogenic potential of HSV-2 has been demonstrated by the *in vitro* transformation of hamster embryo fibroblasts inoculated with UV-inactivated virus (Duff and Rapp 1971). Additional support for the oncogenic role of both type 1 and type 2 herpes simplex viruses has been obtained from studies utilizing various mammalian cell systems (Darai and Munk 1973; Kutinová et al. 1973; MacNab 1974; Kimura et al. 1975). It has been demonstrated that these virus-transformed cells contain viral RNA (Collard et al. 1973) and DNA (Kraiselburd et al. 1975; Frenkel et al. 1976; Minson et al. 1976). In addition, virus-specific proteins (Duff and Rapp 1971, 1973; Darai and Munk 1973; Kutinová et al. 1973; MacNab 1974; Kucera and Gusdow 1976) have been identified. For example, VP143, a nonstructural β-polypeptide of HSV-2 of approximately 143,000 daltons molecular weight, has been identified in HSV-2-transformed cells (Kimura et al. 1975; Melnick et al. 1976). Subsequent studies using antiserum to this protein have demonstrated that the expression of VP143 in the transformed cells is cell-cycle dependent (Flannery et al. 1977).

The result of these and other studies indicate that: (1) the *in vitro* conversion of normal cells to a transformed state is achieved by abolishing viral infectivity (e.g., UV-inactivation of virus) since HSV-2 infection of cells usually results in lysis, (2) variable proportions of the viral genome are retained within HSV-2-transformed cells, and (3) viral transformation is often accompanied by the production of virus-specific proteins either within the cytoplasm or at the cell surface.

I.A.3. Identification of herpes simplex virus markers in cervical tumor cells

Various groups have identified markers of HSV in cervical tumors and tumor-derived cells. Although infectious virus, viral strucural antigens, and HSV-specific cytoplasmic changes have not been localized directly in cervical cancer biopsies (Aurelian et al. 1970, 1972), virus-specific antigens have been observed in exfoliated tumor cells and in tumor cells on the periphery of neoplastic lesions (Aurelian 1972; Aurelian et al. 1972, 1978; Royston and Aurelian 1970).

Hafez, E.S.E., Smith, J.P. (eds.), Carcinoma of the Cervix: Biology and Diagnosis. ISBN-13: 978-94-009-7487-6
© 1982, Martinus Nijhoff Publishers, The Hague/Boston/London.

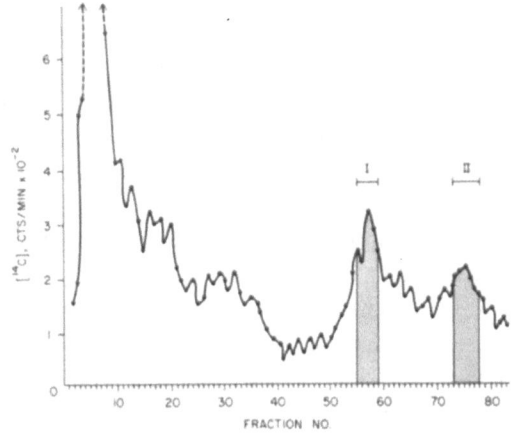

Figure 1. A preparative polyacrylamide gel electrophoresis profile of solubilized HSV-2-infected cell extracts labeled from 4 to 24 hrs. postinfection with [^{14}C]-amino acids. Franctions containing VP143 (pool I) or VP157 (pool II) were pooled, concentrated by vacuum dialysis, and subjected to cylindrical SDS-polyacrylamide gel electrophoresis.

II. IDENTIFICATION OF HERPES SIMPLEX VIRUS ANTIGENS IN HUMAN CERVICAL CELLS

II.A. Rationale for using antisera to individual virus-specific polypeptides

The detection of virus-specific antigens in cervical tumor cells has entailed the use of hyperimmune rabbit or hamster antisera to HSV in immunofluorescence staining. The reproducibility and sensitivity of these methods, however, have proved less than ideal. Furthermore, the identification of the viral gene products within cells and biopsy material has involved the use of antibodies to whole virus-infected cell extracts or fractions thereof. The employment of antisera to multiple antigens precludes identification of individual virus polypeptides and limits definition of the spectrum of virus gene expression within lytically-infected and virus-transformed cells. Therefore, research in this laboratory has focused on the application of hyperimmune antisera to individual HSV polypeptides in concert with highly sensitive immunoenzyme staining to identify virus-specific gene products in cervical tissue and cervical explant cultures of individuals with squamous metaplasia, various grades of dysplasia, CIS, and invasive squamous cell carcinoma.

II.B. Preparation of antisera

II.B.1. Polyacrylamide gel electrophoresis (PAGE)

Antisera to VP143, a nonstructural β-polypeptide of HSV-2, and to VP157 (M.W. 157,000), a structural γ-polypeptide which comprises the major capsid protein of that virus, were prepared in rabbits using procedures initially reported by Courtney and Benyesh-Melnick (1974) with modifications. HSV-2 infected rabbit kidney cells were harvested at 24 hr postinoculation, solubilized in sodium dodecyl sulfate (SDS)-urea and mercaptoethanol (ME), and subjected to preparative polyacrylamide gel electrophoresis (PAGE) using a 'Poly-Prep' apparatus (Buchler Instruments, Fort Lee, NJ). Select cultures were labeled with [^{14}C]amino acids in order to facilitate monitoring of virus polypeptides. Electrophoretic profiles were etablished following liquid scintillation (Figure 1) and fractions containing VP143 or VP157 were pooled, concentrated by

Figure 2. A cylindrical SDS-polyacrylamide gel depicting polypeptides present in pool I following electrophoresis and staining with Coomassie brilliant blue. Portions of replicate unstained gels containing the VP143 band were cut out and employed to inoculate rabbits. Similar procedures were utilized for purification of, and subsequent injection of rabbits with, VP157.

vacuum dialysis, and further purified by cylindrical PAGE (Figure 2).

II.B.2. Immunization of rabbits

Antiserum to HSV-2 was prepared by inoculating rabbits with homogenized virus-infected rabbit kidney cells. Antisera to VP143 and VP157 were prepared by injecting the animals with gel plugs containing the respective polypeptide emulsified in complete Freunds adjuvant. Animals were bled following a regimen of three successive inoculations conducted at two week intervals.

II.B.3. Titer and specificity of antisera

Antisera were examined for titer and specificity by immunofluorescence staining of cultured HSV-2-infected cells. The staining patterns in infected cells obtained with anti-HSV-2, anti-VP143, and anti-VP157 were abolished following immunoprecipitation of antisera with whole virus-infected cell extracts. The specificity of the anti-VP143 and anti-VP157 was further established following analysis of autoradiograms of immunoprecipitates. Briefly, antisera were incubated with [^{35}S]-methionine-labeled HSV-2-infected whole cell extracts containing 0.02% Nonidet P40 following which staphyloccal protein A was added. The resultant precipitate was solubilized in SDS-mercaptoethanol and subjected to analytical PAGE. Autoradiograms were screened for protein band homogeneity in analytical gels using a Corning 750 densitometric system (Corning Medical, Medfield, MA).

II.C. Cervical biopsies and explant cultures

Cervical biopsy specimens were obtained from patients exhibiting squamous metaplasia (5) chronic cervicitis (6), mild to severe dysplasia (45), CIS (14), and invasive squamous cell carcinoma (17). Particular attention was paid to acquisition of biopsies from areas of the cervix exhibiting punctation, white epithelium, or mosaicism. Additional biopsies shown to be negative for dysplasia (3) or from individuals with adenocarcinoma (2) were employed in control studies. Fragments of each biopsy were processed for standard light and electron microscopic evaluation. Additional biopsy fragments were minced in medium. In addition, cervical swab material obtained at time of biopsy was suspended in

medium. Following sterilization by filtration, media was inoculated onto Vero cell monolayers in order to determine whether infectious HSV was resident in biopsy tissues or being shed into the vagina at time of biopsy. Select cervical fragments, also, were explanted on sterile coverslips in petri plates containing L15 medium. Cell outgrowth was monitored using an inverted microscope. When outgrowth reached the periphery of coverslips, cultures were harvested and processed for standard histological and immunocytochemical studies.

II.D. Immunoperoxidase staining for virus-specific antigens

II.D.1. Staining procedure

HSV-2-infected Vero cells, HSV-2-transformed hamster embryo fibroblasts (Duff and Rapp 1971), and cryostat sections of cervical biopsies were examined for the presence of HSV-2 antigens using an indirect immunoperoxidase procedure (Cabral et al. 1978). Adjacent frozen sections from each biopsy were stained with hematoxylin and eosin and employed for confirmation of histopathological diagnosis. All sera were extensively absorbed with Vero cells (10^8/ml serum) and with rabbit liver powder before use. Frozen sections were fixed in acetone, incubated with normal goat serum to eliminate interaction of globulins with viral-induced Fc receptors, treated with anti-HSV-2, anti-VP143, or anti-VP157, and immersed in absolute methanol 0.03% hydrogen peroxide to eliminate endogenous cellular peroxidase activity. Sections, then were incubated with goat anti-rabbit IgG conjugated to horseradish peroxidase, reacted with Hanker-Yates reagent (Hanker et al. 1977), and mounted in Permount.

II.D.2. Expression of antigens in cultured productively-infected and virus-transformed cells

In cells productively infected with HSV-2, VP143 (Figure 3a) and VP157 were identified within nuclei as early as 3 hr and 6 hrs postinfection, respectively. VP157 was also localized within the cytoplasm at time periods extending from 9 hrs postinfection (Figure 3b). In contrast, in HSV-2-transformed cells, staining for VP143 was dispersed in a perinuclear arrangement within the cytoplasm rather

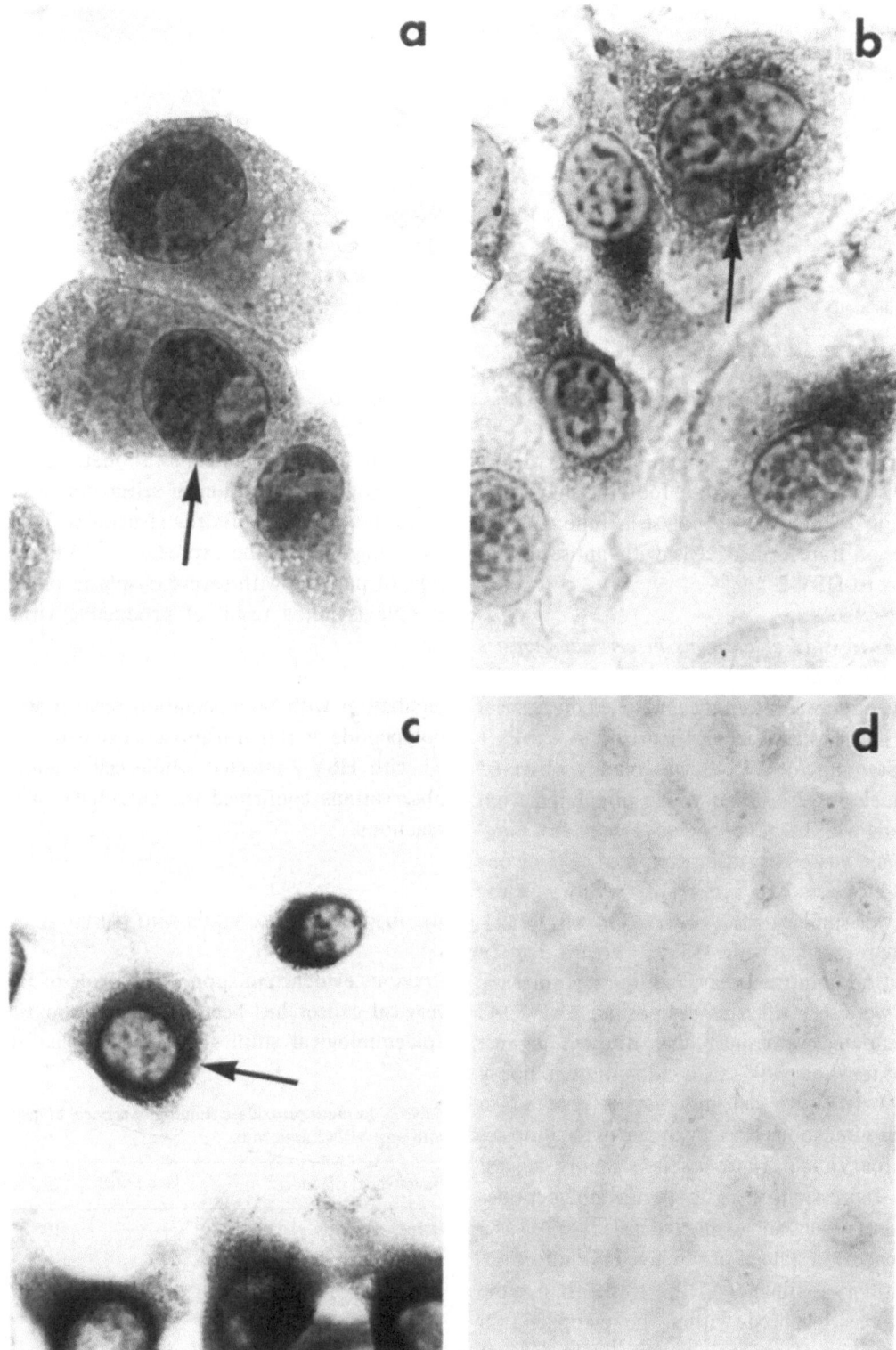

Figure 3. Immunoperoxidase staining of cultured cells for HSV-2-specific polypeptides. (a) Vero cells infected with HSV-2 and examined at 6 hrs postinfection for VP143. Staining is found in large inclusions within the nucleus (arrow), × 990; (b) HSV-2-infected cell examined at 8 hrs postinfection for VP157, the major viral capsid protein. Staining is present throughout the nucleus in fine granules and also within the cytoplasm (arrow), × 990; (c) HSV-2-transformed cells stained for VP143. The protein is found primarily in the cytoplasm in a perinuclear arrangement (arrow), × 990; (d) HSV-2-transformed cells treated with normal rabbit serum as a control. No staining is apparent, × 200.

132

Table 1. Immunoperoxidase staining of cervical biopsy sections with anti-VP143 antiserum.

Histological diagnosis	No. tested	% positive[a]
Herpes cervicitis	2	100
Squamous metaplasia	5	0
Adenocarcinoma	2	0
Mild dysplasia	11	0
Moderate dysplasia	21	5
Severe dysplasia	13	31
Carcinoma *in situ*	14	29
Invasive squamous cell carcinoma	17	41

[a] VP143 was identified in the cytoplasm in all cases except for herpes cervicitis in which the protein was limited to the nucleus.

than within the nucleus (Figure 3c). The distribution of the protein generally took the shape of a 'signet-ring'. Staining was not seen following incubation of transformed cells with antiserum to VP157 or to HSV-2.

II.D.3. Expression of antigens in cervical biopsies and explants

Results of immunostaining conducted on cervical biopsies and explants are summarized in Tables 1 and 2. Staining for VP143 was readily observed within nuclei of 2 biopsies which originated from individuals with herpes cervicitis (Figure 4a). Similar staining was observed in explanted cells of one of these biopsies. The pattern of the intranuclear staining was similar to that observed in cells lytically infected *in vitro* with HSV-2 (Figure 3a). In addition, both intranuclear and intracytoplasmic staining were seen when tissues positive for VP143 were incubated with antibodies directed against VP157 or to whole HSV-2. Co-cultivation of biopsy extracts with Vero cell monolayers resulted in isolation of infectious HSV from one of the biopsies positive for VP143. These results strongly suggest that the expression of virus-specific polypeptides within these tissues and explanted cells resulted as a consequence of a state of productive HSV infection.

In contrast, staining for VP143, rather than in the nucleus, was localized within the cytoplasm in frozen sections of cervical biopsies from 31% of women with severe dysplasia, 29% of patients with CIS, and 41% of individuals with invasive squamous cell carcinoma (Table 1). The protein was dispersed in a perinuclear pattern (Figures 4c and 5b,c) similar to that observed in cells transformed

in vitro by HSV-2 (Figure 3c). Similar staining for VP143 was observed in cervical cells from one individual with moderate dysplasia. Results of immunoperoxidase staining of explants of cervical biopsies with anti-VP143 antiserum (Table 2) were in accord with those derived from staining of sections of cervical tissues. In all cases, staining was observed only in explants originating from those biopsies which were shown to be positive for VP143. Staining was not seen in tissues or explants following incubation with antibodies to VP157 or to HSV-2. In no case was infectious virus isolated from the above tissues as a result of inoculation of Vero cell cultures with extracts of minced cervical fragments or with cervical swab material. Electron microscopic examination of select samples did not reveal the presence of virus structures. Thus, these data suggest that the expression of VP143 within cells of patients with severe dysplasia or with carcinoma is not a result of productive virus infection.

Staining was not observed in tissues following incubation with preinoculation sera or with anti-polypeptide or antiviral antisera extensively absorbed with HSV-2-infected whole cell lysates. These observations confirmed the specificity of staining reactions.

III. HERPES SIMPLEX VIRUS AND CERVICAL CANCER

Previous evidence in support of a role of HSV-2 in cervical cancer has been obtained primarily from epidemiological studies in which higher titers of

Table 2. Immunoperoxidase staining of cervical biopsy explants with anti-VP143 antiserum.

Histological diagnosis[a]	No. tested	% positive[b]
Herpes cervicitis	1	100
Squamous metaplasia	5	0
Mild dysplasia	4	0
Moderate dysplasia	10	10
Severe dysplasia	10	40
Carcinoma *in situ*	6	33
Invasive squamous cell carcinoma	5	40

[a] Histological diagnosis as determined following examination of biopsy of origin.
[b] VP143 was identified in the cytoplasm in all cases except for herpes cervicitis in which the protein was limited to the nucleus.

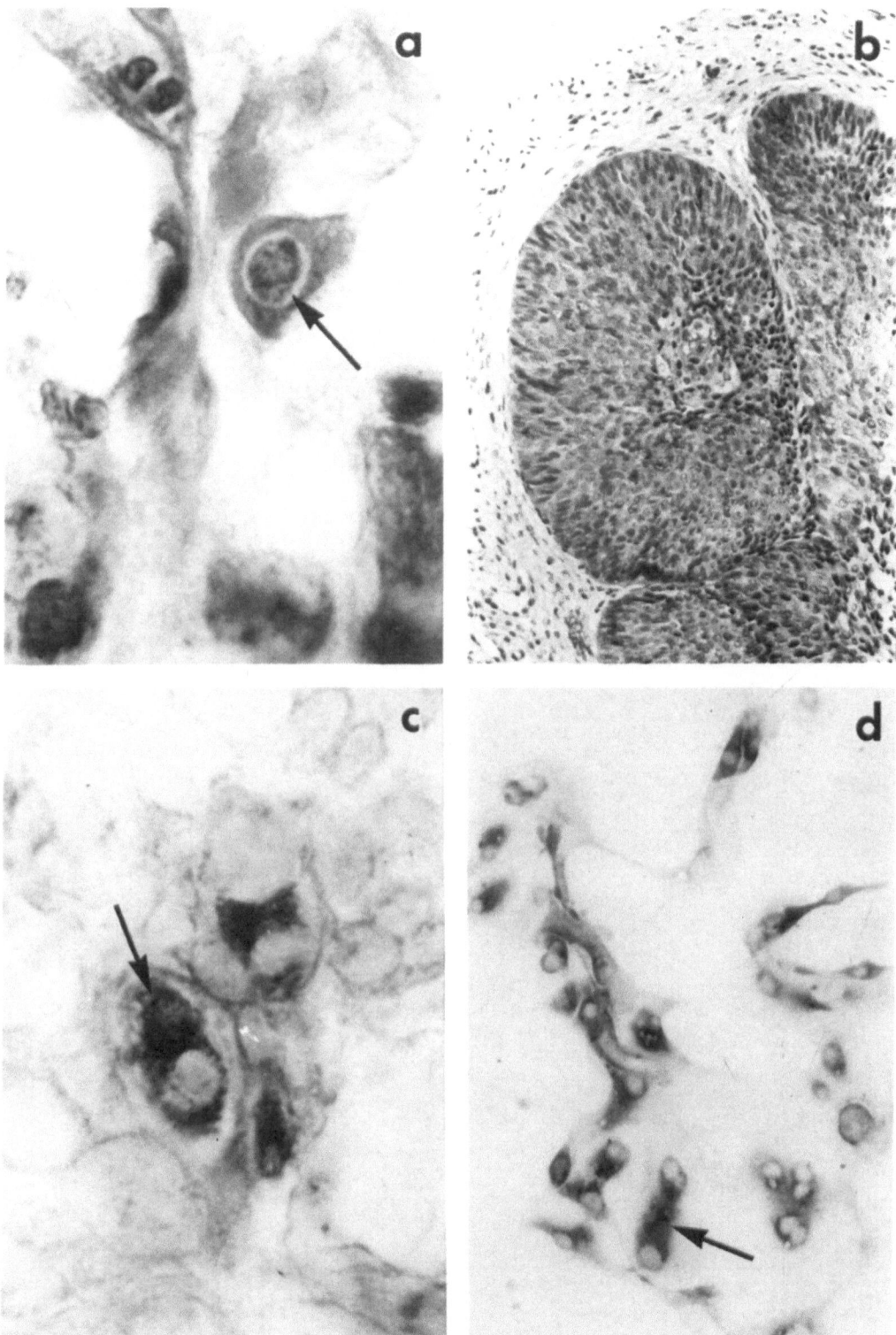

Figure 4. (a) Biopsy from individual with herpes cervicitis. Immunoperoxidase staining for VP143 is intranuclear, × 1900; (b) *In situ* squamous cell carcinoma of the cervix stained with hematoxylin and eosin, × 200; (c) Immunoperoxidase staining of same biopsy material for VP143. Note the pattern of perinuclear staining within the cytoplasm, × 1900; (d) Immunoperoxidase staining for VP143 in an explant of tissue from a patient with CIS. Staining for the protein is limited to the cytoplasm (arrow), × 200.

134

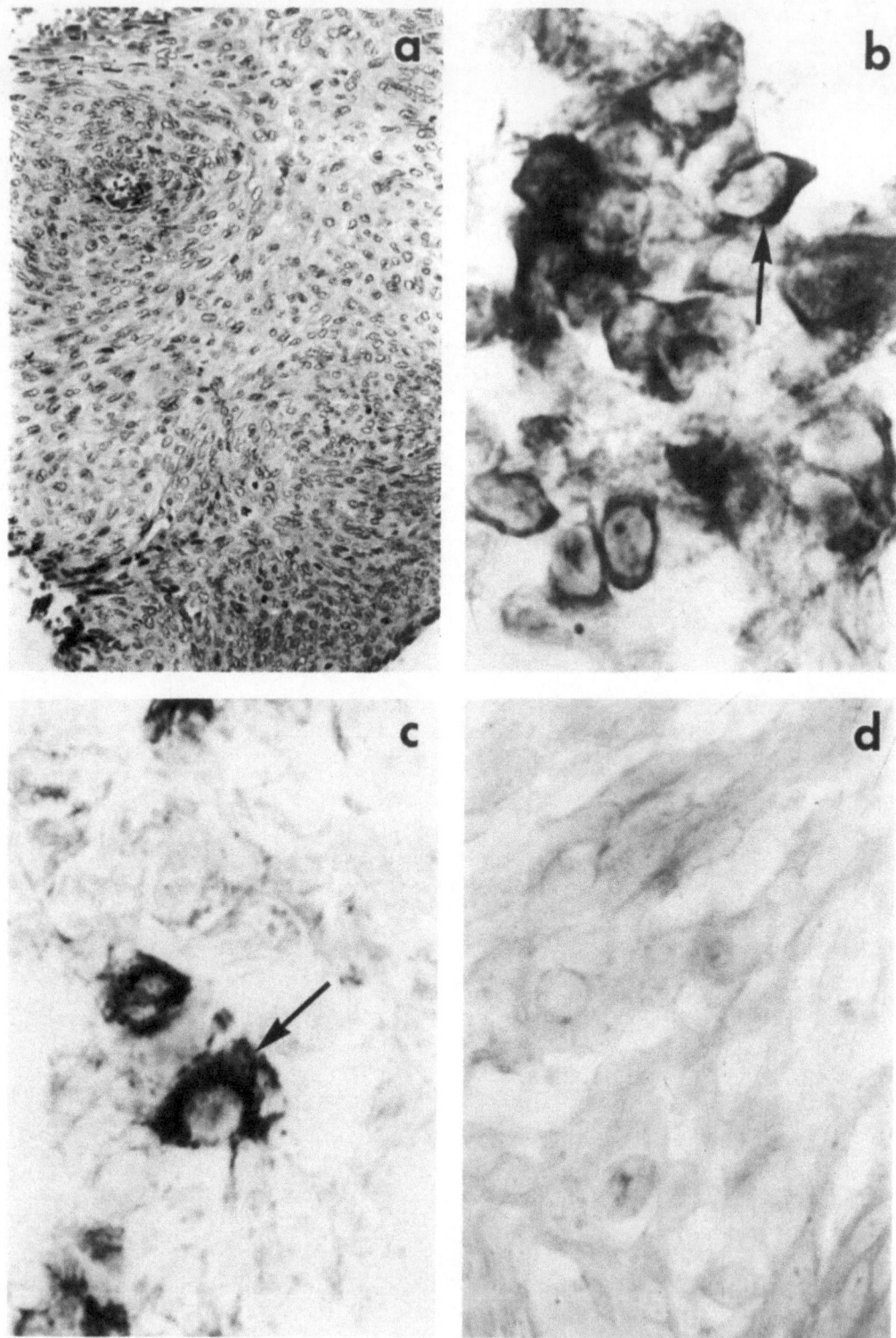

Figure 5. (a) Invasive squamous cell carcinoma of the cervix stained with hemotoxylin and eosin, × 200; (b) Immunoperoxidase staining of same biopsy for VP143. Note the cytoplasmic pattern of staining, × 1900; (c) Invasive squamous cell carcinoma from a biopsy of a second patient depicting cytoplasmic staining for VP143, × 1900; (d) Replicate frozen section from the same patient incubated with normal rabbit serum. Significant staining is absent, × 1000.

antibodies to this virus have been identified in women with premalignant and malignant cervical disease when compared to matched controls. For example, patients with cervical cancer have circulating antibodies which react by complement fixation with early HSV-2 induced polypeptides extracted from virus-infected cells (Anzai et al. 1975). These individuals also contain antibodies which react with an HSV-specific antigen which is produced in HSV-infected cells as early as 4 hours postinfection (Aurelian et al. 1973). The antigen has been designated AG4 and is distinct from viral structural proteins involved in neutralization of HSV-2 infectivity. Antibodies to AG4 have been detected in sera of women with cervical cancer and are present in higher frequency in women with more advanced stages of the disease. In contrast, antibodies to AG4 have not been identified in the majority of matched controls, in sera of patients who had undergone successful therapy for cervical carcinoma, or in sera of women with carcinomas unrelated to cervical cancer. In addition, AG4 reactivity has been demonstrated in extracts of cervical cancer biopsies and in cell cultures derived from two different cervical carcinomas.

Further support for an association between HSV-2 and cervical cancer has resulted from recent reports describing direct localization within premalignant and malignant cells of HSV-specific genetic material or gene products. Ag-e, an antigen consisting of an $0.4M$ phosphate buffer eluate from a calcium phosphate chromatogram of total HSV-2 antigens, has been observed by fluorescence in Pap smears of 80.8% of women with atypia and of 100% of women with CIS or invasive carcinoma (Aurelian et al. 1978). In contrast, the antigen was not identified in exfoliated cells of normal women or of women with benign conditions such as squamous metaplasia. In more recent studies, in situ cytological hybridization using nick-translated ^{3}H-HSV-2 DNA, has been employed to detect HSV RNA in cells undergoing neoplastic change (McDougall et al. 1980). However, viral transcripts were not detected in cells of fully developed squamous-cell cancers using this technique. It was suggested, therefore, that in cells of fully developed tumors either virus-specific transcription was at a reduced level undetectable by the in situ hybridization technique, or virus DNA sequences had been lost.

In the present study, hyperimmune antisera to two HSV-2 polypeptides were used in concert with highly sensitive immunoperoxidase staining to examine cervical biopsy material and cervical explants for HSV-specific antigens. These monospecific antisera represent highly sensitive probes for detection of viral gene expression since viral proteins reflect a natural amplification of viral genetic information. Furthermore, identification of individual viral-specific polypeptides allows for valuable insight as to which viral DNA sequences may be resident in the cell. In cultured cells infected with HSV-2, VP143 was identified within the nucleus as early as 4 hrs postinfection. VP157, the major capsid protein, was observed within the nuclear compartment as early as 6 hrs postinfection and after that time was dispersed both within the nucleus and the cytoplasm. These observations are compatable with those noted in productive lytic HSV-2 infection in vitro. Such patterns of staining were noted in frozen sections and explanted cells of cervical biopsies originating from patients with herpes cervicitis and are consistent with a state of lytic HSV infection.

In contrast, in cells transformed by HSV-2 in vitro, VP143 was found in the cytoplasm in a perinuclear arrangement. This distribution of VP143 is in accord with that noted by immunofluorescence in synchronized HSV-2-transformed cells (Flannery et al. 1977). It has been determined that the hamster cells, transformed by UV-irradiated HSV-2, retain a fraction (8–32%) of viral DNA sequences (Frenkel et al. 1976). Thus, although the role of VP143 in the transformation process remains to be defined, the expression of the protein in the absence of apparent viral infection may serve as a specific marker of integrated HSV-2 DNA sequences within potentially malignant cells. In this respect, VP143 was observed in a perinuclear arrangement within the cytoplasm of cervical cells from 29% to 41% of individuals with severe dysplasia, CIS, and invasive squamous cell carcinoma. This pattern of staining was similar to that observed in the HSV-2 transformed cells in vitro. Staining for VP157 and for HSV-2 was not noted. Furthermore, isolation of infectious HSV from extracts of biopsies or cervical swab material was not achieved. These observations contrast with those derived from in situ hybridization studies (McDougall et al. 1980) in which HSV-RNA was identified only in cells undergoing neoplastic change, since a viral-specific gene product (i.e., VP143) was identified also in fully developed squamous cell cancers. Thus, the identification of HSV-specific information within the cancer cells may have resulted as a consequence of the inherent sensitivity of an assay which employs hyperimmune and monospecific antiserum in concert with immunoenzyme staining.

The results of this study suggest that the expression of HSV-2 polypeptides within cervical cells from individuals with severe dysplasia, CIS, and invasive squamous cell carcinoma are not resultant of productive lytic infection. Rather, as in the case of cells transformed by UV-irradiated HSV-2, a fraction of viral DNA sequences is retained within premalignant and malignant cervical cells, the expression of which results in the production of at least one viral gene product, namely, VP143. Thus, the recognition of a strong correlation between the differential pattern of expression of VP143 and premalignant and malignant cervical disease provides further evidence for a role of HSV-2 in the etiology of cervical cancer. In addition, these data indicate that hyperimmune and specific antiserum to VP143, in concert with highly sensitive immunoenzyme staining, may prove useful in the histological diagnosis of cervical cancer.

ACKNOWLEDGEMENTS

The authors gratefully acknowledge the excellent technical assistance provided by Mr. A Morris Patterson, Ms. Marquita Kirkland, and Mrs. Bernadine Hensley, R.N. This study was supported by NCI Grant No. CA21, 801.

REFERENCES

An SH: Herpes simplex virus infection detected on routine gynecological cell specimens. Acta Cytol 13: 354, 1969.

Anzai T, Dreesman GR, Courtney RJ, Adam E, Rawls WE, Benyesh-Melnick M: Antibody to herpes simplex virus type 2-induced nonstructural proteins in women with cervical cancer and in control groups. J Natl Cancer Inst 54: 1051, 1975.

Aurelian L, Gupta PK, Frost JK, Rosenheim N, Mantione J: Immunologic markers for cervical histopathology. Acta Cytol Baltimore 22: 606, 1978.

Aurelian L, Schumann B, Marcus RL, Davis HJ: Antibody to HSV-2 induced tumor specific antigens in serums of patients with cervical carcinoma. Science 181: 161, 1973.

Aurelian L, Strandberg JD, Davis HJ: HSV-2 antigens absent from biopsied cervical tumor cells: A model consistent with latency. Proc Soc Exptl Biol Med 140: 404, 1972.

Aurelian L, Royston I, Davis HJ: Antibody to genital herpesvirus: Association with cervical atypia and carcinoma in situ. J Natl Cancer Inst 45: 455, 1970.

Beilby JOW, Cameron CH, Catterall RD, Davidson D: Herpesvirus hominis infection of the cervix associated with gonorrhea. Lancet 1: 1065, 1968.

Cabral GA, Gyorkey G, Gyorkey P, Melnick JL, Dreesman GR: Immunohistochemical and electron microscopic detection of hepatitis B surface and core antigens. Exp Molec Pathol 29: 156, 1978.

Collard W, Thornton H, Green M: Cells transformed by human herpesvirus type 2 transcribe virus-specific RNA sequences shared by herpesvirus types 1 and 2. Nature New Biol 243: 264, 1973.

Courtney RJ, Benyesh-Melnick M: Isolation and characterization of a large molecular weight polypeptide of herpes simplex virus type 1. Virology 62: 539, 1974.

Darai G, Munk K: Human embryonic lung cells abortively infected with herpesvirus hominis type 2 show some properties of cell transformation. Nature New Biol 24: 268, 1973.

Duff R, Rapp F: Oncogenic transformation of hamster embryo cells after exposure to inactivated herpes simplex virus type 1. J Virol 12: 209, 1973.

Duff R, Rapp F: Properties of hamster embryo fibroblasts transformed in vitro after exposure to ultraviolet-irradiated herpes simplex virus type 2. J Virol 8: 469, 1971.

Flannery VL, Courtney RJ, Schaffer PA: Expression of an early, nonstructural antigen of herpes simplex virus in cells transformed in vitro by herpes simplex virus. J Virol 21: 284, 1977.

Frenkel N, Locker H, Cox B, Roizman B, Rapp F: Herpes simplex virus DNA in transformed cells: sequence complexity in five hamster cell lines and one derived hamster tumor. J Virol 18: 885, 1976.

Hanker JS, Yates PE, Metz CB, Rustioni A: Aldehyde blockage and periodate oxidation. Histochem J 9: 789, 1977.

Jordan SW, Evangel E, Smith NL: Ethnic distribution of cytologically diagnosed herpes simplex genital infection in a cervical cancer screening program. Acta Cytol 16: 363, 1972.

Kessler II: Perspectives on the epidemiology of cervical cancer with special reference to the herpesvirus hypothesis. Cancer Res 34: 1091, 1974.

Kimura S, Flannery FL, Levy B, Schaffer PA: Oncogenic transformation of primary hamster cells by herpes simplex virus type 2 (HSV-2) and an HSV-2 temperature- sensitive mutant. Int J Cancer 15: 786, 1975.

Kraiselburd E, Gage LP, Weissbach: Presence of a herpes simplex virus DNA fragment in an L cell clone obtained after infection with irradiated herpes simplex virus. J Mol Biol 97: 533, 1975.

Kucera LS, Gusdon JP: Transformation of human embryonic fibroblasts by photodynamically inactivated herpes simplex virus type 2 at supraoptical temperatures. J Gen Virol 30: 257, 1976.

Kutinová L, Vonka V, Broucek J: Increased oncogenicity and synthesis of herpesvirus antigens in hamster cells exposed to herpes simplex type-2 virus. J Nat Cancer Inst 50: 759, 1973.

MacNab JCM: Transformation of rat embryo cells by temperature-sensitive mutants of herpes simplex virus. J Gen Virol 24: 143, 1974.

McDougall JK, Galloway DA, Fenoglio CM: Cervical carcinoma: detection of herpes simplex virus RNA in cells undergoing neoplastic change. Int J Cancer 25: 1, 1980.

Melnick JL, Courtney RJ, Powell KL, Schaffer PA, Benyesh-Melnick M, Dreesman GR, Anzai T, Adam E: Studies on herpes simplex virus and cancer. Cancer Research 36: 845, 1976.

Minson AC, Thouless ME, Eglin RP, Darby G: The detection of virus DNA sequences in a herpes type 2 transformed hamster cell line (333-8-9). Int J Cancer 17: 493, 1976.

Nahmias AJ, Naib ZM, Josey WE: Epidemiological studies relating genital herpetic infection to cervical carcinoma. Cancer Res 34: 111, 1974.

Naib ZM, Nahmias AJ, Josey WE, Zaki SA: Relation of cytohistopathology of genital herpesvirus infection to cervical anaplasia. Cancer Res 33: 1452, 1973.

Naib ZM, Nahmias AJ, Josey WE, Dramer JH: Genital herpetic infection. Association with cervical dysplasia and carcinoma. Cancer 23: 940, 1969.

Naib ZM, Nahmias AJ, Josey WE: Cytology and histopathology of cervical herpes simplex infection. Cancer 19: 1026, 1966.

Ng ABP, Reagan JW, Yen SSC: Herpes genitalis: Clinical and cytopathologic experience with 256 patients. Obstet Gynecol 36: 645, 1970.

Nowakovsky S, McGrew EA, Medak H, Burlakow P, Nanos S: Manifestations of viral infections in exfoliated cells. Acta Cytol 12: 227, 1968.

Rawls WE, Adam E, Melnick JL: An analysis of seroepidemiological studies of herpesvirus type 2 and carcinoma of the cervix. Cancer Res 33: 1477, 1973.

Royston I, Aurelian L: Immunofluorescent detection of herpes antigens in exfoliated cells from human cervical carcinoma. Proc Natl Acad Sci U.S. 67: 204, 1970.

Wolinska WH, Melaned MR: Genitalis in women attending planned parenthood of New York City. Acta Cytol 14: 239, 1970.

21. IMMUNOLOGICAL ASPECTS OF SQUAMOUS CELL CARCINOMA OF THE UTERINE CERVIX: USE OF LEUKOCYTE ADHERENCE INHIBITION ASSAY

M.M. DINI and I. FAIFERMAN

Worldwide, squamous cell carcinoma of the uterine cervix is the most common gynecologic malignancy. The squamous cell carcinoma of the human uterine cervix can serve as an ideal model to study host-tumor interrelationships. Due to the ease of accessibility of the cervix for inspection and evaluation by colposcopy, cytologic and tissue sampling, the entire spectrum of the malignancy can be studied. Squamous cell carcinoma of the cervix probably starts as intraepithelial neoplastic lesions which will gradually progress into different stages of dysplasia (mild, moderate and severe), carcinoma *in situ*, microinvasive and frankly invasive lesions. By using this spontaneous, dynamic human model, immunologic host-tumor interaction can be easily investigated.

I. TUMOR IMMUNOLOGY

Immune defense and other host factors have been implicated as a possible explanation for the well-documented occurrence of spontaneous tumor regression (Everson and Cole 1966; Currie 1976). The existence of immunologic host responses to human gynecologic cancer has been determined by clinical and experimental studies for example, both intraepithelial and invasive carcinoma of the uterine cervix are more common in women who are immunosuppressed (Porreco et al. 1975). This phenomenon can be due to both immunologic and non-immunologic factors such as: (a) impairment of immunologic surveillance, (b) direct carcinogenicity of chemotherapeutic agents, (c) lowering of the host resistance to oncogenic viruses such as herpes virus type II (Aurelian et al. 1971), and (d) an inadequate host response after exposure to an external carcinogen (Stafl 1974).

I.A. Tumor antigens in animal systems

The presence of neoantigens on tumor cells, capable of inducing an immune response in an autochthonous host has been demonstrated. Pioneering studies in inbred strains of mice have shown that tumors possess antigens which induce immunity as shown by transplantation resistance (Foley 1953; Prehn and Main 1957). Several *in vitro* techniques have since been developed which are capable of detecting tumor antigens.

Tumor Associated Transplantation Antigens are surface antigens capable of inducing an immune tumor rejection. These antigens have been demonstrated in both carcinogen and virally-induced neoplasms (Baldwin et al. 1974). Neoantigens found on the cell surface of experimentally induced and naturally occurring neoplasms (Levy 1974; Herberman 1974), do not appear to function as transplantation antigens. Included in this group are fetal cytoplasmic and nuclear antigens of virus induced tumors.

I.B. Tumor antigens in man

Most, of not all, human tumor cells possess antigens which can induce an immune response as measured by *in vitro* assays. Tumor cells of squamous cell carcinoma of the uterine cervix manifest several antigenic determinants such as: (a) Antigens related to herpes virus, presumably coded by the viral genome resident in these neoplastic cells. Expression of these antigens apparently vary according to the environment of the tumor cells, and the size of the viral genome retained in the nucleus (Aurelian 1974). (b) Carcinoembryonic antigen detected both *in vivo* and *in vitro* in tissue culture (Drysdale and Singer 1970; DiSaia et al. 1972).

Hafez, E.S.E., Smith, J.P. (eds.), Carcinoma of the Cervix: Biology and Diagnosis. ISBN-13: 978-94-009-7487-6

Loss of blood group antigens (A, B, and H) which are normally present on the cell surface of healthy cervical epithelium, has also been reported. This antigenic loss has been considered as a sign of dedifferentiation (Davidson et al. 1973).

I.C. Immune responses to the antigenic expression

(a) *Humoral immune response*. This arm of the immune response is mediated by antibodies. Tumor related antibodies may include cytotoxic antibodies, tumor enhancing or blocking factors (Old and Boyse 1964), and unblocking factors. (b) *Cellular immunity*. This arm is mediated by lymphocytes. These reactions are important in experimental and spontaneous tumor systems (Hellstrom and Hellstrom 1979) of both animal and man. These lymphocytes have specific anti-tumor cytolytic properties (Hellstrom and Hellstrom 1974). (c) *Cytotoxicity by armed macrophages*. 'Arming' can be effected by the following: cytophilic antibodies (Evans and Alexander 1970), endotoxin, double stranded RNA, and lipid A. (d) *Antibody-dependent cell mediated immunity*. This is effected by a non-B, non-T, Killer (K), monocytoid cell (Hersey et al. 1973). This system can be readily blocked by free antigen, immune complexes, and unrelated immunoglobulins (Currie, 1976).

Cell mediated immune responses in patients with malignancy have been demonstrated by the following *in vitro* methods: (a) inhibition of colony formation (Hellstrom et al. 1969, (b) lymphoblastic transformation by autochthonous tumor cells (Stjernsward et al. 1973), (c) leukocyte migration inhibition (Goldstein et al. 1971), (d) cytotoxicity using *in vitro* homologous cell lines (DiSaia et al. 1972; Dini et al. 1980). The latter is probably the most commonly used laboratory method for the detection of cell mediated immune responses in squamous cell carcinoma of the uterine cervix. The unpredictability and difficulties inherent in tissue culturing and the constant concern about the fidelity of these cells in expressing *in vitro*, the actual *in vivo* markers, especially in long-term established cell lines with a tendency to dedifferentiate, make cytotoxicity assays quite inconvenient if not unreliable (Baldwin 1975; Herberman and Oldham 1975). (e) *Leukocyte Adherence Inhibition assay* (LAI as-

say). LAI assay has been used in evaluation of cell mediated immune responses in cancer patients. This test can be of special value in the follow-up and posttreatment surveillance of patients following cancer therapy. Leukocyte Adherence Inhibition (LAI) assay has been employed as an investigational probe in patients with squamous cell carcinoma of the cervix. This assay has proved to be useful in several animal and human tumor systems, because of its sensitivity and reproducibility (Bhatti et al. 1977; Grosser and Thompson 1975; Halliday and Miller 1972). Marked lymphocyte mediated immune responses can be detected in patients with invasive squamous cell carcinoma of the uterine cervix.

Using the LAI tube technique, the reactivity of the patients' peripheral blood lymphocytes to the pooled extracts from allogeneic squamous cell carcinoma of the cervix was measured. In the studied series, 87% (28/32) of patients with invasive squamous cell carcinoma reacted strongly to the homologous allogeneic tumor extract (Dini et al. 1980). In contrast the peripheral blood lymphocytes from patients with other unrelated tumors did not react against the cervical tumor extract. There was no significant difference of LAI reactivity in patients with different stages of cervical cancer. A positive correlation has been reported between the intensity of the cell-mediated immune responses determined by migration inhibition, and the clinical stage of the disease (Chiang et al. 1976).

That only 5% (3/54) of patients' peripheral blood lymphocytes reacted positively to the control antigen attests to the specificity of this test. Optimal results were obtained when 10% fetal calf serum and a protein concentration of one mg/ml of tumor tissue extract was used. Bhatti et al. (1977) have used concentrations close to this value. The optimal concentration of tissue extract, for maximum reactivity, should be established independently for each tumor system. This assay clearly demonstrates that the peripheral blood lymphocytes of these patients are sensitized against their squamous cell carcinoma.

Because various assays used in evaluation of cell mediated immunity in cancer patients may lead to dissimilar conclusions, it is unclear whether or not different *in vitro* techniques for detection of cell mediated immune responses measure the same biologic phenomenon.

II. TUMOR GROWTH

It is still not well understood how a malignant cell clone can develop, survive and grow progressively in the face of a specific and potentially cytocidal immune response. The development of a tumor may represent a failure of the immunosurveillance mechanisms (Burnett 1965). The *in vivo* escape mechanism of tumor growth may be due to the following: Immunological enhancement and blocking antibody: Studies in the Maloney sarcoma system indicate that the blocking factors are antibodies which disappear following the onset of tumor regression (Hellstrom et al. 1969). These blocking factors are present in patients with squamous cell carcinoma of the uterine cervix (Dini and Faiferman 1980). Their blocking activity has been identified with the immunoglobulin G and M fraction of sera from patients with invasive squamous cell carcinoma of the cervix. Blocking 'antibodies' may be immune complexes of antibody and shed tumor antigen. The blocking activity may be due to antigen-antibody complexes located on the surface of lymphocytes (Hattler and Soehnlen 1974). The presence of surface-bound immunoglobulins or immune complexes on tumor cells have been demonstrated in both animal and human tumor systems. They have been identified with the *in vivo* manifestation of the *in vitro* blocking effect (Ran and Witz 1972).

Other factors influencing the *in vivo* escape mechanism of tumor growth may include: (1) specific immune tolerance (Currie 1976), (2) non-specific immunodeficiency, (3) immunoselection (Hauschka

et al. 1956), (4) antigenic modulation or shedding of antigen, (5) initial growth in immunologically privileged sites, and (6) emergence of suppressor cells. The paradoxical nature of tumor inception, growth, and progression seems to be dependent on multifactorial phenomena and not on any single factor.

III. CONCLUDING REMARKS

Squamous cell carcinoma of the uterine cervix usually originates in the transitional zone of the squamo-columnar junction. This malignant process probably starts during the teens, passes through the stages of dysplasia (mild, moderate and severe) most commonly during the third decade of woman's life. It presents as carcinoma *in situ* usually in thirties and may culminate in invasive lesions most often during the fifth decade. Different investigators have stated different incidences of progression versus regression in this continuous biologic process. Because of the ease of accessibility of the uterine cervix, this process can be readily studied and therefore may serve as an ideal model in the study of immunological and biological processes as these relate to the genesis of neoplasms from their inception to the often fatal invasive conclusions. The use of this system may help to further clarify questions concerned with tumor immunology and the dynamics of host-tumor relationship. The leukocyte adherence inhibition assay can potentially be a major investigative tool in the study of immunologic aspects of tumor genesis and pathophysiology.

REFERENCES

Aurelian L: Persistence and expression of herpes simplex virus type 2 genome in cervical tumor cells. Cancer Res 34: 1126, 1974.

Aurelian L, Strandberg JD, Melendez LU, Johnson LA: Herpes virus type 2 isolated from cervical tumor cells grown in tissue culture. Science 1974: 704, 1971.

Baldwin RW: *In vitro* assays of cell mediated immunity to human solid tumors. Problems of quantitation, specificity and interpretation. J Natl Cancer Inst 55: 745, 1975.

Baldwin RW, Bowen JD, Embleton KJ, Price MR, Robbins RA: Cellular and humoral immune responses to neoantigens associated with chemically induced tumors. *In* Brent M, Holborrow J (eds): Progress in Immunology II, Vol. 3. New York: Elsevier, 1974, pp 239–248.

Bhatti RA, Guinan PD, McKile OF, et al.: Responsiveness of lymphocytes to soluble extracts of prostatic tumors and abrogation by serum blocking factors. Urology IX (3): 314, 1977.

Burnett FM: Immune surveillance. Brit Med J 1: 338, 1965.

Chiang WT, Wei PY, Alexander ER: Circulatory and cellular immune responses to squamous cell carcinoma of the uterine cervix. Am J Obstet Gynecol 126: 116, 1976.

Currie GA: Immunological reactions in human cancer; malignant melanoma, hypernephroma and neuroblastoma. *In* Symington T, Carter RT (eds): Scientific Foundations of Oncology. Chicago: Yearbook Medical Publish, 1976, pp 544–548.

Davidson I, Norris HJ, Syskal R: Metastatic squamous cell carcinoma of the cervix. The role of immunity in its pathogenesis. Arch Pathol 95: 132, 1973.

Dini MM, Faiferman I: Cytotoxic blocking activity in invasive squamous cell carcinoma of the human uterine cervix. Cancer 46: 2513, 1980.

Dini MM, Jafari K, Faiferman I: Cell mediated cytotoxicity in preinvasive and invasive squamous cell carcinoma of the uterine cervix. Obstet Gynecol 55: 728, 1980.

Dini MM, Nerenberg S, Jafari K, Faiferman I: Leukocyte Adherence Inhibition Assay in Squamous Cell Carcinoma of Cervix (Abstract). Proceedings of the International Symposium on Carcinoma of the Cervix, Biology, Etiology, and Diagnosis, Kiawah Island, Charleston, South Carolina, September 1980.

DiSaia P, Sinkovics JG, Rutledge FN, Smith JP: Cell mediated immunity to human maligant cells: A brief review and further studies with two gynecologic tumors. Am J Obstet Gynecol 114 (7): 979, 1972.

Drysdale JW, Singer RM: Carcinofetal human isoferritin in plasma and HeLa cells. Cancer. 25: 362, 1970.

Evans R, Alexander A: Cellular immunity to nephroblastoma. London: Nature, 1970.

Everson TC, Cole WH: Spontaneous regression of cancer. Philadelphia: Saunders, 1966.

Foley EJ: Attempts to induce immunity against mammary adenocarcinoma in inbred mice. Cancer Res 13: 578, 1953.

Goldstein MS, Shore B, Gusberg B: Cellular immunity as a host response to squamous carcinoma of the cervix. Am J Obstet Gynecol 11: 751, 1971.

Grosser N, Thompson DMP: Cell mediated anti-tumor immunity in breast cancer patients evaluated by antigen induced leukocyte adherence inhibition in test tubes. Cancer Res 35: 2571, 1975.

Halliday WJ, Miller S: Leukocyte Adherence Inhibition. A simple test for cell mediated tumor immunity and serum blocking factors. Internatl J Cancer 9: 477, 1972.

Hattler BG, Soehnlen B: Inhibition of tumor induced lymphocyte blastogenesis by a factor or factors associated with peripheral leukocytes. Science 184: 1374, 1974.

Hauschka TS, Kvedar BJ, Grunel ST, Amos DB: Cytotoxic lymphocytes in melanoma patients. Ann New York Acad Science, 1956, 63.

Hellstrom E, Hellstrom I: Lymphocyte mediated cytotoxicity and blocking serum activity to tumor antigens. Adv Immunol 18: 209, 1974.

Hellstrom KE, Hellstrom I: Enhancement of tumor growth by tumor associated blocking factors. Internatl J Cancer 23: 366, 1979.

Hellstrom I, Hellstrom KE, Evans CA, Heppner GH, Pierce GE, Young PO: Serum mediated protection of neoplastic cells from inhibition by lymphocytes immune to their tumor specific antigens. Proc Natl Acad Science 62: 362, 1969.

Herberman RBE: Cell mediated immunity to tumor cells. Avd Cancer Res 19: 207, 1974.

Herberman RB, Oldham RK: Problems associated with the study of cell mediated immunity to human tumors by micro-cytotoxicity assays. J Natl Cancer Inst 55: 749, 1975.

Hersey P, McClennan ICM: Cellular immunity against tumor specific antigens. Transplantation 16: 9, 1973.

Levy JP: Antigen associated with C-type RNA viruses induced tumors. In Brent L, Holborrow J (eds): Progress in Immunology II, Vol. 3. New York: Elsevier, 1974, p 249.

Old LJ, Boyse EA: Immunology of experimental tumors. Ann Rev Med 15: 167, 1964.

Porreco R, Penn I, Droegemuller W, Greer B, Makowski E: Gynecologic malignancies in immunosuppressed organ homograft recipients. Obstet Gynecol 45: 359, 1975.

Prehn RT, Main JM: Immunity to methylcholantrene-induced sarcomas. J Natl Cancer Inst 18: 769, 1957.

Ran M, Witz IP: Tumor associated immunoglobulins. Enhancement of syngeneic tumors by IgG2-containing tumor eluates. Inter J Cancer 9: 242, 1972.

Stafl A: Vaginal Adenosis: Precancerous lesion. Am J Obstet Gynecol 120: 666, 1974.

Stjernsward JF, Vanky, Klein E: Lymphocyte stimulation by autochthonous human solid tumors. Brit J Cancer 28 (Suppl 1) 72, 1973.

22. HUMAN CELL LINE (SKG-1) DERIVED FROM EPIDERMOID CANCER OF THE CERVIX

S. Nozawa, K. Tsukazaki, Y. Udagawa, I. Ishiwata, H. Oota, S. Kurihara and H. Okumura

I. THE HELA CELL AS CERVICAL CANCER CELL LINE

The HeLa cell line is derived from biopsy specimens of a patient with advanced uterine cervical cancer (Gey et al. 1952). Based on histological and autopsy findings, this cancer was initially identified as anaplastic epidermoid cancer (Leighton 1957). However, the origin of the HeLa cells was reappraised (Jones et al. 1971) and it was suggested that it was adenocarcinomatous with obvious glandular elements. Therefore, the establishment of a cell line derived from epidermoid cancer of the uterine cervix became desirable.

Some investigators (Arata et al. 1969; Friedl et al. 1970; Pattillo et al. 1977; Porter et al. 1978; Ishiwata et al. 1978) have reported such lines. Meanwhile, in this laboratory, several human cancer cell lines have been recently established (Nozawa et al. 1975b, 1976; Ishiwata et al. 1977a, b) including a cancer cell line from human uterine cervical epidermoid cancer (SKG-1). In this report, the process of establishment together with its various cell biological characteristics of the SKG-1 cell line is described.

II. CULTURE MATERIAL

Tumor tissue for culture was obtained aseptically on July 25, 1974, from a radical hysterectomy specimen of a 40-year-old patient with stage II uterine cervical cancer.

II.A. Histopathology

Histologically, moderately differentiated epidermoid cancer cells occupied most of the tumor, but minor components of 'clear cells' with abundant, optically clear cytoplasm and relatively uniform hyperchromatic nuclei were also present (Figure 1A, 1B). The latter could be called 'clear-cell epidermoid cancer' (Abell 1973; Novak and Woodruff 1979). It is necessary to distinguish between clear-cell cancer and 'glassy-cell carcinoma' (Littman et al. 1976) which is considered to be the poorly differentiated type of mixed adenosquamous cancer. For the following reasons, we suggest that the original tumor from which SKG-1 was established was a moderately differentiated epidermoid cancer partially mixed with epidermal clear-cell components:

(1) Most of the tumor was made up of moderately differentiated epidermoid cancer cells, although clear cells were recognized in certain limited areas. (2) In portions in which epidermoid- and clear-cell cancer cells coexisted, a cell type intermediate between these two was observed. In addition, squamous differentiation, in the form of dyskeratotic cells, was recognized in the epidermoid cancer cells. (3) No gland structures were found in the area of clear-cell cancer. (4) Clear cells with abundant intracellular glycogen were present in the original tumor, the cultured cells and in the induced animal tumors.

II.B. Histochemical study of alkaline phosphatase

Alkaline phosphatase (ALP) was examined histochemically using the Azo-dye method with naphthol AS-BI phosphate as the substrate. Simultaneously, the heat-stability test and the L-phenylalanine inhibition test were performed, using the previously reported techniques (Nozawa et al. 1980). Enzyme-histochemically, nonspecific ALP activity was recognized as a red precipitate in cancer cells (Figure 1C). ALP activity persisted after heat inactivation at 65° C for 30 min (Figure 1D), and it

Hafez, E.S.E., Smith, J.P. (eds.), Carcinoma of the Cervix: Biology and Diagnosis. ISBN-13: 978-94-009-7487-6

was abolished by L-phenylalanine treatment (Figure 1E) but not by D-phenylalanine (Figure 1F). The ALP of these cancer cells resembles the Regan isoenzyme found in the placenta, various cancers and in the reserve cells of the normal uterine cervix (Nozawa et al. 1980).

III. ESTABLISHMENT OF THE SKG-1 CELL LINE

III.A. Cell culture techniques and media

For transportation to the culture room, the tumor tissue was placed in Ham's F-12 culture medium (4° C) (GIBCO, N.Y., U.S.A.). It was then washed twice with phosphate-buffered saline (PBS: NaCl, 8 g; KCl, 0.2 g; $Na_2HPO_4 . 2H_2O$, 0.116 g; KH_2PO_4, 0.2 g/liter, pH 7.2–7.4) and finely minced in plastic dishes with a pair of sharp scissors. The minced material was magnetically stirred for 30 min at room temperature in a 0.25% trypsin solution (Nutritional Biochemical Corp., Cleveland, Ohio, U.S.A.) and centrifuged at 900 rpm (150 g ×) for 10 min. The supernatant was discarded and the sediment suspended in Ham's F-12 medium containing 20% newborn calf serum, 100 units penicillin and 100 μg streptomycin per ml. The suspension was adjusted to pH 7.2 with $NaHCO_3$, inoculated into 3.5 or 5 cm diameter plastic dishes (Falcon Plastics Co., Oxnard, Calif., U.S.A.), and cultured at 37° C in a humidified atmosphere (5% CO_2, 95% air).

To obtain pure cancer cells from epithelial cells contaminated with fibroblasts, Okumura's colony isolation technique (Ishiwata et al. 1977b) was used. Briefly, the target colonies were covered for 6–10 min with 2 × 4 mm filter papers that had been soaked in a mixture of 0.02% ethylene-diamine tetraacetic acid (EDTA) and 0.1% trypsin. Cancer cells were separated from colonies contaminated with fibroblasts and transferred, together with the filter papers, to plastic dishes. After the cells became nearly confluent, they were dispersed into a single-cell suspension consisting of PBS, 0.1% trypsin and 0.02% EDTA, in order to obtain a monolayer culture, and then they were placed into a closed-culture system. The cells were transferred to 1:2 or 1:4 dilution, using a 0.25% trypsin solution to free the cells.

III.B. Establishment of cell line

Culture of the present line, SKG-1, was started on July 25, 1974. After a 3-day stationary period, proliferation of the cells was observed. As in the primary culture, the epithelial cells were contaminated with a fairly large number of fibroblasts, the first colony cloning was carried out on August 9, 1974, using the colony isolation technique. Although the number of fibroblasts was decreased, they persisted in the culture, so that the second, third and fourth colony clonings were performed on November 13th and December 5th and 24th, 1974, respectively. After the fourth cloning procedure, the pure epithelial cells were transferred to a closed-culture system on February 10, 1975. Initially, cell growth was rather slow and the cells were passed on April 15th and May 10th and 28th, 1975. The cells were fed at least once a week and passed upon becoming confluent. The subculture has been maintained for a period of more than 6 years and cell growth continues to be stable.

IV. VARIOUS CHARACTERISTICS OF THE CULTURED CELLS

IV.A. Cell biological characteristics

IV.A.1. Growth curve, population doubling time and saturation density. Single-suspension cells of the 20th and 68th generations (5×10^4/ml) were plated onto plastic dishes and incubated for 8 days in a 5% CO_2 incubator. The culture medium (Ham's F-12) was changed every 2 days. The average number of cells was determined daily by counting the cells in 3 dishes and the calculated numbers were recorded on a semilogarithmic graph. One day post-inoculation, these cells grew logarithmically and, after 7 days, they reached a plateau or stationary phase. The population doubling time determined from the growth curve of passage 20 was 35 hr; that of passage 68, 42 hr (Figure 2). The saturation density of these two passage numbers was $3–7 \times 10^4$/cm^2.

IV.A.2. Plating efficiency. The cell suspension was diluted serially and 320 (11th generation) or 100 (38th generation) single-suspension cells were cul-

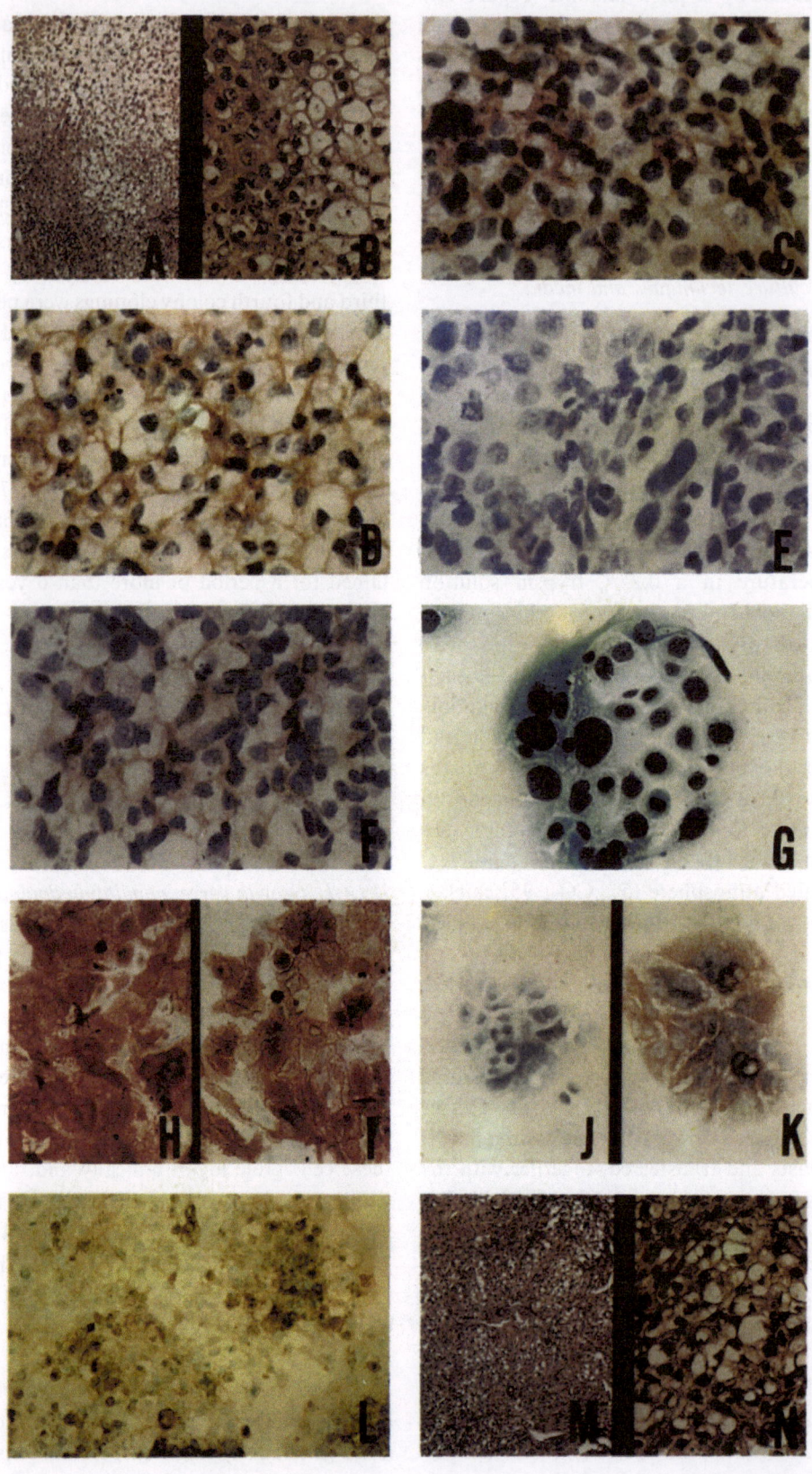

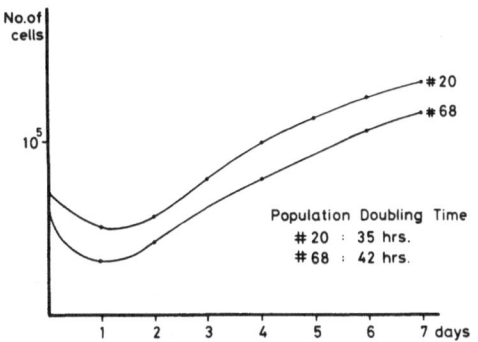

Figure 2. Growth curve of SKG-1 (20th and 68th generations).

tured for 10 days in plastic dishes. Fixed cells were stained with a Giemsa stock solution and visible colonies were calculated manually. Plating efficiency was expressed as the ratio of the number of visible colonies to the total number of inoculated cells. The single-cell rate was 99%. The plating efficiency of passage 11 was 88.4%; that of passage 38, 71.6%.

IV.A.3. Chromosome analysis. Cultured cells of the 11th and 68th generations were used. The monolayer cultured cells were treated for 4–6 hr with 10^{-7} M Colcemid (CIBA Ltd., Basle, Switzerland) at 37° C , placed for 15–20 min in a hypotonic solution (0.2% potassium chloride), fixed for 10 min in an alcohol:acetic acid (3:1) mixture, and refixed for 20 min after changing the fixative. After air-drying, the cells were stained with a 1:10 dilution of a Giemsa stock solution.

About 100 metaphase plates were counted to determine the chromosomal number distribution. These examinations revealed aneuploidy and there was a wide distribution in the chromosome number (range 63 to 238, Figure 3). About 58% of the cells revealed hypertriploidy, and exact counting of this

model range showed that in 9.7% of the cells, the modal number was 74 or 75. Almost the same tendency was observed in passage 68. Karyotypes of 20 metaphase plates were analyzed strictly in accordance with the Paris Conference Recommendations. The structure of Group A, consisting of a total of 8 chromosomes (the largest was metacentric, 2 were submetacentric and 5 smaller chromosomes were metacentric), was common and this structure appeared to be representative of the karyotype of this cell line (Figure 4).

IV.B. Morphology

IV.B.1. Phase contrast microscopy, Giemsa and Papanicolaou stain. The monolayer cultured cells appeared to be epithelial, with a pavement-like arrangement. As the cells became more dense, no contact inhibition was observed and frequent overlapping was noted. The cells were roughly divided into two groups. In one group, they varied in size: they were polygonal with relatively pale, abundant cytoplasm. The nuclei revealed neoplastic features such as bizarre aggregation of chromatin granules,

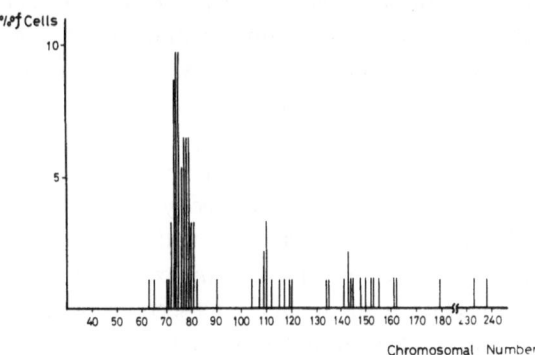

Figure 3. Distribution of the chromosomal number of SKG-1 (11th generation).

Figure 1. (A) Histologically, the original tumor consisted of moderately differentiated epidermoid carcinoma with some clear-cell components. H & E; (B) A higher magnification of Figure 1A; (C) Red precipitate in cancer cells of the original tumor is indicative of alkaline phosphatase (ALP) activity; (D) After heat inactivation (65° C, 30 min), heat-stable ALP activity persisted; (E) After L-phenylalanine inhibition test; (F) After D-phenylalanine inhibition test (control). An obvious difference in inhibition is seen. ALP in these cancer cells resembled the Regan isoenzyme; (G) Cultured cells of SKG-1 colonies were polygonal and revealed anaplastic and pleomorphic features. Fiber-type cells with pyknotic nuclei were also seen. Papanicolaou stain; (H) Strong ALP activity was seen in cultured cells (6th transfer generation); (I) After heat inactivation (65° C, 30 min), heat-stable ALP activity persisted in the cultured cells; (J) After L-phenylalanine inhibition test; (K) After D-phenylalanine inhibition test (control). Marked ALP inhibition was seen. ALP in these cultured cells resembled the Regan isoenzyme; (L) Brown precipitate showed the immunocytochemical localization of placental ALP on cultured cells (indirect peroxidase labelled antibody method); (M) Histologically, tumors induced by heterotransplantation of SKG-1 cells into nude mice resembled the original tumor; (N) A higher magnification of Figure 1 (M).

146

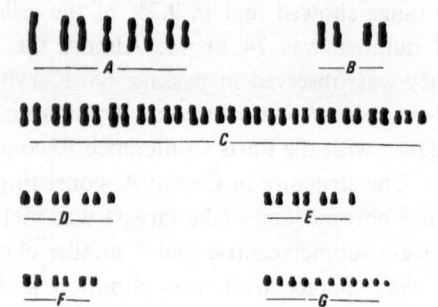

Figure 4. Karyotype analysis of SKG-1 (11th generation).

irregular thickening of the membrane and multiple large nucleoli. Fiber-type cells with pyknotic nuclei were occasionally seen adjacent to polygonal cells (Figure 1G). The second group consisted of relatively large, polygonal cells with abundant cytoplasm and a fine granule appearance with moderately hyperchromatic nuclei. The periodic Acid-Schiff stain revealed small intracytoplasmic glycogen droplets which were digested by diastase. These cells were almost unstainable with mucicarmine.

IV.B.2. Transmission electron microscopy. The cultured cells were fixed for 30 min in 2.5% glutaraldehyde buffered at pH 7.4 with 0.05 M phosphate, washed in 0.1 M phosphate buffer at pH 7.4, postfixed for 1 hr with 1% osmium tetroxide, and dehydrated in a graded series of ethanol. Capsules were then placed directly on the cultured cells and they were polymerized with Epon 812 for 2 days at 60° C. Subsequently, the cells were peeled off the glass at about 90° C, and sections parallel to the glass were stained with uranyl acetate and lead citrate and studied. Electron microscopy revealed that the former group cells were characterized by the abundance of cytoplasmic tonofilaments; the desmosomal junction was seen at the adjacent membrane (Figure 5A). In highly indented nuclei, chromatin clumps and large irregular nucleoli were seen. In the latter group cells, large glycogen deposits in the cytoplasm were revealed, but scarcely any tonofilament was found (Figure 5B). In addition, there were electron-microscopically some cells of an intermediate type; these exhibited a small amount of glycogen and a few tonofilaments.

IV.B.3. Scanning electron microscopy. Specimens were double-fixed with 2.5% glutaraldehyde and 1% osmium tetroxide, dehydrated in a graded series of ethanol and dried by critical-point drying. The samples were then coated with carbon-gold or gold sputter coating in a high vacuum evaporator and examined in a JEOL JSM-35 electron microscope. The cultured cells showed a wide variety of shapes, including thin flat cells, ovoid or spherical cells. The thin cells possessed relatively smooth surfaces covered by a few microvilli or small irregular blebs. At the cell margins, many filopodia extended, their tips touched the surface of the glass (Figure 6A) and, on some occasions, cellular processes with ruffling at the extreme edges were seen. The ovoid or spherical cells were thicker and less extended in any direction. Their surfaces were covered with thick microvilli and many of these cells were probably mitotic (Figure 6B).

IV.B.4. Enzyme- and immuno-cytochemistry of alkaline phosphatase. To demonstrate the localization of ALP in the cultured cells, enzyme-cytochemical study (Nozawa et al. 1980) was performed as well as immunocytochemistry by the immunoperoxidase method. Specific antisera were raised in rabbits immunized with human placental ALP (Iino et al. 1972), and IgG, obtained by purifying these antisera, was labeled with horseradish peroxidase (Nakane and Kawaoi 1974). Simultaneously electron-microscopic enzyme-cytochemical studies of ALP were performed, using the previously reported techniques (Nozawa et al. 1980).

Cells of the 6th and 18th generations were used. Enzyme-cytochemically, nonspecific ALP activity was recognized as a red precipitate in some of the cultured cells (Figure 1H). In cells of the 18th generation, the frequency of nonspecific ALP activity was lower than in the 6th generation. The ALP was heat-stable; it persisted after heat inactivation at 65% C for 30 min (Figure I). ALP activity was abolished by L-phenylalanine treatment (Figure 1J) but not by D-phenylalanine (D-p) treatment (Figure 1K). Therefore, the ALP existing in the cultured cells very closely resembled the Regan isoenzyme found in the original tumor. Electron-microscopic enzyme-cytochemical examinations revealed ALP activity as black dots on the plasma membrane of some cultured cells (Figure

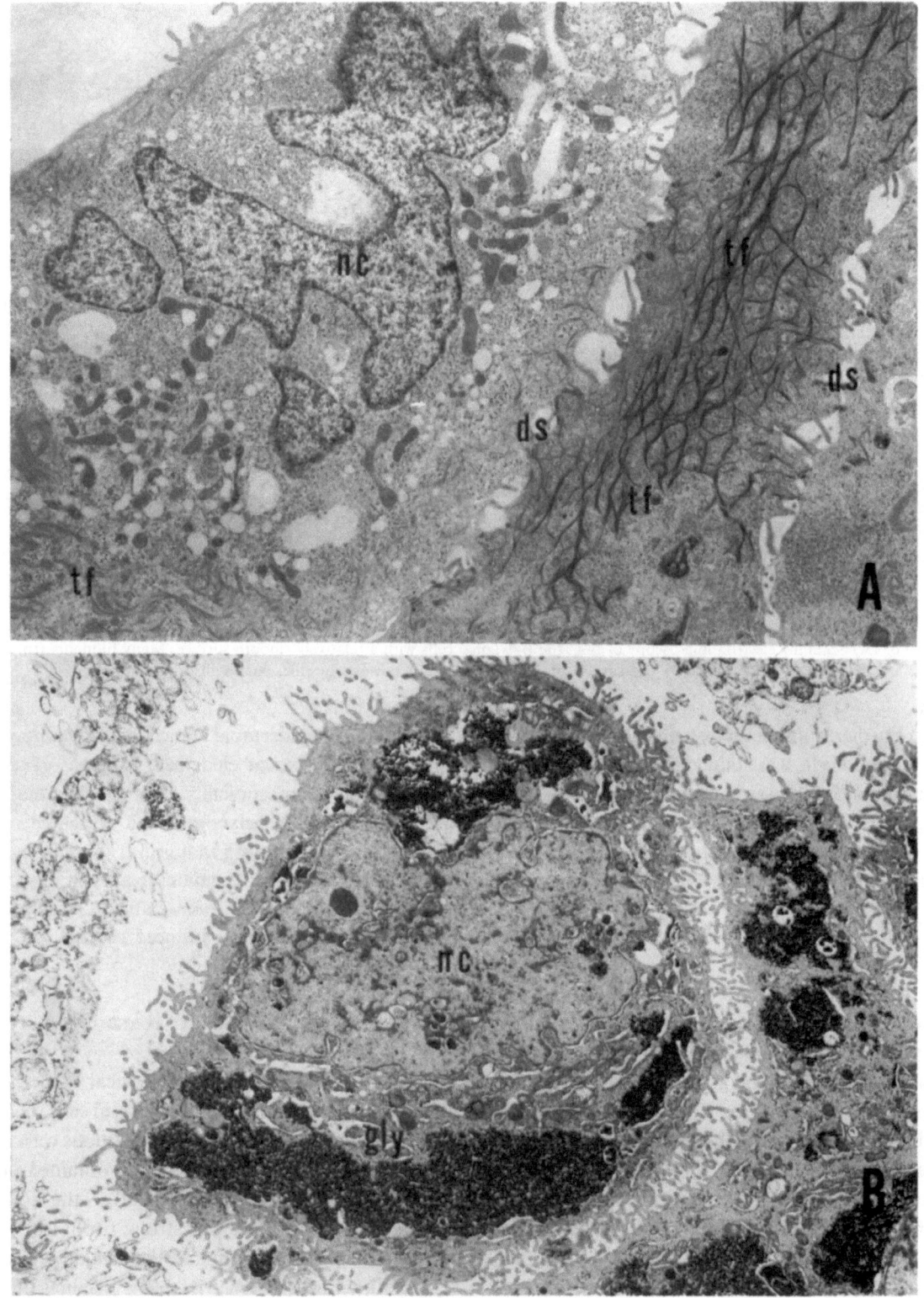

Figure 5. (A) Cultured cells prepared for transmission electron microscopy. Abundant tonofilaments (tf) and desmosomes (ds) were frequently found. nc: nucleus; × 5000); (B) Cultured cells prepared for transmission electron microscopy. Abundant glycogen granules (gly) were found throughout the cytoplasm, × 3000.

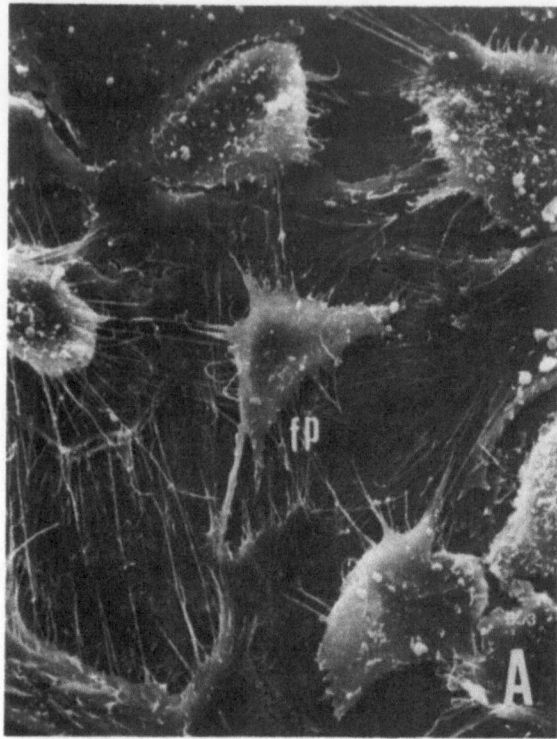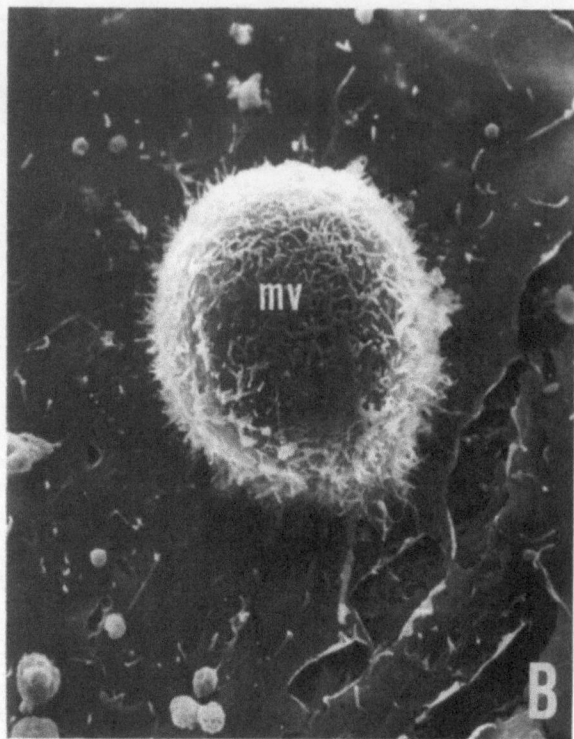

Figure 6. (A) Scanning electron microscopy of thin, flat polygonal cells with a relatively smooth surface. Many filopodia (fp) were noted at the cell margins, × 1400; (B) The surface of spherical cells was covered by thick microvilli (mv), × 5000.

7A). Further, immunocytochemically, a portion of the cultured cells was stained brown, indicating the localization of the same protein as placental ALP (Figure 1L). However, cells exhibiting ALP activity have been decreasing with the passage of generations.

IV.C. Heterotransplantation

Cultured cells (5–7 × 10⁶) were submucosally inoculated into the cheek pouches of Syrian golden hamsters (Nippon Biosupplies Center, Tokyo, Japan) weighing about 50 g. The animals received an injection of 2.5 mg hydrocortisone acetate at one and two weeks after the inoculation. In addition, 8-week-old nude mice (BALB/C Nisseiken Co., Ltd., Tachikawa, Japan) were subcutaneously injected with 5–7 × 10⁶ cells. Injection of these cells into immunosuppressed hamsters or into nude mice resulted in tumor formation. Tumors were extracted from the hamsters 10–14 days, and from the mice 1–3 months, after tumor cell transplantation and morphological observations were made. Histologically, the tumors consisted of moderately

differentiated epidermoid cancer which contained minor components of clear cells (Figures 1M and N). Electron-microscopically, cells which contained a large amount of glycogen and resembled the original tumor operation material (Figure 7B) were present. Enzyme-histochemical examinations confirmed the existence of heat-stable, L-p-sensitive ALP in portions of these induced tumors.

V. IDENTIFICATION OF THE CULTURED CELLS

In primary cultures of uterine cervical cancer, the possibility of contamination by normal cells such as cervical columnar cells, cervical squamous cells and fibroblasts cannot be ruled out. We obtained pure epithelial malignant cells only after the fourth colony cloning, as there was strong fibroblast contamination at the beginning of the primary culture. The cultured cells derived from the original tumor as confirmed by their growth characteristics, chromosomal analysis, morphology, and heterotransplantation: (1) The cells have been growing in multiple layers without contact inhibition for over 6

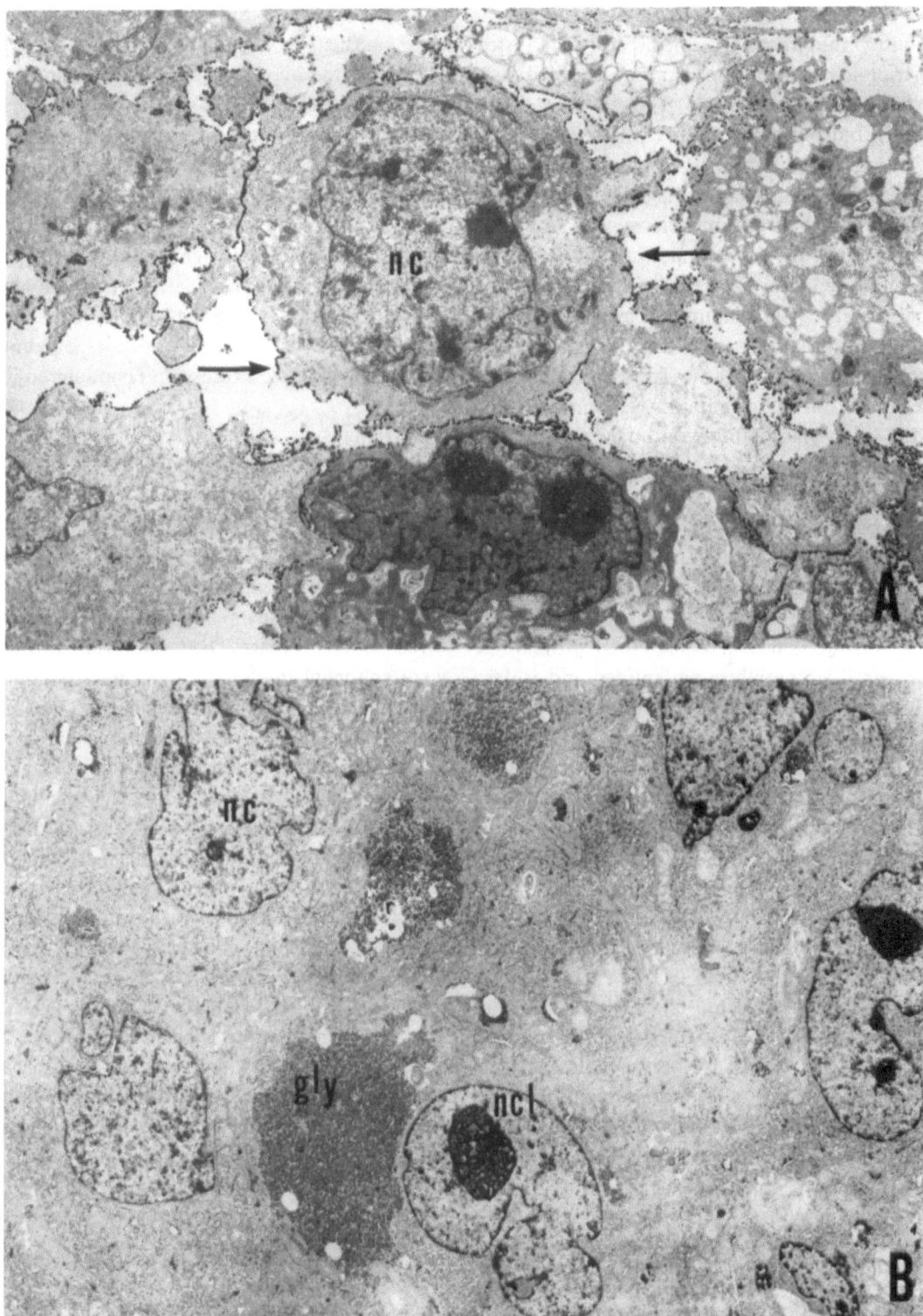

Figure 7. (A) Cultured cells prepared for electron-microscopic enzyme-cytochemistry. Localizations of ALP activity were seen as black dots (arrows) at microvilli and plasma membranes. nc: nucleus, × 4800; (B) Electron micrograph of a tumor produced by heterotransplantation of cultured cells into a nude mouse. Tumor cells contained abundant glycogen granules (gly). ncl: nucleous, × 1400.

years. (2) The chromosomes showed abnormal distribution and about 60% of the cells manifested hypertriploidy. In addition, karyotype analysis revealed abnormal structure. (3) The cells were transplantable and produced tumors which microscopically resembled the original tumor. (4) The cells satisfied criteria of malignancy such as hyperchromasia, nuclear pleomorphism and multiple large nucleoli. (5) Electron-microscopically, many of the cultured cells possessed characteristics of squamous cells such as abundant cytoplasmic glycogen or tonofilaments and the presence of the desmosomal junction at the adjacent cell membrane. Based on these findings, we conclude that the SKG-1 line was established from human uterine epidermoid cancer.

VI. REGAN-LIKE ALKALINE PHOSPHATASE OF THE CULTURED CELLS

Among various kinds of carcinofetal protein, α-fetoprotein, carcinoembryonic antigen and isoferritin are presently being used for biochemical diagnosis. In addition, the Regan isoenzyme (Fishman et al. 1968), a heat-stable and L-p-sensitive ALP which is said to exist only in the placenta and certain types of cancers (Stolbach et al. 1969, Nathanson and Fishman 1977), is thought to be one of the carcinofetal proteins (Fishman 1973). This isoenzyme has attracted attention as one of the markers for abnormalities in phenotypic expression due to gene transformation.

Using enzyme-histochemical techniques, we identified Regan-like ALP in 2 of 83 cases of uterine cervical epidermoid cancer (Nozawa et al. 1975a) as well as in reserve cells of the normal uterine cervix (Nozawa et al. 1980). The present SKG-1 line was derived from the tumor of one of the two invasive cancer patients in whom the Regan-like ALP was recognized. Therefore, this case may be one of the few cases in which ALP isoenzyme, similar to that existing in reserve cells, persisted even after malignant transformation.

Some of the cultured cells exhibit Regan-like ALP on their plasma membrane; furthermore, this ALP was immunocytochemically the same protein as placental ALP. The existence of Regan-like ALP was noted in the tumors induced in the nude mice. Therefore, it is reasonable to conclude that, as far as the ALP is concerned, the characteristics of the original tumor were preserved in the SKG-1 cell line, at least in the earlier generations. As the Regan isoenzyme is one of the carcinofetal proteins, we believe that the establishment of the SKG-1 cell line may facilitate cell biological studies of abnormalities in phenotypic expression encountered in cancers.

VII. CONCLUDING REMARKS

A new cell line, SKG-1, derived from human uterine cervical epidermoid cancer with minor clear-cell components has been successfully cultured for over 6 years. The monolayer cultured cells were epithelial in shape with a pavement-like arrangement, a piling-up tendency and no contact inhibition. Cytology revealed anaplastic and pleomorphic features. Electron-microscopically, two types of cells were distinguished; one type manifested many tonofilaments and desmosomes, the other abundant glycogen in the cytoplasm. Chromosome studies showed aneuploidy; the modal numbers were 74 and 75. There was no apparent marker chromosome. The doubling time was 35–42 hr; the plating efficiency, 70–88%. Heat-stable, L-phenylalanine-sensitive alkaline phosphatase (ALP), Regan-like isoenzyme was found on the cultured cells; enzyme-cytochemical studies revealed that ALP activity was localized on the plasma membrane. The protein was immunocytochemically confirmed to be the same as placental ALP. Transplantation of SKG-1 cells to nude mice and immunosuppressed hamsters induced tumors which resembled the original tumor.

REFERENCES

Abell MR: Invasive carcinoma of uterine cervix. *In* Norris HJ, Hertig AT, Abell MR (eds): The uterus. Baltimore: The Williams & Wilkins Company, 1973, pp 413–456.

Arata T, Ogawa I, Tanaka Y, Hashimoto K: Transplantation of a newly established human cancer cell line. Gann 60: 649, 1969.

Fishman WH, Inglis NR, Stolbach LL, Krant MJ: A serum alkaline phosphatase isoenzyme of human neoplastic cell origin. Cancer Res 28(1): 150, 1968.

Fishman WH: Carcinoplacental isoenzyme antigens. *In* Weber G (ed): Advances in enzyme regulation, Vol. XI. Oxford & New York: Pergamon Press, 1973, pp 293–321.

Friedl F, Kimura I, Osato T, Ito Y: Studies on a new human cell line (SiHa) derived from carcinoma of uterus. Its establishment and morphology. Proc Sci Exp Biol Med 135: 543, 1970.

Gey GO, Coffman WD, Kubicek MT: Tissue culture studies of the proliferative capacity of cervical carcinoma and normal epithelium. Cancer Res 12: 264, 1952.

Iino S, Abe K, Oda T, Suzuki H, Sugimura H: A new method of radioimmunoassay for human placental alkaline phosphatase. Clinica/Chimica Acta 42: 161, 1972.

Ishiwata I, Nozawa S, Nagai S, Kurihara S, Mikata A, Okumura H: Establishment of human leiomyosarcoma cell line. Cancer Res 37: 658, 19777a.

Ishiwata I, Nozawa S, Inoue T, Okumura H: Development and characterization of established cell lines from primary and metastatic regions of human endometrial adenocarcinoma. Cancer Res 37: 1777, 1977b.

Ishiwata I, Nozawa S, Kiguchi K, Kurihara S, Okumura H: Establishment of human uterine cervical cancer cell line and comparative studies between normal and malignant uterine cervical cells in vitro. Acta Obst Gynaec Jap 30: 731, 1978.

Jones HW, McKuick VA, Harper PS, Wuu KD: The Hela Cell and a reappraisal of its origin. Obstetrics and Gynecology 38: 945, 1971.

Leighton J: Contributions of tissue culture studies to an understanding of the biology of cancer: A review. Cancer Res 17: 929, 1957.

Littman P, Clement PB, Henriksen B, Wang CC, Robboy SJ,

Taft PD, Ulfelder H, Scully RE: Glassy cell carcinoma of the cervix. Cancer 37: 2238, 1976.

Nakane PK, Kawaoi A: Peroxidase-labeled antibody. A new method of conjugation. J Histochem Cytochem 22(12): 1084, 1974.

Nathanson L, Fishman WH: New observations on the Regan isoenzyme of alkaline phosphatase in cancer patients. Cancer 27(6): 1388, 1977.

Novak ER, Woodruff JD: Cervical Neoplasia. *In*: Gynecologic and Obstetrics Pathology. Philadelphia: Saunders, 1979, pp 111–156.

Nozawa S, Izumi S, Ohta H, Shinozuka T, Tsutsui F, Kurihara S, Watanabe K: Histochemical studies on alkaline phosphatase in uterine cervical reserve cell, precancerous and cancerous lesions. *In*: Shanmugaratnan K et al. (eds): Proceedings of the 2nd Asian Cancer Conf. Singapore: Stanford College Press, 1975a, pp 324–326.

Nozawa S, Ishiwata I, Kiguchi K, Tguchi J, Tsukahara S, Kurihara S, Komatsu K, Okumura H: Electron microscopic studies on a newly established cell line of human endometrial adenocarcinoma. J Clin Electron Microscopy 8: 442, 1975b.

Nozawa S, Kiguchi K, Ishiwata I, Nagai S, Taguchi S, Tsukahara S, Tsutsui F, Tamura S, Kurihara S, Komatsu N, Okumura H: Electron microscopic studies on a newly established cell line of human uterine cervical cancer. J Clin Electron Microscopy 9: 606, 1976.

Nozawa S, Ohta H, Izumi S, Hayashi S, Tsutsui F, Kurihara S, Watanabe K: Heat-stable alkaline phosphatase in normal female genital organ – with special reference to the histochemical heat stability and L-phenylalanine inhibition test. Acta histochem cytochem 13(5): 521, 1980.

Pattillo RA, Hussa RO, Story MT, Ruckert AC, Shalaby MR, Mattingly RF: Tumor antigen and human chorionic gonadotropin in CaSki cells: A new epidermoid cervical cancer cell line. Science 196: 1456, 1977.

Porter JC, Nalick RH, Vellios F, Neaves WB, MacDonald PC: New tissue culture cell lines derived from human squamous cell carcinoma of the cervix and vagina. Am J Obstet Gynecol 130: 487, 1978.

Stolbach LL, Krant MJ, Fishman WH: Ectopic production of an alkaline phosphatase isoenzyme in patients with cancer. Ann NY Acad Sci 166 (2): 760, 1969.

23. EFFECT OF ORAL CONTRACEPTIVES AND IUDs ON CERVICAL CARCINOGENESIS

U. HERMANNS and E.S.E. HAFEZ

In the late 1950s, two revolutionary developments took place in the field of contraception: the re-introduction of IUDs and the development of oral contraceptives (OCs). OCs first became available for general clinical use in the U.S.A. in 1960 and were rapidly adopted in other countries, being the most popular reversible method of contraception in the world today. It is estimated that up to 40% of women between 15 and 44 years of age in Western Europe and in the U.S.A. use the pill. Two decades after the development of the IUD some 50 to 60 million devices have been in use throughout the world, mostly in China and other developing countries. However, the initial enthusiasm for both contraceptive methods has been tempered by increasing reports of complications. Wide-scale and long-term usage of OCs and IUDs represents a potential health problem in that large numbers of healthy young women are exposed to the effects of these drugs and devices. Particular concern exists between the use of steroid contraceptives or IUDs and an increased risk of developing cancer of the cervix.

Research on the connection between contraceptives and cervical carcinogenesis has focused on morphological observations, experimental studies and four main epidemiological study designs: (i) vital statistics (disease rates and trends), (ii) case reports (tumor registries) (iii) retrospective (case-control) studies and (iv) prospective (cohort) studies. The purpose of this chapter is to summarize and put into perspective the available data of retrospective and prospective studies on the effects of OCs and IUDs on carcinoma of the cervix.

I. ORAL CONTRACEPTIVES

I.A. Steroids and the theory of cervical carcinogenesis

Although sexual transmission of a carcinogenic agent appears to be the central event in cervical cancer development, endocrine factors may play an accessory role. Since the epithelium of the cervix uteri is a target tissue for steroid hormones, OCs are unlikely to be completely without effect on the intra- and intercellular changes of the cervix. The steroid cancer hypothesis postulates that both endogeneous and exogenous steroids play a significant, possibly etiologic role in the pathogenesis of cancer in steroid responsive tissues. The search for a possible relationship of OCs and cervical carcinogenesis is based on the following observations: (1) increase of the incidence of invasive cervical cancer with age and decline after menopause; (2) occurrence of increased levels of circulating estrogen in patients with carcinoma in situ of the cervix (Frazer et al. 1967); (3) high recurrence rate of cervical cancer in women with hyperestrogenized smears (Jordaan 1972); (4) demonstration of estrogen receptors in carcinoma of the cervix (Martin and Hahnel 1978); (5) carcinogenicity of dihydrostilbestrol (DES) in young women after in utero exposure, and (6) occurrence of cytologic, histologic and biochemical alterations in the cervix according to hormonal changes during the menstrual cycle.

The secretory and mitotic activity of the cervical epithelium is clearly responsive to ovarian hormones as well as to exogenous steroids (Hertz 1967). What is true for normal cells might also occur in precancerous tissue. The intensity and especially the imbalance of hormonal stimulation increases the mitotic activity and the duration of

Hafez, E.S.E., Smith, J.P. (eds.), Carcinoma of the Cervix: Biology and Diagnosis. ISBN-13: 978-94-009-7487-6

mitosis, probably leading to the formation of abnormal cells. These cells are characterized by a longer lifetime and a faster reproduction rate than normal cells. In some individuals, particularly susceptible subjects, these alterations may be contributing carcinogenic factors (DeBrux 1972). Even if OCs do not prove to be carcinogenic, they may well be a factor in the biological end transformation that changes cellular replication from a physiological process into a neoplastic one (Jordaan 1972).

I.B. Morphological effects of steroids on the cervix

I.B.1. Histology

A variety of histological changes at the cervix uteri during OC administration have been described, including endocervical erosion, pseudodecidual reaction of the stroma, ectopia, microglandular endocervical hyperplasia and squamous metaplasia (Table 1). Combination contraceptives appear to cause greater histologic changes than sequential agents. Two types of benign atypia are frequently observed in association with OCs.

(a) Epidermialization, a form of squamous metaplasia, is common in women taking sequential OCs. This histological pattern is not specific for exogenous steroid application, but occurs with any relatively unopposed or prolonged estrogen stimulation.

(b) Endocervical microglandular hyperplasia is one of the more specific effects of exogenous steroids on the uterus, and occurs fairly often in patients on combined OCs. There is no statistical connection between microglandular hyperplasia and squamous dyskaryosis or malignancy (Nichols

and Fidler 1971). On clinical examination, the lesions appear polypoid or verrucous and are located at the squamo-columnar junction. Although they rarely appear in a form in which they might be mistaken for malignancy (pseudo-carcinoma), careful examination indicating benign growth is mandatory to avoid needless surgery (Taylor et al. 1967). Discontinuation of the OC usually, but not always, leads to disappearance of the hyperplasia (Seidl 1971; WHO Report 1978). The occurrence of these hyperplastic lesions may be due to the lower dosage of progestin-like agents in current OCs, resulting in a reduction in the anti-estrogenic effect of the component (Taylor et al. 1967).

Both light and electron microscopic studies have failed to detect malignant changes in women using OCs (Gutierrez-Najar et al. 1969; Friedrich 1970). The benign histological changes in women using OCs seem to be an expression of proliferative and functional hyperactivity caused by excessive amounts of potent steroids (Friedrich 1970) and can be compared to the changes occurring during pregnancy (Carbia et al. 1970). It is generally agreed that benign, reversible glandular hyperplasia is the most common histological alteration associated with OCs. Hyperplastic reserve cells, however, may be the origin of severe dysplasia, and incomplete squamous metaplasia could result from the proliferation and abnormal differentiation of the reserve cells (Laguens et al. 1971). This reserve cell theory might explain the development of cancer of the uterine cervix (Coppleson 1970).

The carcinogenic impact of a possible increase of squamous metaplastic activity during OC use (Table 1) is not yet completely understood. Exposure to a carcinogen during a phase of increased

Table 1. Histologic changes during OC administration.

Histologic finding	
Glandular hyperplasia	Attwood 1966; Maqueo et al. 1966; Taylor et al. 1967; Breinl and Warnecke 1967; Kyriakos et al. 1968; Bayer 1968; Kehrer and Mauser 1968; Soost 1968; Candy and Abell 1968; Graham et al. 1968; Talbert and Sherry 1969; Gall et al. 1969; Carbia et al. 1970; Seidl 1971; Fechner 1971; Nichols and Fidler 1971; Mingeot and Fievez 1974; Herting and Schnell 1975
Cervical ectopia	Candy and Abell 1968; Kehrer and Hauser 1968; Gall et al. 1969; Jenson et al. 1970; Dallenbach-Hellweg 1972; Connell 1975
Epidermialization (squamous metaplasia)	Kyriakos et al. 1968; Gall et al. 1969; Carbia et al. 1970; Ide et al. 1972; Mingeot and Fievez 1974; Herting and Schnell 1975

154

metaplastic activity may cause a greater risk of subsequent dysplasia, carcinoma *in situ*, and invasive carcinoma than exposure during a period of metaplastic inactivity (WHO Report 1978). For more detailed information about the specific histological effects of OCs on the genital epithelium, see the review by Fechner (1971). Cytomorphological effects of steroids are reviewed by Dallenbach-Hellweg (1971).

I.B.2. Colposcopy

Leucoplacia, histologically identified as parakeratosis, has most often been reported in connection with oral contraception (Guhr 1965 a,b; Mestwerdt 1972).

Sequential OCs with high-dose estrogen provoke a secretory response, causing hypertrophy of the cervix and its glandular structures. Some eversion of the lower endocervical canal might occur, eventually resulting in metaplasia. Combined OCs do not alter the morphological and dynamic characteristics of the epithelia, other than to increase the production of mucus (Coppleson et al. 1978). Changes at the portio comparable to the appearance during pregnancy have been reported (Soost 1968). Reports indicating a significant increase in the percentage of atypical colposcopic findings during OC administration are rare (Breinl and Warnecke 1967). Most investigators agree that colposcopic follow-ups give normal results (review; see Kaiser 1970).

I.B.3. Cytophotometry

Cytophotometric studies of smears during OC administration reveal that both the DNA of the nuclei and RNA stay within normal ranges (Herzog 1974). However, it has been proposed that contraceptive-hormone therapy frequently leads to a local depletion of folate coenzymes resulting in abnormalities of the DNA synthesis by cervicovaginal cells. The relation to premalignant changes remains controversial (Lindenbaum et al. 1975).

I.C. Experimental steroid application

I.C.1. In vivo studies

Data on animal experiments have been reviewed in detail by Drill (1976). For a summary refer to Population Report of The George Washington University (1977). Various estrogens induce the growth, shorten the induction time and promote the invasiveness of cervical carcinoma in laboratory animals (Kaminetzky 1966, 1973; Myhre and Bjoro 1969; Heston et al. 1973). The administration of high doses of estrogens or of combination OCs (Dunn 1969) for a prolonged period of time increases the occurrence of cervical carcinoma in mice. However, the neoplastic effect of estrogen in animals is strain- and species-dependent. Moreover, Heston et al. (1973) did not find any differences between treated and control animals of the same strain of mouse.

Animal studies relating estrogens with carcinogenesis are inconclusive due to the high dosages used to produce tumors. Mice receiving progestins did not develop cervical cancer (Drill 1975). The progesterone compound seems to protect the cells from carcinogen (Ebner and Sandritter 1968). With very few exceptions, subhuman primates generally appear to be resistant to the carcinogenic effects of steroids indicating that the response obtained in mice is not a general biological phenomenon (Drill 1976). However, malignant uterine mesotheliomas have been demonstrated in squirrel monkeys following estrogen administration (Mc Clure and Graham 1973).

The controversial results in numerous animal species indicate that: (1) dosage, genetic strain, age, and duration of exposure are critical factors in eliciting hormone-induced tumors, and (2) their interpretation with regard to man is difficult. Although most agents that are carcinogenic in man produce malignant tumors in animals, the human population is so heterogenous, that the genetic factor is uncertain (Hertz 1969). Man differs from animals, including other primates, particularly in reproductive functions. Studies in which certain susceptible strains and species are exposed to excessive and continuous dosages cannot be directly related to the effects of OC usage in man, as cervical carcinoma appears to be species-specific. The present knowledge and techniques using animal models in testing sex steroids for carcinogenic effects must be considered to be inadequate.

I.C.2. In vitro studies

Tissue cultures of normal and neoplastic cervical tissue have not undergone any characteristic differentiation when exposed to steroids (Wilbanks 1973; Wolff 1979). There is evidence that synthetic progestogens depress mitosis in uterine cancer cells (Sperling 1975). In view of experimental studies *in vivo* and *in vitro*, it is impossible to draw any firm conclusion about the development of cervical cancer and hormone application.

I.D. Vital and morbidity statistics for carcinoma of the cervix

The results of analyses of death rates for cervical carcinoma during the period of increasing OC use have been controversial. Paffenbarger (1973) concluded from an examination of the death rates for uterine cancer in California for the period 1950–1970, that there is no evidence indicating that OCs induce malignancy in the female reproductive tract. Yet he warned that it may be too early to see such effects, since OCs had been in use for only two decades. Declining death rates for cervical cancer during the time of increased OC use reflect reduced incidence in the disease due to widespread cytological screening (Peckhan 1969; Ravenholt 1972). So far, data from vital or morbidity statistics have yielded relatively little information about a possible connection of OC use and the risk of neoplasia.

I.E. Occurrence of neoplasia during the use of OCs

The occurrence of preclinical and clinical carcinoma of the cervix during the administration of OCs has been observed by several authors (Talbert and Sherry 1969; Diddle et al. 1966; Ayre et al. 1966; Hines and Goldzieher 1968; Cook et al. 1961; Hutcherson et al. 1967; Goldzieher et al. 1968; Laurie and Korba 1971).

As yet, only isolated case reports of cervical adenocarcinoma in connection with oral contraception have been documented (Lauchlan and Penner 1967; Graham et al. 1968; Talbert and Sherry 1969; Czernobilsky et al. 1974; Quizilbash 1975; Gallup and Abell 1977). Adenocarcinomas of the cervix show a greater number of estrogen receptor-positive tumors than squamous carcinomas of the cervix (Martin and Hahnel 1978), indicating that they might be etiologically related to an abnormal response to excessive stimulation by sex steroid hormones (Gallup and Abell 1977).

The results of these tumor registry investigations cannot be evaluated because the incidence of cervical lesions prior to OC use is not known, and the population in the reproductive age range is not given (Ferenczy 1978). As uncontrolled studies they do not provide decisive information about the association between drug exposure and cancer development.

Data relating the occurrence of cervical carcinoma to the use of OCs has shown no marked difference between cervical cancer and control groups (Boyd and Doll 1964). However, in view of reports that occurrence of adenocarcinoma of the cervix is increasing (Gallup and Abell 1977), a careful watch should be kept for evidence of this tendency especially in countries where OCs are widely used.

I.F. Clinical studies

It is generally accepted that cervical cancer progresses from cervical dysplasia to carcinoma *in situ*, and finally to invasive carcinoma. Thus, the clinical evaluation of OCs can be made at different levels, such as on the prevalence of suspicious and abnormal cytological smears, or on the frequency of dysplasia, carcinoma *in situ* and invasive carcinoma (Drill 1975).

I.F.1. Cervical cytology during the administration of OCs

Prevalence. The prevalence rates for suspicious and malignant Papanicolaou (Pap) smears in case-control studies from 1961 to 1975 are summarized in Table 2. This reveals that with few exceptions, the investigations are based on relatively small sample numbers. The studies differ in design, making comparison difficult. In most investigations, case and control groups have not been controlled for some variables which may have had some influence. Although conclusions drawn from the table must be considered with caution for the reasons mentioned above, the studies do not reflect an increase of abnormal smear rates by OC use. Presuming that OCs do not influence cervical cytology, it may be expected on the basis of chance alone that the prevalence rate for OC use will be above the control in about 50% of the studies and below the control in about 50% (Drill 1975). As the prevalence rate for

OC users is slightly below the control rate in 11, equal to the control rate in three and slightly above the control rate in 11 studies, the results only reflect a chance connection.

Combined data from 15 European clinics, (Soost 1968) indicate that the rate of Pap smears of classes III and V is lower in OC users than in non-users. In a comparison of smears from pregnant patients and women receiving high-dose contraception, similar rates of atypical smears were found (de Brux 1974). Cytological examinations of 880 women having used OCs constantly for 8 years did not indicate epithelial atypias (Ebeling et al. 1976). In a mass screening program which included several important variables (age at marriage, number of children, education of the women, and occupation of the husband) Pap smears indicated that women choosing hormonal contraception are not at a higher risk of cervical cancer (Collette et al. 1978).

Incidence. The expected ratio of prevalence rate to annual incidence rate is about 2:1 (Dougherty 1970). However, this was not confirmed by others; in one study, the incidence during use of OCs did not differ significantly from that reported in the literature (Laurie and Korba 1971). Another investigation revealed no difference in the incidence of abnormal smears between the control and study groups (Miller 1973). Pincus and Garcia (1965) found a lower incidence rate in women receiving OCs as compared to those using other forms of contraception.

It has not yet been demonstrated that the incidence of atypical smears for OC users is significantly different from that of a normal screened population. However, differences in the microbiological population of pill users and controls have been reported (Wied et al. 1966). An increase of coccoid bacteria, trichomonas, and fungi in women

Table 2. Prevalence rates for suspicious and malignant cervical smears.

OC users		Controls		Authors
No.	Rate No./100	No.	Rate No./100	
1004	0.4	649	0.6	Tyler 1961
412	0.2	11644	1.1	Pincus 1961
6746	0.8	2510	1.2	Tyler 1964
2850	1.3	2786	3.6	Pincus 1964
270	0.4	3225	0.4	Froewis and Kremer 1965
1346	2.7	4538	3.0	Garcia et al. 1965
490	2.3	500	2.0	Attwood 1966
1628	0.4	19325	0.5	Wied et al. 1966
1000	1.9	200	0.0	Liu et al. 1967
3912	1.0	32046	2.9	Soost and Baier 1967
1031	1.2	32046	2.9	Soost 1968
1746	0.7	?	0.7	Topp and Meissner 1968
2395	0.5	2999	0.4	Andelman et al. 1968
1020	2.6	100000	1.5	Ayre et al. 1969
27508	1.6	6809	0.4	Melamed et al. 1969
2296	2.0	17724	1.0	Kline et al. 1970
4164	0.3	30834	0.6	Chai et al. 1970
1354	9.0	866	5.3 (IUD) 3.1 (diaphragm)	Stern et al. 1970
18380	2.9	127731	1.6	Bibbo et al. 1971
2237	0.9	2000	1.1	Kastner and Holzer 1973
2394	0.6	2294	0.7	Miller 1973
1471	3.9	11654	3.3	Berget and Weber 1974
8366	2.6	?	2.5	Sandmire et al. 1976

using OCs for more than one year suggests that OC administration may account for an increase in atypical cells and class II Pap smears (Scott 1966). Cell abnormalities, corresponding to inflammatory or slight dysplastic changes, are usually spontaneously reversible or regress after cessation of OC use (Favre et al. 1978). Ide et al. (1972) in a prospective study, found different rates of suspicious smears for different types of OCs (1% for sequential OCs, 1% for combined OCs, 0.2% for progestogen OCs).

I.F.2. Dysplasia during the administration of OCs

Cervical dysplasia may be regarded as a transitional state in cervical carcinogenesis, as the majority of new cases of cervical carcinoma originate in a population with dysplastic lesions (Stern 1969).

Prevalence. Prevalence rates for dysplasia in pill users and controls can be seen in Table 3. Bibbo et al (1971) found a rate of dysplasia of 2.3% for OC users as compared to 1.2% in women using no contraception. However, the majority of OC users in this study belonged to certain risk groups. The prevalence of dysplasia was higher in pill choosers than in women preferring other contraceptive methods, before the pill could have had any possible effect (Stern et al. 1970; Ory et al. 1977).

The frequency of dysplasia is apparently influenced by a variety of factors. Choice of contraception as a possible explanatory variable does not seem to be confounded with age at first coitus (Hontz et al. 1974). There are many speculative reasons that might count for this finding, including differences in sexual behavior. Highly significant correlations have been found between: (i) early onset of sexual activity and occurrence of dysplasia, (ii) OC use and occurrence of dysplasia, and (iii) early age as first coitus and OC use.

When correlated for age at first coitus, there was a significantly higher incidence of dysplasia in OC users (Meisels et al. 1977). However, Steps and Finser (1977) did not find a tendency toward promiscuity among aging women using OCs. Hontz et al. (1974), analyzed the age at first intercourse as related to choice of contraceptive methods and did not find any differences between women choosing OCs, IUDs or other methods. Since age at first intercourse is one of the key variables influencing the risk of cervical intraepithelial neoplasia (CIN),

these findings may partly explain the lack of consistently significant differences in the prevalence of CIN between OC and IUD users. Yet, preference for OCs was found among women in lower income groups and among those having been pregnant before the age of 20 (Dubrow et al. 1969).

Incidence. An increased incidence of dysplasia has been reported in women taking the pill (Attwood 1966; Kline et al. 1970). The incidence rates of dysplasia per 1000 women years of follow-up adjusted for age, socio-economic groups, parity, and smoking habits are very similar in the OC and IUD entry groups. Peritz et al. (1977) did not find an association between the incidence of cervical dysplasia and the duration of OC use.

The monitoring of dysplastic changes at the cervix uteri has the advantage of reducing the required sample size, thereby being regarded as a useful tool to study cervical carcinogenesis. However, the number of women with dysplasia progressing to CIN varies according to the technique of diagnosis (cytology versus biopsy), the expertise of diagnosis, the duration of follow-up, and the severity of dysplasia (Richart and Barron 1969). The morphological identification of the various stages of cervical pathology offers room for subjectivity and diagnostic uncertainty. Atypical but benign changes such as atypia associated with inflammation, repair, endocervical hyperplasia etc., are often overdiagnosed as early dysplasia.

The difference between cervical dysplasia and intraepithelial cancer tend gradually to be less and less discernible under the effect of the pill to the extent that in some cases the diagnosis is extremely difficult (Robert and Dupre-Froment 1979). The problem even becomes more complicated when investigators attempt to differentiate not on the basis of histology, but on the cytology alone (Peckhan 1969); this is the case in several studies (Table 2). However, the use of biopsy which is diagnosti-

Table 3. Prevalence rates for dysplasia.

OC users (%)	Controls	Authors
2.2	0.8	Attwood 1966
2.3	3.1 (IUD) 1.2 (No IUD or OC)	Bibbo et al. 1971
0.4	0.5	Berget and Weber 1974

cally more reliable than cytology might remove some of the dysplastic lesions, preventing any meaningful interpretation of follow-up studies (Kline et al. 1970).

Presently, there are no data on which an evaluation of carcinogenic factors on the incidence or progression of early CIN can be based. To meaningfully evaluate the effect of OCs on the incidence of dysplasia, large sample sizes and long follow-up periods are necessary, as carcinoma of the cervix is characterized by both low incidence and a long latency period. According to previous estimates (Richart and Barron 1967; Seigel and Corfman 1968), 60,000 cases and an equal number of controls must be followed for one year in order to detect a doubling of the base incidence of CIN.

A further problem in evaluating the significance of data at present is the unknown prognosis of dysplastic changes. Cervical dysplasia may regress to normal, persist as dysplasia, or progress to carcinoma *in situ*. The frequency with which one stage transforms itself into the next, the rate at which such transformation occurs, and the degree to which the different stages are reversible is difficult to establish.

Several investigators have observed regression of cervical dysplasia during OC use (Ayre et al. 1969; Soost 1968; Kline et al. 1970). Whether the changes can be attributed to the effect of the OCs is highly questionable. Pincus (1965) and Ayre et al. (1969) suggested that OCs may suppress dysplasia. Fuertes de la Haba et al. (1973) reported no significant difference between the patterns of progression and regression of cervical cytological status in users of OCs and vaginal contraceptives. However, this conclusion was based on grouping all women with changes from one diagnostic category of cytological status to another, regardless of whether the change was from normal to atypical or from dysplasia to carcinoma *in situ*. Furthermore, there were no data indicating the degree to which the women studied actually adhered to the method of contraception of which they were originally allocated in this randomized clinical trial. Consequently, the validity of these data remains doubtful. Similar results were achieved by comparing the progression rates among women using either IUDs or OCs or no contraceptives at all (Richart and Barron 1967). However, the percentage of women showing progression or regression will vary considerably depending on such factors as the duration of follow-up, the type of interim treatment used and the severity of the dysplasia (Hall and Walton 1968; Barron and Richart 1970). There is no evidence that the use of OCs is connected with the development of dysplastic changes at an earlier age (Kastner and Holzner 1974; Hertig and Schnell 1975).

I.F.3. Carcinoma in situ during the administration of OCs

Prevalence. The prevalence rates of carcinoma *in situ* in OC users as compared to those in controls are summarized in Table 4. In a case-control study of histologically diagnosed carcinoma *in situ* (Worth and Boyes 1972), there were no significant differences between positive cases and controls in the pattern of OC use. Both groups were comparable with respect to age at marriage and age at first pregnancy, but differed with regard to parity and marital status. In another case-control study, no positive association was shown between the use of either sequential or combination OCs and carcinoma *in situ* (Thomas 1972). No variation was found between patients with intraepithelial neop-

Table 4. Prevalence rates for carcinoma *in situ*.

OC users		Controls		Authors
No.	Rate (No./1000)	No.	Rate No./1000	
27508	6.6	6809	3.8	Melamed et al 1969
4164	1.0	30834	1.7	Chai et al 1970
4455	2.7	5415	3.0 (IUD)	Smithies and Grubb 1970
18380	5.7	127731	3.5	Bibbo et al. 1971
2394	0.8	2394	2.1	Miller 1973
9653	0.5			Vessey et al. 1976
1471	0.2	11654	0.2	Berget and Weber 1974

lasia and randomly selected controls, with regard to OC or IUD use (Sandmire et al. 1976). The study however, did not match for age, parity, and other sex-related variables. Boyce et al. (1977) found both cases and controls to be similar in their current or former use of OCs according to type and mean duration of use. Although the groups in this study were matched for age, ethnic origin, socio-economic status, age at first coitus and age at first pregnancy, the analysis ignored the matched pair design. Results given in Table 5 show that the prevalence rate for carcinoma *in situ* is not influenced by OC administration, although singular studies show opposite conclusions (Wunder 1973; Segal and Anderson 1968).

In a retrospective study comparing OC users to three control groups (postnatal women, IUD users, and women using neither OC nor an IUD), the prevalence rate of carcinoma *in situ* in pill users represented an increase approaching the 5% significance level. Being aware of the deficiencies of a retrospective study, the authors suggested the need for a carefully controlled prospective study (Smithies and Grubb 1970). Melamed et al. (1969) found the prevalence rate for carcinoma *in situ* to be twice as high in OC users as in diaphragm users. This difference can be attributed to either a decreased

prevalence rate for women using a diaphragm or to an increased rate for women using OCs. A lower incidence of cervical carcinoma in women using barrier contraceptive methods has been reported (Boyd and Doll 1964; Worth and Boyes 1972; Boyce et al. 1977; Wright et al. 1978). Thus, diaphragm users cannot be considered as adequate control groups for OC users.

Interpretation of this study is further impaired by the following factors: (i) the sexual behavior of diaphragm users is significantly different to that of OC users (Hertz 1969; Wright et al. 1978). (ii) The population studied included Puerto Rican women who are known to have a higher incidence of cervical cancer (Garcia 1967; Haenszel and Hillhouse 1969). Differences in demographic characteristics between women choosing the pill or the diaphragm have been reported (Dubrow et al. 1969). (iii) The groups were not controlled for major variables, and it cannot be anticipated that OC users and diaphragm users are comparable in all respects except for their choice of contraception. (iv) The rates do not consider variations in cytologic examinations prior to the study, which could significantly affect prevalence rates (Dunn 1969).

Incidence. Keifer and Scott (1975) did not find an increased occurrence of carcinoma *in situ* in OC

Table 5. Studies denying carcinogenecity of IUDs.

No. of subjects	Type of IUD	Duration of use	Findings	Remarks	Authors
72	?	average of 3 years	Most Pap smears of IUD users classified as class I or II		Ishihama and Kagabu 1964
250	Lippes loop	total of 2061 women months	Non of the women wearing an IUD developed malignancy	More than one third of the cases had preinsertional cervical erosion	Shahani et al. 1967
260	Lippes loop	6–7 years	Dysplasia or malignancy was not observed in any one of the smears	Only 12 cases were available for follow-up	Aikat and Aikat 1973
229	Lippes loop	½–8 years	Most dysplasias in IUD users showed regression to normal at follow-up 6–12 months after IUD insertion	Only postinsertional smears were available	Engineer and Misra 1976
193	Lippes loop	1–12 years	Incidence of dysplasia higher in pre than post-insertional smears	Regular follow-up of the IUD users not possible	Engineer et al. 1978
2294	Cu IUD	3 years	More than 80% of dysplasias regressed to normal	Only 46% of initial cases were available for follow-up	Luthra et al. 1977

users. This result was confirmed after controlling their data for the age of the patients (Diddle et al. 1978). The effect to prolonged use of various contraceptives on the early incidence rates of CIN have been evaluated by three major prospective studies: Melamed and Flehinger (1973) reported similar incidence rates of carcinoma *in situ* in women using either OCs, the diaphragm or IUD. Each IUD and diaphragm user was matched with three OC users for age, ethnic origin, age at first pregnancy, number of live births and socioeconomic status. All women were disease-free on admission to the study, and ascertainment of new cases of carcinoma *in situ* during follow-up was provided either cytologically or by biopsy. These cohorts of contraceptive users were followed for 3 years, and there was a steady reduction of subjects from all categories due to loss of follow-up. In another study the rate of CIN during 56,000 women years of prospective observation did not differ significantly between women using OCs and those using IUDs (Vessey et al. 1976). Unlike the study of Melamed and Flehinger (1973), in which more than 70% of the women were lost to follow-up by the end of the observation period, the follow-up in this study was maintained with an annual loss rate of 0.7% to the end of four years of observation. The study of the Royal College of General Practitioners in Britain (1974) produced similar results.

In a case comparison study, the likelihood of occurrence of carcinoma *in situ* increased linearly with the duration of OC use, but there were not any firm biologic interpretations because of the variations in the histological diagnosis of carcinoma *in situ* (Ory et al. 1977). In the Walnut Creek study (Peritz et al. 1977), the incidence of cervical CIN appeared to be initially related to the duration of OC use. Subsequently, after regarding sexual activity, the difference between users and non-users lost its statistical significance, and the association with duration of use was weakened (Ramcharan 1978). Whereas OCs seem to have an initial beneficial effect on cervical dysplasia during the first 6 months of use, life-table analysis reveals a significant increase in progression to carcinoma *in situ* in OC users over a long period of time (Stern et al. 1977). It is suggested that non-reversal of dysplasia within the first 6 months of pill use is predictive of progression after long-term exposure.

I.F.4. *Invasive carcinoma during the administration of OCs*

Lower prevalence rates have been reported for invasive squamous cell carcinoma in OC users as compared to controls using either IUDs or other contraceptive methods (Bibbo et al. 1971; Berget and Weber 1974). This reduced rate for OC users may be explained by more regular check-ups of women taking the pill (Schrage 1965; Courey and Powell 1971). The Royal College of General Practitioners (1974) reported a lower incidence of cervical carcinoma in OC users as compared to non-users, but the numbers were too small to be statistically significant. In a case control study, no association was demonstrated between the use of OCs and the occurrence of cervical carcinoma (Boyce et al. 1972). According to Sandmire et al. (1976), there was no increase in the risk of invasive epidermoid carcinoma in OC users when compared with controls. However, the median age of the study group was lower than that of the controls, thus introducing an age-specific prevalence rate bias.

II. INTRAUTERINE DEVICE

The number of investigations dealing with a possible connection between IUD use and increased risk of cervical neoplasia are limited, as compared to studies on OCs.

II.A. *IUDs and the theory of cervical carcinogenesis*

Theoretically, there are two possible mechanisms that may explain a possible oncogenic potential of IUDs.

II.A.1. *Foreign body reaction*

Since the mechanism of IUD performance consists of a foreign body effect, it may then be compared to other plastic and metallic devices used for prosthetic and cosmetic reasons. After decades of clinical experience, no increase in the incidence of carcinoma in individuals with these devices was detected. If cancer of the uterus is caused by stimulation from a foreign body, it would develop from the endometrium of the uterine cavity which is directly in touch with that foreign body.

II.A.2. Change in cervical secretion

A change in cervical discharge may be a result of altered cell activity and could possibly alter the milieu for the cervical tissue. Changes have been noted in the composition and quantity of cervical secretions among some IUD users, but these changes have not been demonstrated consistently, nor have they been associated with cancerous or precancerous lesions (Moyer and Mishell 1971).

II.B. Morphological effects of IUDs on the cervix

Examinations of colposcopic evaluations of IUD users are limited. In one study, colposcopy was used to determine the site of cervical biopsy, but the colposcopic appearance of the cervix during long-term IUD use was not reported (Medhat, et al. 1980). Whereas changes in the structure of the cervical epithelium have been established by colposcopy during long-term administration of OCs, findings in the cervix of women using IUDs are unremarkable, showing no hyperplastic or hyperemic ectopies (Baader 1974).

II.C. Experimental studies

II.C.1. In vivo studies

In animal experiments, the carcinogenic potential of inert plastic IUDs when embedded subcutaneously has been clearly demonstrated (Oppenheimer et al. 1948; Corfman and Richart 1967). Polyethylene seems to be particularly carcinogenic (Eckardt and Hindin 1973). Uterine epidermoid carcinoma, which seldom occurs spontaneously in rats, was noted after insertion of stainless steel and polyethylene devices (Corfman and Richart 1967). Although experimental findings in animals indicate that the use of IUDs has led either to inflammatory processes or to the development of epidermoid metaplasia followed by squamous epithelioma, similar effects have not been noted in human tissue (Cappelaere 1971).

The oncogenic potential of material used for IUDs has been established in animals, but the results cannot be extrapolated to human conditions. Malignancy after embedding a device subcutaneously is not a true indication of its carcinogenicity inside the uterine cavity.

II.C.2. In vitro studies

Copper ions react with a variety of amino acids and proteins forming chelates which allow the incorporation of the metal into the cell metabolism (Zipper et al. 1971). A decrease in the alkaline phosphatase activity and interference with cellular DNA synthesis may disturb the normal metabolism of human endometrial cells. However, the impact of these results on cervical carcinogenesis has yet to be evaluated.

II.D. Occurrence of neoplasia during the use of IUDs

There are several case reports about the development of cervical neoplasia in women using IUDs (Willson and Ledger 1968; Tietze 1966; Ayre 1965; Sammour et al. 1967; Tichauer and Vargas 1968;

Table 6. Studies indicating carcinogenecity of IUDs.

No. of subjects	Type of IUD	Duration of use	Findings	Remarks	Authors
450	Lippes loop	1–3 months	Marked dysplastic changes developed in few cases after IUD insertion	Pre-insertional smears were available in all women studied. The follow-up rate was 62%	Wahi et al. 1968
637	Cu IUD	2 years	Frequency of dysplasia increases initially during the first 12 months of IUD use	The follow-up rate was 45%	Luthra et al. 1975
152	Lippes loop	3 years	The incidence of dysplasia slightly higher in IUD users than in controls	Pre-insertional smears were available in less than half of the studied women	Misra and Engineer 1976

Phillips and Lu 1970; Shimomura 1972; Goldman and Halbrecht 1973) and it was concluded that the neoplasia cannot be related to the presence of an IUD. However, it is impossible to interpret the results of these studies accurately as the series were small, there were no control groups for comparing results, and details about the population from which the sample was collected were not available. Comparing different types of contraception, the incidence rate of biopsy-proven cervical neoplasia was much lower in diaphragm users than in IUD users (Wright et al. 1978). Diaphragm users however, cannot be regarded as an acceptable control group.

II.E. Clinical studies

II.E.1. Cervical cytology during the use of IUDs

Relevant cervical smear studies are summarized in Table 7. Evaluations of cytology after IUD insertion reveal that prolonged usage of IUDs is often associated with exfoliation of atypical cells which may be mistaken as representing carcinoma (Ayre 1965; Abrams and Spritzer 1966; Sagirogolu and Sagirogolu 1977; Gupta et al. 1971; Ashton and Johnston 1975; Misra and Engineer 1976; Misra et al. 1977; Gupta et al. 1978). Three types of epithelial atypia have been associated with IUDs. (a) Squamous atypia in exfoliative smears occurs more often in IUD users than in the general population; however this is not necessarily significantly related to the IUD. (b) The columnar atypias associated with IUDs are characterized by cells with hyperdistended cytoplasmatic vacuoles. They probably represent atypical secretion associated with inflammation, but may strongly suggest cells shed from an adenocarcinoma. (c) The indeterminate atypia can mimic carcinoma in situ, and must therefore be carefully discriminated from neoplasia. The origin of these atypical cells associated with IUDs is not fully understood, but their identity with metaplastic cells has been proposed (Piver et al. 1966). Marked dysplastic changes reported in some

Table 7. Important findings of cervical smear studies in IUD users.

Type of IUD	Duration of use	Method of investigation	Findings	Authors
Yusie Ring	?	Smear	No significant difference in the incidence of class I–III smears between IUD users and non-users	Hata et al. 1969
Lippes loop	5 years	Smear	No significant difference in the incidence of negative suspicious smears between IUD users and non-users	Ishihama et al. 1970
Cu IUD	½–4 years	Smear	Incidence of dysplasia lower in Cu IUD users than in loop users	Misra et al. 1977
Birnberg bow & Lippes loop	1 year	Smear	Rate of suspicious and atypical smears (class III and IV) in IUD users similar to that in general screening	Piver et al. 1966
Lippes loop & Birnberg bow & Hall and Stone Stainless steel ring	?	Smear/colposcopy	No significant difference in progression rates between IUD users and non-users	Richart and Barron 1967
Lippes loop	2 weeks–4,5 yr	Smear, endometrial washing endometrial biopsy	Marked dysplastic changes in few cases of IUD users	Wahi et al. 1968
Lippes loop	2 weeks–4,4 yr	Smear, cervical biopsy	Higher incidence of dysplasia grade I and II in IUD users than in controls	Luthra and Wahl 1968
Lippes loop	½–1 year	Smear	No increase of suspicious smears in IUD users	Aikat 1968

Lippes loop users were considered severe enough for the IUD to be removed (Wahi et al. 1968). Tietze (1966) observed a 1% increase in dysplasia with inert IUDs.

Several reports indicate that the prevalence of cervical lesions does not increase with the use of copper IUDs (Hegenfeldt 1972; Tatum 1971; Luthra et al. 1975, 1977; Affandi and Virkar 1976). However, in most studies the follow-up period was too short to draw firm conclusions. Exfoliative cytological studies have demonstrated the increased incidence of dysplasia among Lippes loop users to be negligible when compared to the controls (Misra and Engineer 1976). In another study the same authors reported an almost identical incidence rate for both Lippes loop users and controls, with a slightly higher incidence rate of inflammatory changes in the IUD group (Engineer and Misra 1976). When following Lippes loop users for periods ranging from 1 to 12 years, the incidence of dysplasia was higher in pre-insertional smears than in the post-IUD smears (Engineer et al. 1978). A comparison of pre- and post-insertion cytology of inert IUD users revealed only inflammatory changes (Chun and Chung 1965). Until now, no abnormal cytological changes due to the use of copper IUDs have been reported (Tatum 1971; Hegenfeldt 1972). The follow-up period of most studies was short and post-insertional cytology demonstrated a lower incidence of dysplastic lesions among women with copper IUDs as compared to those using Lippes loop (Misra et al. 1977). Despite the experimental results previously mentioned, the copper IUDs may have a protective effect against the occurrence of cervical dysplasia. All studies mentioned thus far have failed to detect any abnormal development of cervical tissue in the presence of inert or copper IUDs. These studies however, have lacked in control groups.

Several studies have compared the cervical cytology in IUD users and non-users in cytologic screening programs (Ishihama and Kagabu 1964, 1965; Dabancens et al. 1974; Piver et al. 1966; Pincus and Garcia 1965; Misra and Engineer 1976; Ishihama et al. 1970). The prevalence rates for cervical lesions in pregnant women, non-pregnant women, current OC users, current IUD users and women using neither OCs or IUDs have been compared which indicate that current IUD users have the highest rate of dysplasia among the six groups (Bibbo et al. 1971). Pincus and Garcia (1965) reported suspicious Pap smears in 5.4% of IUD users, whereas the corresponding rate in non-users was only 2.9%. However, it is not evident from the study that the group of IUD users are a random sample of the total population from which the base rate was estimated (Richart and Barron 1967). Davies and Wardle (1976) found a higher incidence of smears containing malignant or dyskaryotic cells than that reported as the national average. In contrast, case control studies comparing IUD users to women using no contraception at all indicate that use of IUDs does not increase the risk of developing cervical carcinoma (Sandmire et al. 1976).

Most of the studies listed fail to indicate a significant difference in the smears between IUD users and non-users. However, the selection of control groups does not allow any definite conclusions to be drawn from the results, as these groups include women using either OCs or barrier methods or no contraception at all. Furthermore, most studies do not examine long-term effects of IUD use beyond 5 years, although the latent time for cervical cancer is estimated to 7–10 years.

Follow-ups of women using recently developed copper IUDs cannot be regarded as sufficient (Luthra et al. 1975). A combined evaluation of Pap smears, colposcopy and colposcopically directed biopsies of women using IUDs for an average of 5 years and of matched controls did not show significant differences between IUD users and non-users regarding dysplastic and non-dysplastic changes (Medhat et al. 1980).

Ayre (1965) found progressing changes of the cervical epithelium in five women during a short period after IUD insertion. Luthra et al. (1975) observed one case of severe dysplasia progressing to carcinoma *in situ* following the insertion of a copper IUD. However, these findings have not been confirmed by other studies. Follow-up of IUD users and controls showed no significant increase in the rate of progression from cervical dysplasia to carcinoma *in situ* between the two groups (Piver et al. 1966). Richart and Barron (1967) reported in a 3 year study that the life table rates of progression from dysplasia to carcinoma *in situ* were not significantly different for IUD users and non-users.

Wahi et al. (1968) published similar results.

The only prospective study (Tietze 1966), reports a 1% transition from a preinsertional negative smear to dysplasia and appearance of carcinoma *in situ* in four of the 4,800 cases after 6 months of IUD use. In two-thirds of these cases, the dysplastic changes showed regression. A long-term study in Lippes loop users achieved similar results: in the majority of cases, preinsertional dysplasia regresses to normal during the postinsertional period instead of advancing towards malignancy (Misra and Engineer 1976; Engineer et al. 1978). Aikat and Aikat (1973) reported similar results. Analysis of yearly incidence of dysplasia indicated a declining trend with prolonged use of Lippes loop (Misra and Engineer 1976). Long-term follow-up studies reported almost normal smears in the majority of women using inert IUDs for more than 5 years (Lippes 1967; Hill 1969; Sagiroglu and Sagiroglu 1970). The accumulated data fail to indicate any progression of dysplasia with prolonged retention of an IUD, and should be considered as insufficient.

III. CONTRACEPTION AS A VARIABLE IN CERVICAL CARCINOGENESIS

Epidemiological evidence supports the concept that cervical precancerous lesions and carcinoma are coitally related, specifically with age at first coitus and the number of sexual partners (Rotkin 1967, 1973; Martin 1967; Moghissi and Mack 1968; Barron and Richart 1970). Although the sexual transmission of a carcinogen appears to be the key variable, endocrine factors may play an accessory role. Endocrine imbalance may increase mitotic activity and lengthen duration of mitosis, probably leading to the production of abnormal cells. These changes may have a direct correlation to carcinogenic potential in certain sensitive individuals (de Brux 1972). Contraceptives may promote cervical carcinogenesis indirectly since variables accounting for differences in risk of cervical carcinoma may at the same time characterize groups using certain contraceptive methods. Promiscuous young women have an increased incidence of metaplasia apparently initiated and maintained by coitus (Coppleson 1970). Coital

frequency in both OC and IUD users exceeded that of other contraceptive users, even when age, race, education, and religion were controlled variables (Westoff et al. 1969). Sexually active women have an increased incidence of cervical ectopy (Moghissi 1973).

Eversion of endocervical columnar epithelium to the vaginal environment induces squamous metaplastic transformation, probably a precursor of cervical neoplasm (Coppleson 1970). Reliable contraception may be associated with a more permissive attitude of decreasing the age at first coitus and increasing the frequency of intercourse, probably with several partners, thus playing its part in the development of cervical atypia. However, OCs may block the passage of sexually transmitted mutagens by making cervical mucus thick and impenetrable (Singer and Jordan 1977). OC administration may also lead to more regular examinations by Pap smear, thereby increasing the probability of early diagnosis of cervical lesions (Thompson 1969; Courey and Powell 1971; Diddle et al. 1978). Although, the screening of a population generally lowers the mortality rate, it is not known whether systematic screening of patients using contraceptives (motivated toward by either selecting contraception or cancer screening) will lower the mortality rate from cervical cancer. For further understanding of the relationship between OCs and cervical carcinoma, see the review by Wolff (1979) and Moghissi (1977).

IV. METHODOLOGY IN CANCER RESEARCH

Due to apparent conflicts in the available data and difficulties in interpreting certain findings, it is necessary to consider some technical issues.

IV.A. Problems of data collection

IV.A.1. General problems

As yet, there is no suitable animal model for testing cervical carcinogenesis, and extrapolation of conclusions from one species to another has dubious validity. The double blind clinical trial for the assessment of a carcinogenic effect of a drug or device is impossible for contraceptives since it is unlikely that adequate numbers of women would accept the random allocation of various contraceptive methods. Furthermore, random allocation as carried out during the original studies in Puerto Rico is not ethically acceptable. Evaluation must then depend on observational studies, mainly case control and cohort studies. Most investigators have studied fairly highly-selected biased population samples from which general conclusions could not be made. Even considering known differences between case and control groups, the problem of self-selection in a non-randomized study is never completely resolved. A further problem, inherent in the sample itself, is the follow-up: users of contraceptives tend to belong to unstable populations in which contraceptive methods are often discontinued or changed. Women who were not using contraception at the beginning of the study may have started later, thus altering the control group. Studies with an extensive follow-up period are needed to evaluate long-term effects of steroid contraceptives. Available data only relate to a relatively limited time of the reproductive period, and it is currently impossible to predict long-term sequelae of steroid contraceptive use.

The time required may be reduced by studying the rates of progression from dysplasia to carcinoma *in situ*. This approach, based on the assumption that such progression rates are indicators of carcinogenesis, has been attempted for the study of both OCs and IUDs.

IV.A.2. Problems of prospective studies

Prospective studies, although desirable, are difficult and costly to perform because of the rare occurrence, the long latency period of cervical carcinoma, and the requirement of a large sample size. Based on a yearly incidence rate of 0.3% for carcinoma of the cervix, 60,000 women using OCs and a control group of the same size would have to be followed for one year in order to establish a twofold increase of the base incidence of CIN. To reduce the sample size to 35,000, the study would have to be continued for 10 years (Richart and Barron 1967; Stern et al. 1970; Seigel and Corfman 1968). The required numbers are reduced if the study is extended over a longer period of time since the incidence of cancer increases with age. This advantage is however, counterbalanced by the problems associated with prolonged follow-up.

IV.A.3. Problems of retrospective studies

Retrospective studies require much smaller sample sizes than prospective studies. Criticism of the retrospective approach includes the hazards of bias in the choice of study cases and controls, and in obtaining histories. Users of contraceptives are self-selected and undergo further screening by their physicians on the basis of their medical histories. In addition, the pattern of contraceptive practice in a given population varies over time and women may have problems in recalling the types of contraceptives used in the past and the duration of different episodes of use.

Both type and dose of steroids in contraceptives have been greatly altered over the past decade. Doses of estrogens and progestogens in combined OCs have been progressively reduced. All of the new formulations introduced in the U.S. during the last 9 years contain less than 50 ug of ethinyl-estradiol and less than 1 mg of norethindrone. New progestogens are being introduced, while others (17-hydroxyprogesterones) are being withdrawn. Sequential pills for instance have been taken off the market in some countries. Experience with recently introduced OCs such as the mini-pill, is sufficient. As a woman may be exposed to a variety of preparations and dosages during her reproductive period, it is difficult to associate exposure of one specific OC with cervical carcinogenesis thus restricting generalization from currently available research data (WHO Scientific Group 1978; Seigel and Corfman 1968).

IV.B. Problems with interpretation of results

There are several factors contributing to the controversy about any association of cervical carcinoma with OCs and IUDs in the current literature. Inconsistent design of the statistical approach does not allow a comparison of different studies. Prevalence rates can only be determined by cytological examinations performed for the first time in the study group which is unlikely to occur in a mass screening program. In reports on the determination of incidence rates of cervical carcinoma, it usually remains uncertain as to whether the patients were adequately screened before entering the study. Patients with suspicious smears were either admitted to follow-up studies or the initial cytological status was not indicated. Only a few investigations are restricted to one type of IUD or OC; therefore, the variety of OC formulations and IUD materials may mask or confuse factors contributing to carcinogenesis. Most studies do not control for key variables such as age at first coitus, age, ethnic background, frequency of sexual activity, number of sexual partners, parity and socioeconomic status.

Most published results are derived from routine cervical cytology or screening programs which are not specifically designed to test the effects of the pill or IUD on women using these methods over a 5 year period or more. As long as it is not known whether or not OCs and IUDs are positively related to cervical cancer and whether the diaphragm has a protective effect, it is impossible to have women using any other kind of contraception as a control group. Failure to select comparable controls or to correct for differences between cases and controls during analysis, decreases the confidence of case control studies. Cohort studies are easier to interpret than case-control studies since standardized incidence rates among different groups can be directly estimated. However, losses to follow-up, particularly if they are numerous or selective, reduce the validity of these studies.

IV.C. Inconsistent diagnostic methodology

The terminology, diagnostic criteria and methods of precancerous and cancerous lesions differ enough to affect interpretations of results. It is questionable whether there are adequate confirmations of Pap smears and histologic diagnosis in all studies. Even if apparently causal associations between OC use and precancerous lesions are demonstrated; these findings may not necessarily imply an increased risk of subsequent invasive carcinoma. These aspects are important for the evaluation of the current data because virtually all studies consider dysplasia and carcinoma *in situ* rather than invasive carcinoma. The determination of progression rates from dysplasia to carcinoma in cohort studies does not solve the question of initiation of malignant growth by contraceptives. Conclusions from case control studies are usually expressed as relative risk or risk ration, based upon the ratio between the incidence among the case and

control group. However, comparing the ratio of disease incidence among users versus non-users in case control studies reveals the relative risk which is an index of association only. Proof of a causal connection would require further evidence (WHO Report 1978). Methodological gaps may or may not account for the conflicting results of retrospective studies. Again prospective studies are rare because they require large sample sizes, long-term follow-up, and a very stable population. What is true for studies on OCs can basically be applied to those on IUDs An aggravating factor in IUD research however, is the limited number of studies carried out so far. These problems have confronted investigators since the use of OCs and IUDs has become widespread. The large-scale use of these contraceptives in Asia means risking, in effect, a worldwide uncontrolled experiment.

V. FUTURE RESEARCH

Further basic research is needed on oncogenesis, particularly with regard to the role of steroids and IUD materials. Ultrastructural investigations, in addition to the conventional light microscopy studies, might be useful. Research on larger and better-controlled samples is required to assess the validity of the trends reported in previous studies. Prevalence and incidence rates of cervical carcinoma in users and non-users of contraceptives must be clarified. Observations of progression rates may answer the question as to wheter women with dysplasia may have an increased risk of cancer associated with OC use. Any consideration of the problem must take into account the biased choice of contraceptives among population groups with different probabilities of developing carcinoma of the cervix. Attention must be given to contraceptive use in relation to key life events such as adolescence and childbirth. Changes in exposure related to age and parity may alter the risk of carcinogenesis associated with OCs or IUDs. The multiple-risk factors contributing to cervical carcinogenesis, which themselves may influence the use of contraception, must be considered. Contraception and its inter-relationship with other variables needs further investigation as it may only affect the risk of neoplasia in the presence of predisposing factors.

The effects of contraceptives among subgroups with risk factors known to affect the risk of neoplasia should likewise be studied. A variety of issues remain to be solved by specially designed studies:

1. The dose effect of steroid hormones on the cervical epithelium, including the cumulative effect of prolonged or repeated OC exposure.

2. The time effect of contraception on cervical tissue, including the time of first exposure (teenage versus adult) and duration of use (short-term versus long-term).

3. The influence of contraception on the usual procedures for determining and curing precancerous conditions (eventually increased frequency of visits to the physician, increased vigilance of the physician, increased frequency of biopsies because of dysplasia etc.).

International studies employing common protocols and research instruments are necessary to facilitate conclusive interpretation and generalization of findings. It is hoped that specific documentation about the type and pattern of contraceptive practice will accompany future studies in order to allow differentiation. In view of the impact of any statement on a relationship between contraception and the occurrence of cervical carcinoma, future studies require a high confidence level. Preliminary reports, helpful as they may be for the initiation and design of further studies, should be restricted in a matter of similar popularity as contraception, thus preventing further confusion about the problem in question. The need for long-term funding of follow-up studies is obvious, and it is felt that drug companies should initiate the necessary funding for at least part of the pre- and post-marketing research. Drugs with less potentially adverse effects, utilizable in small dosages and improved contraceptive devices need to be developed through continuing research.

VI. CONCLUDING REMARKS

Unfortunately, the vast amount of literature on possible relationships between the use of estrogens and cervical carcinoma does not clarify the issue but causes confusion and brings an occasional lack of objectivity to the controversy. A relationship between steroid hormones and carcinogenesis has often been suspected, but never proved. Efforts to resolve the issue by animal experiments fail to give conclusive results, mainly due to difficulties in extrapolating findings. Tissue cultures of normal and neoplastic cervical epithelium exposed to steroids have not undergone any characteristic differentiation. Neither light and electron-microscopic nor biochemical observations have yielded any information.

Increased frequency of invasive carcinoma following certain forms of contraception has not been demonstrated, but suspicious cytological and histological findings, suggestive of precancerous conditions, have been reported. Although some studies have linked OC use with an increased incidence of cervical cancer, the interpretation of their results is difficult. Case reports reviewed thus far, have proved to be somewhat exaggerated, and the conclusions drawn are only partially true. Currently, available epidemiological data do not provide a sound statistical basis. Prospective studies have encountered difficulties, such as evaluation of all the major co-variables and high dimensionality of the data.

In most studies conducted prior to 1975, there is no direct check for possible confounding between OC use and age at first coitus or number of sexual partners. Use of other variables to indirectly check for possible confounding between contraceptive methods and sexual behavior may be insufficient. Re-analysis of several studies taking these factors into account have altered the previous conclusions.

Despite the long history of IUD development and its widespread use, systematic studies on the effects of the IUD on the cervix uteri have not been carried out. The data available do not suggest an etiologic role of IUDs in the development of cervical carcinoma or any contribution to a more rapid progression of dysplasia to cancer. However, epidemiologic literature on the association of cervical carcinoma with IUD use gives inconclusive evidence of a direct connection as the most important variable, age at first coitus, is not considered in any of the studies. Whereas, the preponderance of data indicates that inert IUDs do not have any effect on the cervical epithelium, studies describing the effect of copper on the cervical epithelium with regard to dysplasia cannot be regarded as efficient. As yet, data to evaluate the question of whether and how

OCs and IUDs interact with other risk factors in influencing cervical carcinogenesis is insufficient. Studies examining the question, whether by choosing to use OCs, a woman identifies herself as being at higher risk of developing dysplasia or carcinoma *in situ*, came to different conclusions. Increased risk of cervical dysplasia and carcinoma *in situ* may be associated with OC administration, especially long-term use by women with predisposing factors. Very few data are currently available concerning the effect of contraceptive methods on the risk of invasive carcinoma of the cervix. Recommendations for future research are outlined. Popularity of the controversy about contraception in the medical journals as well as in the lay press calls for conclusive comments. However, for reasons mentioned above, any final conclusions must be deferred. Lack of conclusive data gives way to more or less speculative thoughts about the role of contraceptives among factors of cervical carcino-genesis. The present state of knowledge emphasizes the responsibility of physicians prescribing contraception to monitor their clients carefully and to make their data quickly available to the scientific community. The fundamental question for patient and physician is whether the need for OC and IUD is great enough to require daily ingestion of a potent drug or permanent insertion of an intrauterine device; either of which, may or may not have the potential for causing or advancing cancer. According to common statements in previous reviews, the risks of contraception are low as compared to those of unwanted pregnancies. However, only the individuals concerned can decide whether the benefit is worth the risk. The principal of public health, that a drug or device be proven safe before and not after it is marketed, needs to be observed more strictly. The remaining unfortunate question is how long women will be willing to continue serving as guinea pigs for contraceptive research.

REFERENCES

Abrams RY, Spritzer T: Endometrial cytology in patients using intrauterine contraceptive devices. Acta Cytol 10, 240, 1966.

Affandi MZ, Virkar KD: Cytological follow up of 200 women using copper devices for contraception. Contraception 13, 739–746, 1976.

Aikat M: Cytological study in women with Lippes loop. *In* Laumas KR (ed): Review of Research Work in India on Intrauterine Contraceptive devices. New Delhi: Indian Council of Medical Research, pp 65Ø73, 1968.

Aikat M, Aikat BK: Long term effect of Lippes loop on cervical epithelium and endometrium. Indian J Med Res, 61, 1313, 1973.

Andelman MB, Zackler J, Slutsky HL, Jacobson MM: Family planning and public health. Int J Fertil 13, 405, 1968.

Ashton PR, Johnston WW: Cytopathologic alterations associated with intrauterine contraceptive devices. Acta Cytol 19, 583, 1975.

Attwood ME: Cytology and contraceptive pill. J Obstet Gynaecol Br Commonw 73, 662, 1966.

Ayre JE: Human precarcinogenic cell manifestations associated with polyethylene contraceptive device. Ind Med Surg 34, 394, 1965.

Ayre JE, Hillemanns HG, LeGuerrier J, Arsenault J: Influence of morethynodrel and mestranol upon cervical dysplasia and carcinoma *in situ*. Obstet Gynecol 28, 90, 1966.

Ayre JE, Reyner FC, Fagundes WB, LeGuerrier JM: Oral progestins and regression of carcinoma *in situ* and cervical dysplasia. Obstet Gynecol 34, 545, 1969.

Baader O: Colposcopic findings in contraception. J Reprod Med 12, 186, 1974.

Barron BA, Richart RM: An epidemiologic study of cervical neoplastic disease. Cancer 27, 978, 1970.

Bayer R: Vergleichsuntersuchungen mit Ovulationshemmern zur Darstellung der direkten und indirekten Auswirkungen auf Portio und Scheide. Gynaekol 90, 552, 1968.

Berget A, Weber T: Influence of oral contraceptives on cytology and histology of the cervix uteri. Dan Med Bull 21, 172, 1974.

Bibbo M, Keebler CM, Wied GL: Prevalence and incidence rates of cervical atypia. J Reprod Med 6, 184, 1971.

Boyce JG, Lu T, Nelson JH Jr, Fruchter RG: Oral contraceptives and cervical carcinoma. J Obstet Gynecol 128, 761, 1977.

Boyce JG, Lu T, Nelson JG, Joyce D: Cervical carcinoma and oral contraception. Obstet Gynecol 40, 139, 1972.

Boyd JT, Doll R: A study of the aetiology of carcinoma of the cervix uteri. Br J Cancer 18, 419, 1964.

Breinl H, Warnecke W: Langzeitbehandlung mit Ovulations-hemmern. Med Klin 62, 1835, 1967.

Candy J, Abell MR: Progestogen induced adenomatous hyperplasia of the uterine cervix. J Am Med Assoc 203, 323, 1968.

Cappelaere P: Contraception et risques cancérigènes. Lille Médicale, Series 3, 16 (Special Issue), 45, 1971.

Carbia E, Rubio-Linares G, Alvarado-Duran A, Lopez-Llera M: Histologic study of the uterine cervix during oral contraception with ethynodiol diacetate and mestranol. Obstet Gynecol 35, 381, 1970.

Chai MS, Johnson WD, Tricomi V: Five years experience with contraceptive pills: Cervical epithelial changes. N.Y. State J Med, 70, 2663, 1970.

Chun D, Chung HK: Vaginal cytology in women using intrauterine device. *In* Intrauterine Contraception. Proc Second Int Conference, New York. SJ Seagal, AL Southam KD Shafer (eds). Excerpta Medica, Amsterdam pp 157–158, 1965.

Collette HA, Linthorst G, Waard F: Cervical carcinoma and the pill. Lancet 1, 441, 1978.

Connell EB: The pill revisited. Fam Plann Perspect 7, 62, 1975.

Cook HH, Gamble CF, Satterthwaite AP: Am J Obstet Gynecol 82, 437, 1961.

Coppleson M: The origin and nature of premalignant lesions of the cervix uteri. Int J Gynaecol Obstet 8, 539, 1970.

Coppleson M, Pixley E, Reid B: Colposcopy, a Scientific and Practical Approach to the Cervix and Vagina in Health and Disease. Thomas, Springfield, IL, p 116, 1978.

Corfman PA, Richart RM: Induction in rats of uterine epidermoid carcinoma by plastic and stainless steel intrauterine devices. Am J Obstet Gynecol 98, 987, 1967.

Courey NG, Powell AS: The pill, the smear and cancer. NY State J Med 71, 2513, 1971.

Czernobilsky B, Kessler I, Lancet M: Cervical adenocarcinoma in a woman on long term contraceptives. Obstet Gynecol 43, 517, 1974.

Dabancens A, Prado R, Larraguibel R, Zanartu J: Intraepithelial cervical neoplasia in women using intrauterine devices and long-acting progestogens as contraceptives. Am J Obstet Gynecol 119, 1052, 1974.

Dallenbach-Hellweg G: Differentiation of normal and carcinomatous vaginal epithelial cell. Normal, abnormal and atypical differentiation processes. Cytological criteria of the malignant cell. Beitr Pathol 147, 71, 1971.

Davies M, Wardle C: The effect of the intrauterine device and oral contraceptives on the cervical smear. Acta Cytol 20, 493, 1976.

DeBrux J: Oestro-progestatifs oraux et col utérin. Pathol Eur 7, 283, 1972.

DeBrux J: Les Lésions du col utérin au cours de la contraception orale. Sem Hôp Paris 22, 1491, 1974.

DeLignières B: Les estroprogestatifs de synthèse; risques et contre-indications. Synthetic estroprogestational agents: risks and contraindications. Gaz Méd Fr 85, 3117, 1978.

Diddle AW, Gardner WH, Williamson PJ, Johnson JR, Hemphill JL, Goodwin CW: Oral contraceptive steroids and dysplasia and carcinoma of the cervix uteri. J Tenn Med Assoc 71, 725, 1978.

Diddle AW, Watts GF, Gardner WH, Williamson PJ: Oral contraceptive medication: A prolonged experience. Am J Obstet Gynecol 95, 489, 1966.

Dougherty M: Cervical cytology and sequential birth control pills. Obstet Gynecol 36, 741, 1970.

Drill VA: Oral contraceptives; relations to mammary cancer, benign breast lesions, and cervical cancer. Annu Rev Pharmacol 15, 367, 1975.

Drill VA: Effect of estrogens and progestins on the cervix uteri. J Toxicol Environ Health 1, 193, 1976.

Dubrow H, Melamed MR, Flehinger BJ: A study of factors affecting choice of contraceptives. Obstet Gynecol Surv 24, 1012, 1969.

Dunn TB: Cancer of the uterine cervix induced in Balb mice by an antifertility drug. Proc Am Assoc Cancer Res 10, 21, 1969.

Ebeling K, Ruckhaberle B, Kuhndel K, Schulz S, Kronert M: Ergebnisse zytologischer und histologischer Untersuchungen der Cervix uteri nach längerer Einnahme hormoneller Kontrazeptiva. Z Gynaekol 7, 385, 1976.

Ebner HJ, Sandritter W: The effects of norprogesterone on experimental cancer of the cervix. Ger Med Mon 13, 41, 1968.

Eckardt RE, Hindin R: The health hazards of plastics. Med Res Div, Esso Res Engineering Co, Linden NJ, J Occup Med 15, 808, 1973.

Engineer AD, Mistra JS: Cytological studies in women using intrauterine contraception. Indian J Med Res 64, 1255, 1976.

Engineer AD, Mistra JS, Tandon P: Cervical studies in Lippes loop users. Indian J Med Res 67, 953, 1978.

Favre J, Siebert S, Drevet N: Oral oestroprogestative concentration and cervical and vaginal cytology. Archs Anat Cytol

Pathol 26, 234, 1978.

Fechner RE: The surgical pathology of the reproductive system and breast during oral contraceptive therapy. Pathol Annu 6, 299, 1971.

Ferenczy A: Steroid contraception and cervical and ovarian neoplasia. *In* Risks, Benefits and Controversies in Fertility Control. JJ Sciarra, J Zatuchni, JJ Spiedel (eds) Harper & Row, New York, pp 194–210, 1978.

Frazer RC, Cudmore DC, Melanson J, Morse W: The metabolism and production rate of estradiol 17 B in premenopausal women with cervical carcinoma. Am J Obstet Gynecol 98, 509, 1967.

Friedrich ER: Do oral contraceptives cause premalignant endocervical changes? Int J Gynaecol Obstet: 8, 114, 1970.

Froewis J, Kremer H: Zur Frage der kanzerogenen Wirkung von oral wirksamen Oestrogen-Gestagen-Hormonkombinationen. Wien Klin Wochenschr: 77, 792, 1965.

Fuertes-de la Haba A, Pelergrina I, Bangdiwala IS, Hernandez-Cibes JH: J Reprod Med: 10, 3, 1973.

Gall SA, Bourgeois C, Maguire R: The morphologic effect of oral contraceptive agents on the cervix. J Am Med Assoc: 207, 2243, 1969.

Gallup DG, Abell MR: Invasive adenocarcinoma of the uterine cervix. Obstet Gynecol: 49, 000, 1977.

Garcia CR: The oral contaceptive. An appraisal and review Am J Med Sci: 253, 718, 1967.

Garcia CR, Incus G, Rocamora H, Wallach EE: Proc 6th Panam Congr of Endocrinol Int Congr Ser 112 Excerpta Medica, Amsterdam pp 138–149, 1965.

Goldman JA, Halbrecht I: Invasive epidermal carcinoma of the cervix in a woman with an IUD; a case report. Contraception 7, 227, 1973.

Goldzieher JW, Maas JM, Hines DC: Seven years of clinical experience with a sequential oral contraceptive. Int J Fertil: 13, 399, 1968.

Graham J, Graham R, Hirabayashi K: Reversible cancer and the contraceptive pill. Report of a case. Obstet Gynecol: 31, 190, 1968.

Guhr O: Kolposkopische, cytologische und histologische Portiobefunde bei ovulationshemmenden Medikamenten. Arch Gynaekol: 202, 205, 1965a.

Guhr O: Kolposkopische, zytologische und histologische Portiobefunde unter ovulationshemmender Medikation. Muenchen Med Wochenschr: 107, 485, 1965b.

Guiterrez-Najar A, Giner-Valazquez J, Martinez-Manautou J: Role of cervical mucus in contraception with the continuous chlormadinone acetate method. Adv Plann Parenth: 4, 97, 1969.

Gupta PK, Burroughs F, Luff RD, Frost JK, Erozan YS: Epithelial atypias associated with intrauterine contraceptive devices (IUD). Acta Cytol: 5, 286, 1978.

Gupta PK, Malkani PK, Bhasin K: Cellular response in the uterine cavity after IUD insertion and structural changes of the IUD. Contraception: 4, 375, 1971.

Haenszel W, Hillhouse M: Uterine cancer morbidity in New York City and its relation to the pattern of regional variation within the United States. J Natl Cancer Inst: 22, 1157, 1969.

Hall JE, Walton L: Dysplasia of the cervix. A prospective study of 206 cases. Am J Obstet Gynecol: 100, 662, 1968.

Hata Y, Ishihama A, Kundo N, Nakamura Y, Miyai T, Makino T, Kagabu T: The effect of long term use of intrauterine devices. Int J Fertil: 14, 241, 1969.

Hegenfeldt K: Studies on the mode of action of the Cu-T device. Acta Endocrinol (Suppl): 71, 165, 1972.

Herting W, Schnell JD: Morphologische Veränderungen an

170

Zervix-Schleimhaut und Plattenepithel der Portio bei Frauen mit und ohne Einnahme von Ovulationshemmern. Fortsch Med: 4, 176, 1975.

Hertz R: The role of steroid hormones in the etiology and pathogenesis of cancer. Am J Obstet Gynecol: 98, 1013, 1967.

Hertz R: Report of the task force on carcinogenesis. In United States Food and Drug Administration. Advisory Committee of Obstetrics and Gynecology. Second report on the oral contracepives. Government Printing Office, 1969.

Herzog RE: Zytophotometrische und interferenzmikroskopische Untersuchungen über die mögliche Karzinogenität von Ovulationshemmern. Arch Gynakol: 217, 443, 1974.

Heston WE, Vlahakis G, Desmukes B: Effects of antifertility drug Enovid in five strains of mice, with particular regard to carcinogenesis. J Natl Cncer Inst: 51, 209, 1973.

Hill AM: Contraception with Grafenberg ring. Am J Obstet Gynaecol: 103, 200, 1969.

Hines DC, Goldzieher JW: Large scale study of an oral contraceptive. Fertil Steril: 19, 841, 1968.

Hontz AC, Balin H, Merritt CG: Dysplasia and the pill. A progress report on the American Women's Health Program. J Reprod Med: 13, 101, 1974.

Hutcherson WP, Schwartz HA, Weathers W, McGuire JE: Long term evaluation of two oral contraceptives. Fertil Steril: 18, 616, 1967.

Ide R, Wijnants P, Bonte J: Observations cytologiques de frottis cervico-vaginaux sous contraception hormonale. Cytologic observations of cervicovaginal smear during hormonal contraception. Rev Cytol Clin: 5, 105, 1972.

Ishihama A, Kagubu T: On the cytological and histological studies after long insertion of intrauterine contraceptive device (IUD), Yokohama Med Bull: 15, 201, 1964.

Ishihama A, Kagubu T: Cytological studies after insertion of intrauterine contraceptive devices. Am J Obstet Gynecol: 9, 576, 1965.

Ishihama A, Kagabu T, Imai T, Shima M: Cytologic studies after insertion of intrauterine contraceptive devices. Acta Cytol: 14, 35, 1970.

Jensen HK, Hansen PA, Blom J: Incidence of Canadida albicans in women using oral contraceptives. Acta Obstet Gynecol Scand: 49, 293, 1970.

Jick H: Estrogens and increased endometrial cancer. Fact or Antifact? Ca 29, 250, 1979.

Jordaan HV: How dangerous are oral contraceptives? South Afr Med J: 46, 1215, 1972.

Kaiser P: Colposcopic, cytologic and histologic findings on the portio in contraceptive therapy using Ovosiston. Z Gynaekol: 28, 92, 1970.

Kaminetzky HA: Merthycholanthrene- induced cervical dysplasia and the sex steroids. Obstet Gynecol: 27, 489, 1966.

Kaminetzky HA: Sex steroids and experimental carcinoma of the uterine cervix. Excerpta Med Internat Congr Ser: 279, 155, 1973.

Kastner H, Holzner E: Zytologische Portiobefunde unter ovulationshemmender Medikation. Wiener Klin Wochenschr: 11, 175, 1973.

Kastner H, Holzer E: Cervical cytology in women using oral contraceptives. Wiener Klin Wochenschr: 85, 175–178, 1974.

Keifer WS, Scott JC: A clinical appraisal of patients following long term contraception. Am J Obstet Gynecol: 122, 446, 1975.

Kerhrer B, Hauser GA: Häufigkeit und Auftreten der Portio-ektopien unter Ovulationshemmern. Gynaecologia: 165, 209, 1968.

Kline T, Holland M, Wemple D: Atypical cytology with contraceptive hormone medication. Am J Clin Pathol: 53, 215, 1970.

Kyriakos M, Kempson RL, Konikow NF: Clinical and pathologic study of endocervical lesions associated with oral contraceptives. Cancer: 22, 99, 1968.

Laguens RP, Lagrutta J, Quijano F: Fine structure of reserve cell hyperplasia and incomplete squamous metaplasia of the uterine cervix. Int J Gynaecol Obstet: 9, 41, 1971.

Lauchlan SC, Penner DW: Simultaneous adenocarcinoma in situ and epidermid carcinoma in situ. Cancer: 20, 2250, 1967.

Laurie RE, Korba VD: Cervical cytology and histology in patients treated with a combination oral contraceptive in low dosage. Contraception: 3, 415, 1971.

Lindenbaum J, Whitehead N, Regner F: Oral contraceptive hormones, folate metabolism, and the cervical epithelium. Am J Clin Nutr: 28, 346, 1975.

Lippes J: Observations after four years of experience with the intrauterine plastic loop at the Buffalo Planned Parenthood Center. Sex Res: 3, 323, 1967.

Liu W, Koebel L, Shipp J, Prisby H: Cytologic changes following the use of oral contraceptives. Obstet Gynecol: 30, 228, 1967.

Luthra UK, Wahi PN: IUCD and tissue reacion with special reference to endometrium and cervix. In Review of Research work in India on Intrauterine Contraceptive Devices.KR Laumas (ed). Indian Council of Medical Research, New Delhi, pp 54–65, 1968.

Luthra UK, Mitra AB, Bhinder G, Bhatnagar P, Saxena NC: Surveillance for carcinogenesis in women using Cu-IUD for contraception. Indian J Med Res: 63, 1787, 1975.

Luthra UK, Mitra AB, Prabhakar AK, Bhatnagar P: Cytological monitoring of female genital tract in women using Cu IUD. Indian J Med Res: 66, 216, 1977.

Maqueo M, Azuela JC, Calderon NN, Goldzieher JW: Morphology of the cervix in women treated with synthetic progestins. Am J Obstet Gynecol: 96, 994, 1966.

Martin CE: Marital and coital factors in cervical cancer. Am J Public Health: 57, 803, 1967

Martin JD, Hahnel R: Oestrogen receptor studies in carcinoma of the endometrium, carcinoma of the uterine cervix and other gynaecological malignancies. Austr. N.Z. J Obstet Gynaecol 18, 55, 1978.

McClure HM, Graham CE: Malignant uterine mesotheliomas in squirrel monkeys following diethylstilbestrol administration Lab Anim Sci: 23, 493, 1973.

McQueen EG: Hormonal steroid contraceptives. IV: Adverse reactions and management of the patient. Durgs: 2, 138, 1971.

Medhat J, Boyce J, Sillman I, Waxman M, Fruchter R: A colposcopic study of the effect of IUDs on cervical epithelium. Int J Gynaecol Obstet: 17, 440, 1980.

Meisels A, Begin R, Schneider V: Dysplasias of uterine cervix. Cancer: 40, 3076, 1977.

Melamed MR, Flehinger BJ: Early incidence rates of precancerous lesions in women using contraceptives. Gynecol Oncol: 1, 290, 1973.

Melamed MR, Koss LG, Flehinger BJ, Kelisky RP, Dubrow H: Prevalence rates of uterine cervical carcinoma in situ for women using the diaphragm or contraceptive oral steroids. Br Med J: 3, 195, 1969.

Mestwerdt G: Praemaligne Dysplasien nach Ovulationshemmern. Münch Med Wochenschr: 16, 771, 1972.

Miller DF: The impact of hormonal contraceptive therapy on a community and effects on cytopathology of the cervix. Am J Obstet Gynecol: 115, 978, 1973.

Mingeot R, Fievez C: Endocervical changes with the use of synthetic steroids. Obstet Gynecol: 44, 53, 1974.

Misra JS, Engineer AD: Long term effect of IUDs. Cyto-morphological and cytohormonal study. J Obstet Gynecol India: 26, 394, 1976.

Misra JS, Engineer AD, Tandon P: Cytological studies in women using copper uterine devices. Acta Cytol: 21, 514, 1977.

Moghissi KS, Mack HC: Epidemiology of cervical cancer study of a prison population. Am J Obstet Gynecol: 100, 607, 1968.

Moghissi KS: The effect of steroidal contraceptives on the reproductive system. In Human Reproduction. E.S.E. Hafez and T.N. Evans (eds). Harper & Row, New York, pp 559–587, 1973.

Moghissi KS: Oral contraceptives and endometrial and cervical cancer. J Toxicol Environ Healh: 3, 243, 1977.

Moyer DL, Mishell DR: Reactions of human endometrium to the intrauterine foreign body II. Long term effects in the endometrial histology and cytology. Am J Obstet Gynecol: 111, 66, 1971.

Myhre E, Bjoro K: Oral contraceptives and cervical cancer. A preliminary report of an experimental study. Acta Pathol Microbiol Scand: 76, 495, 1969.

Nichols TM, Fidler HK: Microglandular hyperplasia in cervical cone biopsies taken for suspicious and positive cytology. Am J Clin Pathol: 56, 424, 1971.

Oppenheimer BS, Oppenheimer ET, Stout AP: Sarcomas in-duced in rats by implanting cellophone. Proc Exp Biol Med: 67, 33, 1948.

Ory HW, Conger BS, Naib Z, Tyler CW, Hatcher RA: Pre-liminary analysis of oral contraceptive use and risk of devel-oping premalignant lesions of the uterine cervix. In Pharma-cology of Steroid Contraceptive Drugs. Raven Press, New York, p 211, 1977.

Paffenbarger RS: Surveillance for carcinogenesis from steroid contraceptives. In Host–Environment Interactions in the Etiology of Cancer in Man. R. Doll and I. Vodopya (eds). Int. Agency for Research on Cancer, Lyon, p 183, 1973.

Peckhan B: Implications of contraception. B. Cancer and contra-ceptive devices. J Med Educ 44, Suppl 2, 68, 1969.

Peritz E, Ramcharan S, Frank J, Brown WL, Huang S, Ray R: The incidence of cervical cancer and duration of oral contra-ceptive use. Epidemiol: 106, 462, 1977.

Phillips E, Lu W: Case report of the reliability and hazards of intrauterine devices. Zbl Gynaekol: 94, 1569, 1970.

Pincus G: Modern Trends in Endocrinology (second series), H. Gardiner-Hill ed., Hoeber, New York, p 231–245, 1961.

Pincus G: Clinical control of fertility. In Advances in Chemistry, RF Gould, (ed), Vol 45, pp 177–189, 1964.

Pincus G: In The Control of Fertility. Academic Press New York, pp 240–255, 1965.

Pincus G, Garcia CR: Studies on vaginal cervical and uterine histology. Metabolism: 14, 344, 1965.

Piver MS, Whiteley JP, Bolognese RJ: Effect of an intrauterine contraceptive device upon cervical and endometrial exfoliative cytology. Obstet Gynecol: 28, 528, 1966.

Population Reports. Oral contraceptives, No. 4 Series A. George Washington University,Washington, DC pp. 1–74, 1977.

Quizilbash AH: In situ and microinvasive adenocarcinoma of the uterine cervix. Am J Clin Pathol: 64, 155, 1975.

Ramcharan S: Walnut Creek Study of OC use, sexual behavior, and cervical cancer. Cited in: Population Reports. Oral Contraceptives, No. 5, series A, George Washington Times, Washington, DC, A–166, 1978.

Ravenholt RT: Oral contraceptives and prevention of cancer of the uterus and breast. Paper presented at the Sixteenth International Congess of the International Confederation of Midwives, Washington, DC, 1972.

Richart RM, Barron BA: The intrauterine device and cervical neoplasia. A prospective study of patients with cervical dysplasia. J Am Med Assoc: 199, 817, 1967.

Richart RM, Barron BA: A follow-up of patients with cervical dysplasia. Am J Obstet Gynecol: 105, 386, 1969.

Robert HG, Dupre-Froment J: Of the cervix, intraepithelial cancer in pill users and non-users. Contracept Fertil Sex: 7, 9, 1979.

Rotkin ID: Adolescent coitus and cervical cancer: associations of related events with increased risk. Cancer Res: 27, 603, 1967.

Rotkin ID: A comparison review of key epidemiological studies in cervical cancer related to current searches for transmissible agents. Cancer Res: 33, 1353, 1973.

Royal College of General Practitioners. Oral Contraceptives and Health. Pitman, New York, pp. 1–78, 1974.

Sagiroglu N, Sagiroglu E: The cytology of intrauterine devices. Acta Cytol: 14, 58, 1970.

Sammour MB, Iskander SG, Rifai SF: Combined histologic and cytologic study of intrauterine contraception. Am J Obstet Gynecol: 98, 946, 1967.

Sandmire HF, Austin SD, Bechtel RC: Carcinoma of the cervix in oral contraceptive steroid and IUD users and nonusers. Am J Obstet Gynecol: 125, 339, 1976.

Scott RB: Report of the task force on carcinogenic potential. In United States. Food and Drug Administration. Advisory Committee on Obstetrics and Gynecology. Report on oral contraceptives. U.S. Government Printing Office Washing-ton, DC, pp 21–32, 1966.

Schrage R: Die Zusammensetzung der weiblichen Klientel bei Krebsfrüherkennungsuntersuchungen. Frauenarzt: 4, 266, 1965.

Segal SJ, Anderson RK: Oral contraceptives and cervical cancer. Memorandum to the Population Council Field Staff, pp 1–2, 1968.

Seidl S: Atypical cervical hyperplasias in hormonal contra-ception. Geburtshilfe Frauenheilkd: 31, 1006, 1971.

Seigel D, Corfman P: Epidemiological problems associated with studies of the safety of oral contraceptives. J Am Med Assoc: 203, 950, 1968.

Shahani SM, Dandekar PV, Chikhlikar AR: Intrauterine de-vices: effectiveness and changes in the genital tract. Excerpta Medica International Congress Series No. 133, 1138, 1967.

Shimomura T: Contraceptive ring inserted for a long period. Kitano Byoin Itano Hosp J Med: 17, 69, 1972.

Singer A, Jordan JA: Oestrogen-like activity and cervical atypias (letter) Lancet: 2, 359, 1977.

Smithies A, Grubb CK: The cytology of patients on oral contraceptives. A preliminary study. Cited in: FA Langley proferred papers. Acta Cytol: 14, 156, 1970.

Soost H: Atypical changes in cervical epithelium following application of ovulation inhibition. Acta Cytol: 12, 294, 1968.

Soost HJ, Baier W: Einfluss der Ovulationshemmer auf das Gebaermutterhalsepithel. Dtsch Med Wochenschr: 40, 1799, 1967.

Sperlng MA: Complications of systemic oral contraceptive therapy: Neoplasm breast, uterus, cervix and vagina. West J Med: 122, 42, 1975.

Steps H, Finser HK: Zytologische Befunde bei jungen Frauen unter Berücksichtigung des Sexualverhaltens. Fortschr Med: 11, 739, 1977.

Stern E: Epidemiology of dysplasia. Obstet Gynecol Surv: 24, 711, 1969.

Stern E, Clark V, Coffelt CF: Contraceptives and dysplasia:

172

higher rate for pill choosers. Science: 169, 497, 1970.

Stern E, Forsythe AB, Coffelt CF: Steroid contraceptive use and cervical dysplasia; increased risk of progression. Science: 196, 1460, 1977.

Talbert JR, Sherry JB: Adenocarcinoma-like lesion of cervix–a pill induced problem? Am J Obstet Gynecol: 105, 117, 1969.

Tatum HJ: Intrauterine contraception using the copper seven device. Cited in: J Newton, J Elias and McEdwany. Lancet: 1, 951, 1971.

Taylor HB, Irek NS, Norris HJ: Atypical endocervical hyperplasia in women taking oral contraceptives. J Am Med Assoc: 202, 637, 1967.

Thomas D: Relationship of oral contraceptives to cervical carcinogenesis. Obstet Gynecol: 40, 508, 1972.

Thompson DW: Oral contraceptives and cervical atypia: a plea for objective appraisal. Can Med Assoc J: 101, 285, 1969.

Tichauer RW, Vargas BE: Pilot study with Lippes loop in La Pez, Bolivia, J Med Woman Assoc: 23, 456, 1968.

Tietze: Contraception by intrauterine devices. Am J Obstet Gynecol: 96, 1043, 1966.

Topp G, Meissner H: Results of colposcopic, cytologic and histological studies after treatment with ovulation inhibitors. Zentralbl Gynaekol: 90, 1778, 1968.

Tyler ET: Oral contraception. J Am Med Assoc: 175, 225, 1961.

Tyler ET: Current status of oral contraception. J Am Med Assoc: 187, 562, 1964.

Vessey M, Doll R, Peto R, Johnson B, Wiggins P: A long term follow up study of women using different methods of contraception. An interim report J Biol Soc Sci: 8, 375, 1976.

Wachtel E, Husain OAN: Contraceptives and cervical carcinoma. Br Med J: 3, 412, 1969.

Wahi PN, Lahiri VL, Mali S, Lathra UK: Study of cervical epithelial changes in women using Lippes loop. Indian J Med Res: 56, 294, 1968.

Westoff CF, Bumpass L, Ryder NB: Oral contraception, coital frequency, and the time required to conceive. Soc Biol: 16, 1, 1969.

Wied GL, Davis E, Frank R, Segal PB, Meir P, Rosenthal E: Statistical evaluation of the effect of hormonal contraceptives on the cytologic smear pattern. Obstet Gynecol: 27, 327, 1966.

Wilbanks GD: The effect of hormones on human carcinoma in situ in tissue cultures. VIIth World Congress of Obstet. Moscow. Excerpta Medica: 279, 173, 1973.

Willson JR, Ledger WT: Complications associated with the use of intrauterine contraceptive device in women of middle and upper social economic class. Am J Obstet Gynecol: 100, 649, 1968.

Wolff JP: Contraception and cancer of the cervix. In Regulation of Fertility. Evaluation and Perspectives INSERM: Paris, pp 159–168, 1979.

World Health Organization (WHO). Steroid contraception and the risk of neoplasia. Report of a WHO Scientif Group. Geneva (WHO Technical Report Series 619), pp 1–54, 1978.

Worth AJ, Boyes DA: A case control study into possible effects of birth control pills on preclinical carcinoma of the cervix. J Obstet Gynecol Br Commonw: 79, 673, 1972.

Wright NH, Vessey MP, Kenward B, McPherson K, Doll R: Neoplasia and dysplasia of the cervix uteri and contraception: a possible protective effect of the diaphragm. Br J Cancer: 38, 273, 1978.

Wunder G: Carcinoma in situ und Karzinom der Zervix unter Einnahme oraler Kontrazeptiva. Fortschr Med: 9, 1082, 1973.

Zipper J, Medel M, Pastene L, Rivera M, Tatum HJ: Human fertility control through the use of endouterine metal antagonisms of trace elements (EMATE). In E. Diczfalusy and U. Borell, eds. Control of Human Fertility. Proceedings of the 15th Nobel Symposium, Sodergarn, Lidingo, Sweden, May 27–29, 1970. John Wiley, New York, pp 199–218, 1971.

IV. DIAGNOSIS AND PROGNOSIS

24. DIAGNOSTIC DILEMMA OF RECURRENT CERVICAL CARCINOMA

J.H. Shepherd, H. Praphat, E. Ruffolo and D. Cavanagh

Early squamous cervical carcinoma responds well to both primary surgical treatment in the form of radical hysterectomy, and also to adequate radiotherapy: cure rates in terms of 90 percent are expected. However, recurrent or residual disease has a much more sinister prognosis so that only 10 percent will be alive 2 years after diagnosis of the recurrence (Calame 1969). The detection and subsequent management of such recurrence can be very difficult, especially after radiotherapy. From the natural history of the disease it can be seen that the majority of recurrences will manifest themselves during the first 2 years following treatment and deaths due to the disease will in the main have occurred during the first 5 years. To give these cases a chance for survival, they must be detected as early as possible.

I. RECURRENCE

I.A. Sites and incidence

Recurrence may be central, on the lateral pelvic side walls, or at more distant sites (Table 1). As would be expected it is more common to get recurrence after radiotherapy not because the treatment is less effective, but because the more advanced lesions are treated by this modality. The later the stage of the disease, the higher the incidence of recurrence; central recurrence occurs in 2.5 percent of patients with stage I and II disease, in 7 percent of patients with stage III, and in up to 38 percent of those with stage IV disease (Paunier et al. 1967). As far as prognosis is concerned, primary tumor size gives a better indication of tumor behavior than does clinical staging and constitutes an objective method of classifying tumors that the latter cannot do

(Burghardt and Pickel 1978). In view of the fact that this particular cancer metastasizes mainly by direct spread and lymphatic channels, many of these cases have either pelvic side-wall involvement or more distant spread. It is, however, the central recurrences that can be offered surgical extirpation and perhaps pose the greatest problem with early detection.

I.B. Symptoms and signs

Certain symptoms should be carefully inquired about, such as pain, particularly of sciatic, obturator or pelvic distribution, lower limb edema, vaginal bleeding or discharge, a persistent cough, and also weight loss. The occurrence of anemia, jaundice, lymphadenopathy, ascites, hepatomegaly, or deep venous thrombosis are signs that on general examination might be found. Frequent pelvic assessments may well detect any change that arises, especially the appearance of friability of the vaginal

Table 1. Sites of recurrence in cervical carcinoma.

1.	Central, including bladder	21%	
	vagina	20%	
	rectum	19%	60%
2.	Lateral pelvic side wall lymph nodes		60%
3.	Distant lymph nodes:		
	para-aortic		33%
	inguinal		7%
	supraclavicular		1%
4.	Liver		16%
5.	Skeleton (including vertebral column 9%)		16%
6.	Lung		14%
7.	Vulva (including distal urethra)		3%
8.	Skin		2%
9.	Brain		1%

Based on data from autopsies on treated patients (Henriksen 1949).

Hafez, E.S.E., Smith, J.P. (eds.), Carcinoma of the Cervix: Biology and Diagnosis. ISBN-13: 978-94-009-7487-6

vault, and nodularity of the parametrial and paravaginal tissues or uterosacral ligaments. Induration and fibrosis of the pelvic tissues often associated with vaginal stenosis makes interpretation and even examination very difficult however. This is especially so after radiotherapy to a bulky tumor, even though techniques are improving with the introduction of megavoltage linear accelerators and after-loading techniques.

I.C. The need for regular follow-up

Although the question has been raised as to whether there is a difference in survival rates between cervical carcinoma patients followed by routine examination and those patients not regularly followed (Van Voorhis 1970), the time interval between each examination is important. In the past, the majority of recurrences have been detected by physical examination and cytologic methods, although a few were also detected by intravenous pyelography (Calame 1969). Most oncologists agree that in order to detect at an early stage the salvagable central recurrence, a careful surveillance is warranted. At least 10 percent of patients initially responding to primary treatment will develop a central pelvic recurrence; one third of these may expect to be successfully treated (Kottmeier 1969).

II. ANCILLARY METHODS OF DETECTING RECURRENCE

A battery of routine diagnostic tests constitute the traditional oncological survey, namely chest roentgenography, intravenous pyelography, barium enema, cystoscopy, proctoscopy and bone scan. To this list may be added the sophisticated radioisotope scanning techniques, ultrasonography, and computerized axial tomography (CAT scan) that are now available.

II.A. Chest roentgenography and intravenous pyelography

These two particular studies, chest films and intravenous pyelograms, are important as baselines for the follow-up of treated cancer patients, as well as for prognostic purposes (Shingleton et al. 1971). Periodic repetitions of these two examinations are

of significant benefit, aiding in the detection of recurrence and should be routine (Photopulos et al. 1977). They may be performed six-monthly for 2 years, and then yearly.

II.B. Further investigations

Other radiographic studies, such as regular skeletal surveys or barium examinations of the gastrointestinal tract are unlikely to be rewarding. Although individual patients with late disease may have abnormalities demonstrable by cystoscopy or proctosigmoidoscopy, these uncomfortable procedures are also not routinely informative. Specific symptoms, such as bone pain, hematuria, or an alteration in bowel habit, perhaps associated with the sudden appearance of a hernia, should on the other hand, be fully evaluated. Further investigations may then be undertaken depending on the individual problem.

II.C. Computerized axial tomography

Recently, computerized axial tomography has been used extensively in an attempt to diagnose a multitude of lesions, not the least of which is recurrent cancer. Great enthusiasm may accompany this technique, and certainly select centers may provide excellent results with the CAT scan. It is possible to define solid tumors, cystic masses and alterations in the size or shape of pelvic structures. Retroperitoneal tumors and non-functioning kidneys may be examined also (Abrams et al. 1978). However, interpretation of equivocal induration and fibrosis in a post-radiation patient, especially after an initially bulky tumor, is very difficult. Similarly, the accuracy of the CAT scan in demonstrating lymph node metastases in patients with cervical carcinoma is not as good as it is in patients with lymphomas (Lee et al. 1978). Brain, lung, and upper abdominal lesions may be well outlined, but the efficiency and cost effectiveness of this modality has not yet been proved in dealing with recurrent pelvic malignancies, and continues to be investigated.

II.D. Ultrasonography

Ultrasonography appears to be the non-invasive scanning technique of choice, and Donald first illustrated the value of ultrasonic echoes in obstetric and gynecologic diagnoses (Donald 1965). More recent reviews have confirmed this (Alberts et al. 1978). Ultrasound study provides a somewhat better differentiation of solid from cystic lesions than the CAT scan, although the latter denotes to best advantage the anatomy of the area, providing a means of viewing bone as well as soft tissue detail (Carter et al. 1976). Considering the greater cost and time requirement for CAT scans, ultrasonography is a more efficacious method of following abdominal and pelvic tumor size in patients on therapy (Nash et al. 1979).

A problem arises with the interpretation of clinical and radiological suspicious yet equivocal findings and perhaps simultaneous real-time ultrasonic scanning and pelvic examination might be applicable (Platt et al. 1980). Add to this a directed biopsy technique to yield histologic proof for a definite diagnosis and then a satisfactory and indisputable answer would result.

This has been tried with some success using various radiologic guidance methods including the CAT scan, ultrasonography and fluoroscopy (Ferrucci et al. 1980). Although contact B-scan ultrasonography affords a flexible approach for tumor localization in transverse, longitudinal, and oblique scanning planes, it is the recent introduction of high resolution real-time transducer systems that holds promise for improved ultrasonic guidance. The ultrasound method should be preferred whenever possible because of its simplicity of performance and lack of ionizing radiation.

II.E. Lymphangiography

Lymphangiography has had its protagonists. With regard to primary diagnosis, although a good correlation between lymphangiography and para-aortic lymph node biopsy proved metastases has been demonstrated (Piver and Barlow 1973), this is by no means generally accepted (Berman et al. 1977). In fact, the specificity of lymphangiography examinations is not accurate enough to be of clinical significance in the detection of para-aortic lymph node metastases (Brown et al. 1979). As far as detecting recurrence following radiotherapy or surgery, even allowing for recanalization of lymphatic vessels, there is no good evidence to suggest

that this technique has a feasible role to offer.

II.F. Radio-isotope studies

Radio-isotope studies of the liver and brain, as well as of bone, may on occasions have a place, but not as a routine. Specific indications and suspicions may arise to necessitate such investigations however.

III. HISTOLOGIC DIAGNOSIS

There can be no doubt that the most definite method of diagnosing a recurrence is to prove the presence of malignant cells when viewed down a microscope. Only thus may the necessary knowledge be provided so that a final therapeutic decision may then be taken. Although the diagnosis of gynecological malignancies may on occasions be obvious, and biopsy specimens obtained easily, this is by no means always the case. Thus, if the tumors are not accessible, clinical impressions may dictate the necessity for further operative procedures in order to obtain material for examination. Even laparotomy may be necessary to meet this requirement, if cytology and superficial biopsy specimens yield negative results in a highly suspicious situation.

III.A. Needle biopsy

Ever since Mr. Stanley needled a tumor arising from the liver in 1833 at St. Bartholomew's Hospital in London, needle biopsy and aspiration has developed into an accepted and efficient diagnostic aid. Numerous modifications of the instrument and procedure have resulted in disposable biopsy needles such as the Tru-cut variety being produced.

A recent series has shown this needle biopsy to be an extremely useful tool in the armamentarium of the gynecologic oncologist (Shepherd et al. 1980). It may be used for primary diagnoses as well as for diagnosing recurrent cervical tumors, both in the pelvis and at more distant sites. Recto-vaginal examination allows the instrument to be guided by the opposite hand to the center of a suspicious lesion. This procedure has proved to be safe as long as central masses only are biopsied and the needle is kept away from the pelvic side walls. It is the post-radiotherapy group of patients that are most troublesome and require some further investigation, such as biopsy, to fully evaluate the significance of a mass or induration with fibrosis, even many years after treatment.

III.B. False negative cytology and histology

A significant number of cases have negative Pap smears and vault punch biopsies, and yet needle biopsies from the deeper tissues of the parametria or vault prove positive (Table 2). This is not surprising in view of the fact that a comparatively small number of patients will exhibit superficial vaginal recurrence, but a much larger number will have deeper central pelvic disease (Table 1). Highly satisfactory specimens may be obtained for both frozen section and conventional permanent paraffin sectioning and microscopic interpretation. Figures 1 and 2 show such examples in cases when vault punch biopsies were non-contributory but tumor was demonstrable in the needle biopsies.

III.C. Aspiration cytology

The value of the needle biopsy is that it may obviate the need for more major and invasive methods to make a diagnosis so that appropriate management may be planned. An alternative method may be the use of fine needle aspiration cytology which may predict the histologic picture of various lesions with a high degree of accuracy (Sevin et al. 1979). Not as much material is available for study with this method as by needle biopsy, and therefore malignant cells in association with fibrosis or fluid may not be picked up, especially following radiation therapy or chemotherapy.

IV. FURTHER MANAGEMENT

IV.A. Curative

Having diagnosed the recurrence, then appropriate management may be instituted, depending on the particular situation. If surgery has been the primary treatment, then radiotherapy to the whole pelvis should be the next choice. The question as to whether exploratory laparotomy with selective para-aortic lymph node biopsies should be performed is open to debate. It seems only logical, however, to be sure of the extent of the spread of disease so that adequate treatment with radiotherapy to the upper abdomen may be given if necessary.

Radical hysterectomy for post-radiation or residual cancer is an acceptable procedure for early disease. On occasion, small cervical or vaginal post-radiation neoplasms may be successfully managed by more conservative procedures, such as simple hysterectomy and partial vaginectomy (Adcock 1979).

IV.B. Exenteration

More often, however, an exenterative procedure needs to be considered. A careful pre-operative assessment, as well as exploratory laparotomy, is vital in order to select patients who might be candidates for this procedure. In the past, five year survival rates in the range of 10 to 20 percent have been commonly quoted, along with a similar operative mortality (Brunschwig 1965; Symmonds et al. 1968). There can be little merit in submitting an unsuitable patient to such a massive procedure when the disease cannot be totally extirpated. However, with careful selection and preparation, the salvage rate can be greatly improved, and approach a 50 percent–5 year survival (Symmonds et al. 1975). Thus, a real chance of cure may be offered, but the keystone must remain early detection.

IV.C. Chemotherapy

If the disease is not resectable, then chemotherapy is the next line of attack. As yet, there is no dramatically successful regimen available for this squamous

Table 2. Relative accuracy of cytologic and histopathologic methods for the diagnosis of recurrent cervical carcinoma.

Method	Accuracy
Papanicolaou smear	69%
Punch biopsy	82%
Needle biopsy	96%

Source: Shepherd et al. 1980.

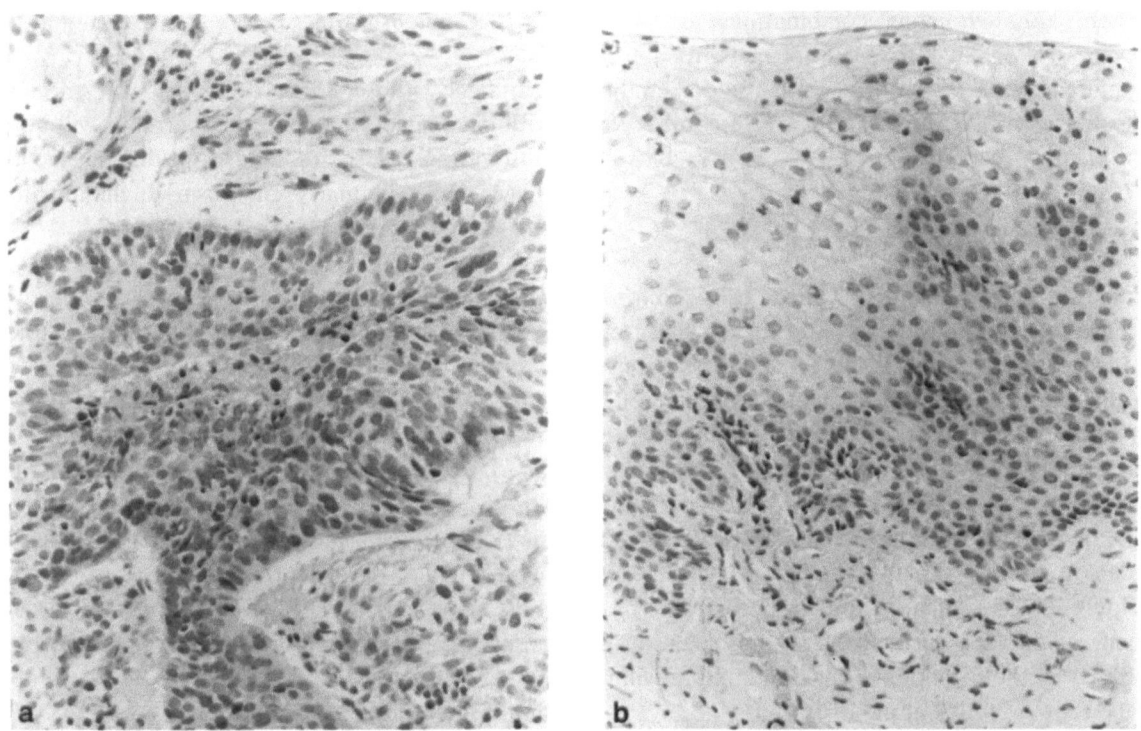

Figure 1. (a) Microscopy of needle biopsy specimen showing recurrent invasive cervical squamous cell carcinoma despite: (b) A benign appearing vaginal punch biopsy.

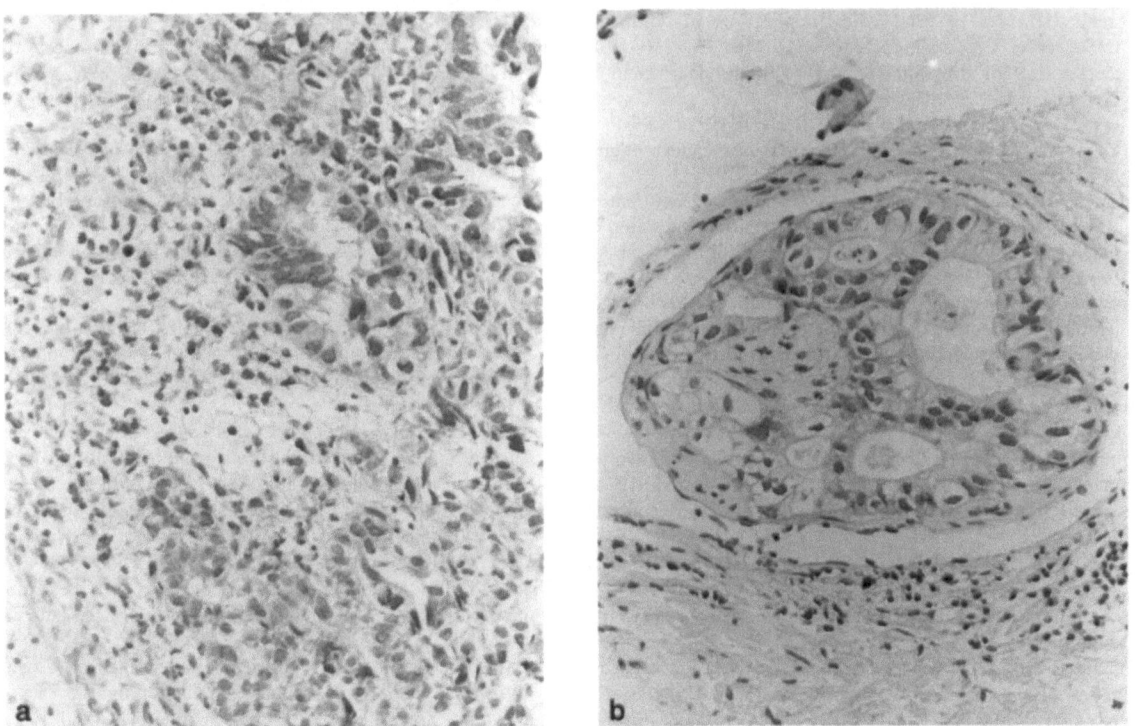

Figure 2. (a) Microscopy of needle biopsy specimen demonstrating recurrent adenocarcinoma of the endocervix. (b) As above, demonstrating invasion of perineural space.

lesion, although many combinations are under review. Now that tumor culture methods are becoming established, perhaps a fuller understanding of kinetics will result in new ways to combat this problem.

IV.D. Palliation

Palliative surgery may on occasions be called for to relieve intestinal obstruction, to divert urine from either a vesicovaginal fistula or obstructed ureter, to ligate the hypogastric arteries in an attempt to staunch hemorrhage, or even simply to ease the discomfort from abdominal ascites or a malignant pleural effusion. Palliation in the form of radiation therapy to painful bony metastases may be dramatic in its effect. Finally, the terminal patient will require much sympathy and symptomatic treatment. Eventually such analgesia and sedation as offered by the Brompton's cocktail mixture will be called for (Melzack et al. 1976).

IV.E. Cause of death

Ultimately, those 85 percent who will succumb within a year of diagnosis of recurrence will do so with various deaths ranging from uremia, hemorrhage, and pulmonary embolism to malnutrition and cachexia.

V. CONCLUSION: THE NEED FOR EARLY DETECTION

Thus, in conclusion, it may be seen that this disease, eminently curable in the early stages, must be compulsively followed to detect recurrence if any hope of salvage is to exist. Managing such patients may often present a clinical dilemma for diagnosis before palliative or further curative surgery is thought necessary. These points apply to cervical carcinoma more than to any other gynecologic cancer and useful aids such as the needle biopsy should be utilized accordingly.

REFERENCES

Abrams HL, McNeil BJ: Medical implications of computed tomography (CAT scanning). N Engl J Med 298: 310, 1978.

Adcock LL: Radical hysterectomy preceding pelvic irradiation. Gyn Oncol 8: 152, 1979.

Alberts DS, Woolfenden JM, Haber K, Giles HR, Galendo J: Comparison of ultrasonic and indium-III-bleomycin scanning of gynecologic tumors. Gyn Oncol 6: 145, 1978.

Berman ML, Lagassee LD, Watring WG, Ballon SC, Schlesinger RE, Moore JG, Donaldson RC: The operative evaluation of patients with cervical carcinoma by an extraperitoneal approach. Obstet Gynecol 50: 658, 1977.

Brown RC, Buchsbaum HJ, Tewfik HH, Platz CS: Accuracy of lymphangiography in the diagnosis of para-aortic lymph node metastases from carcinoma of the cervix. Obstet Gynecol 54: 571, 1979.

Brunschwig A: What are the indications and results of pelvic exenteration? J Am Med Assoc 194: 204, 1965.

Burghardt E, Pickel H: Local spread and lymph node involvement in cervical cancer. Obstet and Gynecol 52: 138, 1978.

Calame RJ: Recurrent carcinoma of the cervix. Am J Obstet Gynecol 105: 380, 1969.

Carter BL, Kahn PC, Wolpert SM, Hammerschlag SB, Schwartz AM, Scott RM: Unusual pelvic masses: A comparison of computed tomographic scanning and ultrasonography. Radiology 121: 383, 1976.

Donald I: Ultrasonic echo sounding in obstetrical and gynecological diagnosis. Am J Obstet Gynecol 93: 935, 1965.

Ferrucci JT, Wittenberg J, Mueller PR, Simeone JF, Harbin WP, Kirkpatrick RH, Taft PD: Diagnosis of abdominal malignancy by radiologic fine-needle aspiration biopsy. Am J Roentgenology 134: 323, 1980.

Henriksen E: The lymphatic spread of carcinoma of the cervix and body of the uterus: a study of 420 necropsies. Am J Obstet Gynecol 58: 924, 1949.

Kottmeier HL: Evaluation of treatment of recurrences after surgery and radiotherapy for carcinoma of the cervix. Cancer of the Uterus and Ovary. Chicago: Year Book Medical Publishers, Inc, 1969, p 283.

Lee JKT, Stanley RJ, Sagel SS, McClennan BL: Accuracy of C.T. in detecting intraabdominal and pelvic lymph node metastases from pelvic cancers. Am J Roentgenol 131: 675, 1978.

Melzack R, Ofiesh JA, Bount BM: The Brompton mixture: effects on pain in cancer patients. Can Med Assoc J 115: 125, 1976.

Nash CH, Alberts DS, Suciu TN, Giles HR, Tobias DA, Waldman RS: Comparison of B-mode ultrasonography and computed tomography in gynecologic cancer. Gyn Oncol 8: 172, 1979.

Paunier JP, Delclos L, Fletcher GH: Causes time of death and sites of failure in squamous cell carcinoma of the uterine cervix on intact uterus. Radiology 88: 555, 1967.

Photopulos GJ, Shirley REL, Ansbacher R: Evaluation of conventional diagnostic tests for detection of recurrent carcinoma of the cervix. Am J Obstet Gynecol 129: 533, 1977.

Piver MS, Barlow JJ: Para-aortic lymphadenectomy, aortic node biopsy and aortic lymphangiography in staging patients with advanced cervical cancer. Cancer 32: 367, 1973.

Platt LD, Manning FA, Hill LM: Simultaneous real-time ultrasound scanning and pelvic examination in assessment of pelvic disease. Am J Obstet Gynecol 136: 693, 1980.

St Bartholomew's Hospital (Report): Abscess of the liver with hydatids: operation. Lancet 189: 1833-4,

Sevin B, Greening SE, Nadji M, Ng AB, Averette HE, Nordqvist

SRB: Fine needle aspiration cytology in gynecologic oncology, cervical aspects. Acta Cytologica 23: 277, 1979.

Shepherd JH, Cavanagh D, Praphat H, Ruffolo E: The value of needle biopsy in the diagnosis of gynecologic cancer. Gynec Oncol 11: 309, 1981.

Shingleton HM, Fowler WC, Koch GC: Pretreatment evaluation in cervical cancer. Am J Obstet Gynecol 110: 388, 1971.

Symmonds RE, Pratt JH, Welch JS: Exenterative operations Am J Obstet Gynecol 101: 66, 1968.

Symmonds RE, Pratt JH, Webb MJ: Exenterative operations: experience with 198 patients. Am J Obstet Gynecol 121: 907, 1975.

Van Voorhis LW: Carcinoma of the cervix. II A critical evaluation of patient follow-up. Am J Obstet Gynecol 108: 115, 1970.

25. PROGNOSTIC FACTORS IN CARCINOMA OF THE CERVIX

H.R.K. BARBER, S. SOMMERS and A. ROMOFF

It is estimated that there will be 16,000 new cases of invasive cancer of the cervix in 1981. Most of these cases will be detected in stages I and II. Although the survival rate in stage I ranges from 80 to 90 percent in most series, a constant re-evaluation is indicated in the hope that modifying the plan of treatment will result in an improved survival. In a previous report a number of parameters were explored with this purpose. This report includes an additional three years in the study.

The main goal of oncology is prevention of cancer and failing in this, the next goal is to achieve early detection. However, among patients who have developed invasive cervical carcinoma, different parameters have been studied in order to predict prognosis. This report has been directed to a study of the stromal reaction and vascular invasion as a prognostic factor in stage IB cancer of the cervix.

In a previous report, 110 stage IB cancers of the cervix were reported. Among those patients with pelvic lymph node metastases and/or blood vessel invasion, 59.4 percent survived 5 years after radical hysterectomy and 50 percent after radiation therapy. However, when the lymph nodes and blood vessels were not involved the results were 90% and 50.4% respectively. The histologic and nuclear grades and stromal reactions showed no statistical relationship to survival.

I. HISTOLOGIC GRADING

The tumors were graded from I to III with grade I being the most differentiated and grade III the most immature. The neoplasm is named from its most differentiated portion and graded from its least differentiated parts. The classification is based on the uniformity or lack of uniformity of the cells, whether the nucleus is regular or not, the ratio between the nucleus and cytoplasm, the number and size of the nucleoli, and the number of mitoses per high power field.

II. NUCLEAR GRADE

The nuclei of the tumor cells were graded from 1 to 3. Grade 1 is the most abnormal. The nuclei are markedly enlarged, irregular in outline with chromatin clumping and prominent nucleoli; grade 2, intermediate degree of differentiation; grade 3, similar in size and appearance to each and to normal cervical tissue when present.

III. STROMAL REACTION

The stroma of each cervical cancer was graded according to the number of lymphocytes, plasma cells, and polymorphonuclear leukocytes present. Lymphocytes, plasma cells, and polymorphonuclear infiltration in the stroma and around small veins were graded 0 to 3: 0 = none, 1 = minimal, 2 = moderate, and 3 = marked.

Between 1976 and late 1979, 74 untreated cancers of the cervix were admitted. There were 39 in stage 1B, 25 in stage II and 10 in stage III.

There were 39 patients treated for stage 1B evaluated. Of this number, 23 had blood vessel and/or lymph node or lymphatic involvement, 13 had no involvement and 3 were undetermined. There were 23 patients with lymphatic and/or vascular invasion. Among these 14 were alive at 3 years. Among 13 patients in whom there were

Hafez, E.S.E., Smith, J.P. (eds.), Carcinoma of the Cervix: Biology and Diagnosis. ISBN-13: 978-94-009-7487-6

no lymphatic/vascular invasion 11 were alive at 3 years. The three undetermined included cases where the original slides were returned to the hospital in which the biopsies were taken and it was not possible to get them for review. This is an important observation and it differs from the previous report in that those with lymphatic/ vascular invasion had a 59.4 percent 5-year survival whereas those patients in whom there was no lymphatic/vascular invasion had a 90 percent 5-year survival. It was during the second part of this study that intravenous chemotherapy was given to patients with lymphatic/blood vessel invasion.

Three modalities of treatment were employed in this series. Twenty-seven patients received a radical hysterectomy and pelvic node dissection; 11 radiation therapy, and 1 a total hysterectomy. Among those treated by radical hysterectomy and pelvic lymph node dissection, 2 died in the first year and 1 was lost to follow-up, while none died in the second and third years but 12 were lost to follow-up. The results from radiation therapy show that out of 11 patients, 4 died and 2 were lost to follow-up. The patients receiving radiation therapy had medical complications and/or a large lesion.

The results of 26 patients with a positive stromal reaction and 10 that had a poor infiltration of lymphocytes and polymorphonuclear leukocytes showed no difference in survival. Three patients had no stromal grading on the original specimen.

Among patients with a positive stromal response, 17 of 26 were alive at three years while 8 of 10 with a negative stromal response were alive at three years. Host resistance is considered an important factor in cancer control. This can be studied by examining the lymphocytes and plasma cells that infiltrate the area where the tumor is growing. A marked lymphocyte and plasma cell response is interpreted as the body mounting a defense against the cancer. In certain tumors, especially breast cancer, this has been repeatedly confirmed. In the present series the number of lymphocytes and plasma cells were not as great in stage I as anticipated, expecially since this stage had the best survival rate. However, in another study reported by the authors, the number

of lymphocytes and plasma cells increased as the disease became more advanced and may indicate that the tumor has to grow to a certain volume or a given potency before it can stimulate a local immune response. If a correlation is observed between lymphocytes and plasma cell response and long-term survival when large series are accumulated, perhaps immunotherapy can then be employed to stimulate an immune response of this type.

The nuclear grade reveals that in patients with grade 1 the 3-year survival is 83.1%, with grade 2, 78.1% and grade 3, 100%. Among those with histologic grade 1, the 3-year survival is 66.7%, grade 2, 81.1% and grade 3 is 85.7%. It is generally reported that histologic grade III is a more potent tumor stage for stage than is a grade I or II tumor. However, in this small series the patients with grade III have done better than those with grade I or II. The explanation may be the result of selecting the more aggressive tumors for intravenous anticancer chemotherapy. However, the histologic grading takes precedence over the nuclear grading for identifying the most aggressive tumor in this series.

Table 1 summarizes the material from this study. The direct method for calculating a survival rate does not utilize all information available. The actuarial, or life table, method utilizes all survival information accumulated up to the closing date of the study and describes the manner in which the patient group was depleted during the total period of observation. This provides a better insight into the nature of the disease and the effect of therapy than does one specific endpoint. As example, using the overall 5-year survival, the direct method, does not tell whether all patients died at 1 year or 3 years or by a fixed percentage rate for each year during the period studied. However, with the use of the life-table method it is obvious to determine the number that died each year. Six died during this period and 14 withdrew from the series. The original chemotherapeutic regimen using Bleomycin accounted for much of this. However, by using Mitomycin and 5-FU all have continued in the series. In a small series this number withdrawing from the protocol has a great influence on the cumulative proportion surviving.

IV. CONCLUDING REMARKS

The interpretation of data is difficult and limited by the small number of cases. However, as the material accumulates and is reported by stage, grade and histologic criteria a meaningful and profitable study will result.

The material reviewed indicates that staging and grading are both important and should be used to establish therapy. These parameters are not competitive but rather complementary. In general, stage of the disease was more important than histologic or nuclear grades. There are varying degrees of malignancy in groups of a particular stage. Therefore, it is important to examine tumor tissues microscopically to determine their grade or degree of malignancy according to histologic and nuclear grade as well as the stromal reaction. Staging is determined clinically and estimates the extent of disease and the size of the tumor, whereas histologic type and grading provide the microscopic character. Since there is a considerable variation in the potency of tumors within a given stage, it is important to tailor treatment to the cancer rather than the stage of disease.

Host resistance is considered an important factor in cancer control. This can be studied by examining the lymphocytes and plasma cells that infiltrates the area where the tumor is growing. A marked lymphocyte and plasma cell response is interpreted as the body mounting a defense against the tumor. Infiltrates of lymphoid cells are present at the tumor site in most neoplasms and plasma cells are consistently and characteristically associated with squamous cell carcinomas of va-

rious organs (Ioachim 1976). No attempt was made to identify cells separately but were grouped as lymphocytes. Although reports indicate that the best survival is found among patients with a good stromal response, occasionally this is not confirmed. It may be that the lymphocytes are suppressor or tolerant rather than helper and therefore work to the disadvantage of the host. It will take time to study stromal response in greater detail.

The chromosomal region that encodes for the glycoproteins that function as strong histocompatibility antigens includes other genetic loci as well. In mice, genes exist that determine whether the animal makes very little or a great deal of antibody in response to certain kinds of antigens. Genes that appear to govern the level of immune responsiveness to antigens in this manner are called Ir genes. Analysis of segregant populations of mice reveals that some Ir genes are closely linked to genes encoding for major histocompatibility complex (MHC). The MHC, therefore, includes several different kinds of genes: those that encode for histocompatibility antigens important in allograft immunity, those that govern the amount of antibody produced in response to antigenic challenge, termed Ir genes, and genes governing susceptibility to oncogenic viruses. When this can be easily applied clinically and antisera is available to identify helper, suppressor and tolerant T cells as well as plasma cells, the role of local immunity will be clarified.

The poor results following vascular and/or lymphatic invasion reported in the previous study is not confirmed in this paper. Statisticians maintain that the numbers are too small to be signifi-

Table 1. Cancer of the cervix, survival - stage IB.

Years after treatment	Alive at beginning of treatment	Died during interval	Lost to follow-up	With-drawn alive during interval	Effective number exposed to the risk of dying	Proportion dying	Proportion surviving	Cumulative proportion surviving from beginning of treatment through end of interval
0–1	39	3	1		38.5	0.078	0.922	0.922
1–2	35	1		6	32	0.031	0.969	0.893
2–3	28	2		8	24	0.083	0.917	0.818

cant. However, the authors of this paper believe that it may be the result of treating this high risk group with prophylactic chemotherapy. It is suggestive, but not conclusive, that this may be the reason for improvement among patients with vascular invasion. The study will continue and hopefully the accumulation of more data will continue to show the initial improved survival among these high risk patients.

The authors continue to identify patients whose cervical cancer shows vascular invasion to be at high risk. It is the opinion of the authors that this group should receive chemotherapy prophylactically. The lack of success of chemotherapy has been shown for a mass of squamous cell cancer, but little has been done to evaluate its use prophylactically. Until a method of monitoring the tumor is available, the prophylactic treatment must be structured on an empirical basis

and evaluated in a retrospective manner. Several regimens have been tried and for a variety of reasons discontinued. Currently Mitomycin, 20 mg is given as a bolus followed by 1500 mg 5-FU given as a continuous infusion over 24 hours and continued for 5 days. This is repeated at 4-week intervals if the blood count is not suppressed. Chemotherapy was selected over radiation therapy on the assumption that invasion of a vascular channal may have a higher disproportion for metastatic disease outside of the local area.

ACKNOWLEDGEMENT

The authors wish to express their thanks to Marcia Miller and Ruzena Danek for preparation of this manuscript.

REFERENCES

Barber HRK, Sommers SC, Rotterdam H, Kwon T: Vascular invasion as a prognostic factor in stage IB cancer of the cervix. Obstet Gynec 52(3): 343, 1978.

Barber HRK, Sommers SC, Snyder R, Kwon T: Histologic and nuclear grading and stromal reactions as indices for prognosis in ovarian cancer. Am J Obstet Gynec 121: 795, 1975.

Black M, Speer FD: Nuclear structure in cancer tissues. Surg Gynec Obstet 105: 97, 1957.

Burnet FM: The concept of immunological surveillance. Prog Exp Tumor Res 13: 1, 1970.

Chabon AB, Takenchi SJ, Sommers SC: Histologic differences in breast carcinoma of Japanese and American women. Cancer. 33: 1577, 1974.

Friedell GH, Steiner G, Kistner RW: Prognostic value of blood vessel invasion in cervical cancer. Obstet Gynec 29: 855, 1967.

Gusberg SB, Herman GG: Radiosensitivity and virulence factors in cervical cancer. Am J Obstet Gynec 100(5): 627, 1968.

Gusberg SB, Yannopoulos K, Cohen CJ: Virulence indices and lymph nodes in cancer of the cervix. Am J Roentgen Rad Ther 111(2): 273, 1971.

Ioachim HL: Guest Editorial: The stromal reaction of tumors: An expression of immune surveillance. JNCI 57: 465, 1976.

Ioachim HL, Dorsett B, Paluch E: The immune response at the tumor site in lung carcinoma. Cancer 38: 2296, 1976.

Laroye GJ: Immunological surveillance against cancer: Critique of an established hypothesis. Med Hypotheses 1: 43, 1976.

Riotton G, Christopherson WM: Cytology of the female genital tract. International Histological Classification of Tumors No. 8. Geneva: World Health Organization, 1973.

van Nagell JR, Rayburn W, Donaldson ES, Hanson M, Gay EC, Yoneda J, Marayuma Y, Powell DF: Therapeutic implications of patterns of recurrence in cancer of the uterine cervix. Cancer 44: 2354, 1979.

van Nagell JR, Donaldson ES, Wood BS, Parker JC: The significance of vascular invasion and lymphocytic infiltration in invasive cervical cancer. Cancer 41: 228, 1978.

26. COLPOSCOPY AND CYTOLOGY FOR THE DIAGNOSIS OF EARLY CERVICAL CARCINOMA

U. HERMANNS*, H. AMIRIKIA and E.S.E. HAFEZ

Lack of clinical signs in the intraepithelial phases of cervical carcinoma require routine surveillance techniques to detect these early lesions. Using cytology as the most easily applied economical and effective tool of cancer detection is advantageous in all countries establishing cancer screening programs. Colposcopy was introduced in the United States 5 years after its development in 1925 by Hinselmann, yet these efforts were largely unsuccessful. With the exception of Australia, colposcopy was not initially introduced to English speaking countries due to language barriers. In the 1940s, acceptance of colposcopy in American gynecologic practice was further impeded by the introduction of the Papanicolaou (Pap) smear used as a screening method.

Colposcopy and cytology have been considered as competitive methods until it was realized that both gave comparable results. Because colposcopy requires considerable expense and time, the value of this method as a mass screening device has been questioned. Many clinicians believe that preclinical cervical carcinoma can be accurately diagnosed by the combined use of cytology and biopsy while ignoring the difficulties in the interpretation of cellular and tissue specimens. The advantages and disadvantages of cytology and colposcopy are thereby discussed with sepcial reference to their concomitant use as a basis for additional diagnostic procedures.

I. SEPARATE USE OF CYTOLOGY AND COLPOSCOPY

Extensive investigations have been conducted on

carcinoma *in situ* and early invasive lesions of the uterine cervix using cytology, whereas studies involving cervical cancer detection by colposcopy are more limited.

I.A. Cytology in early cancer detection

In contrast to colposcopy, the Pap smear technique is easy and requires no expensive instrumentation. Cytological screening detects cellular changes of cervical cancer at an early stage, but its accuracy is often over-emphasized (Denzler 1978). The Pap smear is not a definitive technique to detect cervical cancer and false-negative results are often reported.

Invasive cancers of the cervix occurring in a screened population is clearly an indication of false-negative cytology results. Two cervical smears taken sequentially increse the detection of abnormal cytology by 86% (Shulman et al. 1975), indicating that in a high percentage of cases, a single smear does not precisely reflect the histologic state of the abnormal cervix. Re-screening shows evidence of disease that should have been detected at the first screening (Coppleson and Brown 1974).

There is a wide range from 1.8% to 30% in the incidence of false-negative smears (Soule and Dahlin 1960; Maisel et al. 1963; Navratil 1964; Richart 1964; Griffiths and Younge 1967; Christopherson 1970; Pedersen et al. 1971). Several authors compared the results of Pap smears and histology for dysplasia, carcinoma *in situ* and invasive carcinoma of the cervix (Table 1). Besides the relatively high incidence of false-negative results, there is a so-called doubtful group with a rate between 0.5% and 6.0% (Stafl and Friedrich 1973), which may contain a significant number of early preclinical malignancies.

* Fellowship of Deutscher Akademischer Austauschdienst (DAAD).

Hafez, E.S.E., Smith, J.P. (eds.), Carcinoma of the Cervix: Biology and Diagnosis. ISBN-13: 978-94-009-7487-6
© 1982, Martinus Nijhoff Publishers, The Hague/Boston/London.

I.B. Colposcopy in early cancer detection

The time required for colposcopic evaluation depends on the skill of the examiner. Its accuracy in the diagnosis of cervical cancer has been well documented (Donohue and Meriwether 1972; Ortiz and Odel 1970; Stafl and Mattingly 1973; Tredway et al. 1972), and is found superior to cytology in the detection of cervical dysplasia (Kioko 1979). The colposcopic grading system allows correct prediction of histological diagnosis in preclinical invasive carcinoma, carcinoma *in situ*, or major dysplasia, in about 95% of grade III atypias (Coppleson et al. 1978).

The overall incidence of false-negative colposcopic findings varies from 2 to 26% (Table 2). Reports claiming that the false-negative rate of colposcopy is greater than that of cytology (Olson and Nichols 1960; Kern et al. 1964; Navratil 1964;

Crapanzano 1972), do not differentiate between 'negative' and 'unsatisfactory' colposcopy. When the squamo-columnar junction is not visible, colposcopy procedure is defined as 'unsatisfactory' (Committee on terminology, 1976); its incidence is about 5–45% (Table 3). Excluding unsatisfactory cases with an error rate of about 20% (Feldman et al. 1976), the accuracy of colposcopy increases to 90% (Table 2). There are three main reasons for false-negative results:

1. The lesion is exclusively located high in the cervical canal.

2. The increased vascularity due to acute cervicitis may mask the underlying malignant epithelium.

3. The transformation zone recedes into the cervical canal in postmenopausal women.

The main disadvantage of colposcopy is its lack of specificity. Although a relationship exists between the colposcopic finding and the degree of cytologic

Table 1. Diagnostic accuracy of cervical carcinoma without colposcopy.

		Cytology		Undirected biopsy	
Overall	Correct diagnosis	44–79%	Dolan et al. 1975; White et al. 1976; Tovell et al. 1976; Swan 1976; Ronk et al. 1977; Knutzen and Sherwood 1977; Pang et al. 1977	50–94%	Sabatelle et al. 1969; Krumholz and Knapp 1972; Selim et al. 1973
	Underdiagnosis	6–34%	Kolstad 1970; Martin 1972; Selim et al. 1973; Dolan et al. 1975; Selim et al. 1977; Fritsches and Busch 1977		
Dysplasia	Correct diagnosis	40–93%	Wied et al. 1962; Chao et al. 1969; Cecchini et al. 1978; Satoh 1978	35%	Satoh 1978
	Underdiagnosis	12–14%	Chao et al. 1969; Kioko 1979	20–52%	Sabatelle et al. 1969; Chao et al. 1969
Carcinoma *in situ*	Correct diagnosis	68–95%	Wied et al. 1962; Chao et al. 1969; Van Nagell et al. 1976; Cecchini et al. 1978; Satoh 1978; Naujoks et al. 1979	70–95%	Chao et al. 1969; Griffiths and Younge 1967; Satoh 1978
	Underdiagnosis	1–22%	Chao et al. 1969; Griffiths and Younge 1967; Stafl and Mattingly 1973; Naujoks et al. 1979	15%	Villasanta and Durkan 1966; Anderson and Linton 1967
Invasive carcinoma	Correct diagnosis	18–98%	Wied et al. 1962; Chao et al. 1969; Van Nagell et al. 1976; Cecchini et al. 1978; Satoh 1978	58–100%	Griffiths and Younge 1967; Satoh 1978
	Underdiagnosis	0%	Chao et al. 1969		

Table 2. Diagnostic accuracy of cervical carcinoma with colposcopy.

	Colposcopy		Target biopsy	
Correct diagnosis	42–89%	Stafl and Mattingly 1973; Kanka et al. 1974; Dolan et al. 1975; Swan 1976; Tovell et al. 1976; Hovadhanakul et al. 1976; Knutzen and Sherwood 1977; Kohan et al. 1977; Ronk et al. 1977; Selim et al. 1977; Pang et al. 1977	73–100%	Crapanzano 1972; Dolan et al. 1975; Boelter and Newman 1975; Cruikshank et al. 1976; Hovadhanakul et al. 1976; White et al. 1976; Benedet et al. 1977; Knutzen and Sherwood 1977; Pang et al. 1977; Ronk et al. 1977; Kirkup et al. 1980
Underdiagnosis	2–26%	Kolstad 1970; Stafl and Mattingly 1973; Tovell et al. 1976; Fritsches and Busch 1977; Ronk et al. 1977; Kohan et al. 1977; Kirkup et al. 1980; Allahverdian et al. 1980	0.3–21%	Ortiz et al. 1969; Hollyock and Chanen 1972; Stafl and Mattingly 1973; Dolan et al. 1975; Knutzen and Sherwood 1977; Pang et al. 1977; Kirkup et al. 1980

atypia, the malignancy index of all colposcopic atypias is between 6 and 14%, thus suggesting a high false-positive rate (Coppleson et al. 1978). The major factors responsible for false-positives include benign lesions of the cervix (i.e., papillomas, syphilitic ulcers, and benign granulomatous lesions), in which colposcopic differentiation from a malignant lesion is extremely difficult (Stafl and Mattingly 1973).

In colposcopic technique, the entire transformation zone and the entire cervical lesion must be visualized (Lang 1976). Although dysplasia of the cervix and carcinoma *in situ* mainly occur within the confines of the colposcopic transformation zone (Selim et al. 1977), carcinomatous lesions may rarely be located in the endocervix, beyond colposcopical visibility.

About 80 to 90% of patients are suitable for colposcopic examination (Townsend et al. 1970; Donohue and Meriwether 1972; Stafl and Mattingly 1973; Benedet et al. 1976). In one-fourth of the cases, metaplastic epithelium as the potential precursor of squamous carcinoma is entirely within the cervical canal.

II. CONCOMITANT USE OF CYTOLOGY AND COLPOSCOPY

Cytology and colposcopy techniques have their own specific advantages and limitations. By the combined use of both techniques, the diagnostic accuracy for preclinical cervical carcinoma reaches 98–99% (Gronrovs et al. 1967). Use of colposcopy in addition to cytology positively influences both initial diagnosis and further diagnostic measurements.

II.A. *Effect of colposcopy on the initial diagnosis*

The addition of colposcopic screening to smear screening may discover preclinical cancer in 1 out of 700 cases with negative cytology (Hill 1966). In many cases, however, dysplasia appears cytologically negative and colposcopically positive, and in those cases, a change to neoplasia could be detected by periodic cytologic follow-up at a very early stage (Odell 1976). Use of colposcopy renders optical evidence predominantly in young women of intraepithelial lesions that precede positive cytology for years (Stafl and Mattingly 1975; Herbeck 1979). This adds an additional 5–15% security to the 80%

Table 3. Rate of unsatisfactory colposcopy in the diagnosis of cervical carcinoma.

Rate	Author
5–10%	White et al. 1976; Krumholz and Talebian 1976; Swan 1976; Talebian et al. 1977; Akerele 1977; Kirkup et al. 1980.
11–15%	Coppleson 1960; Donohue and Meriwether 1972; Stafl and Mattingly 1973; Hovadhanakul et al. 1976
16–44%	Ostergard and Gondos 1973; Chanen and Hollyock 1974; Dolan et al. 1975; Ronk et al. 1977.

detection rate already reached by cytology (Herbeck and Menken 1977).

Besides the problems in establishing an efficient screening program, there are many difficulties associated with proper handling of patients with suspicious or positive smears. Among them are questionable accuracy of blind biopsy, extent of cone biopsy, complications of conization – especially during pregnancy – diagnosis, and follow-up of young patients who desire having children.

II.B. Effect of colposcopy on further diagnostic procedures

II.B.1. Follow-up of abnormal cytology without colposcopy

II.B.1.a. Repeated cytology. Class II smears (inflammatory atypia smears) cannot be regarded as a negative group because of a 2–36% incidence of more advanced lesions in subsequent tissue diagnosis (Hulka 1968; Stafl and Mattingly 1973; Kohan et al. 1977; Younglove and Newman 1978). Traditionally, patients with Pap smears labeled as inflammatory atypia are treated for the infection and followed by repeated cytology until the results are definitely negative or positive (Dunn 1979). However, repeat cytology is of no value in short-term follow-up of cervical intraepithelial neoplasia (CIN) (Deppe et al. 1978).

Second cytology examination alone, categorized 62% of atypical smears as 'suspicious', whereas, cytology combined with colposcopy and target biopsy proved 79% of the preliminary atypical smears to be dysplastic (Allahverdian et al. 1980). Although such lesions may become evident by persistent abnormal cytology, a delay in the diagnosis of carcinoma *in situ* may result in the loss of follow-up or continued advancement of the neoplasia (Stafl and Mattingly 1973).

II.B.1.b. Cervical biopsy. The likelihood of finding carcinoma is 70–80% with a class III smear, 80–95% with a class IV smear, and about 100% with a class V smear (Singleton and Rutledge 1968). The final diagnosis of carcinoma *in situ* or invasive cancer prior to any therapy depends on histology. Before the renaissance of colposcopy in the diagnosis of cervical cancer, the management of an abnormal Pap smear invariably included random biopsies or conization of the cervix (Hulka 1968). Most gynecologists perform cone biopsy following a cytology report indicating either dysplasia, pre-invasive or early invasive cancer in the non-pregnant and pregnant patient, regardless of the stage of pregnancy (Rogers and Williams 1967).

1. *Random or multiple quadrant biopsy.* Cervical lesions are most likely found on the portio vaginalis (Selim et al. 1977), yet the most significant lesion may be missed by a non-directed biopsy (Sabatelle et al. 1969). In the absence of visible lesions, a random or multiple-quadrant biopsy is inadequate as a definitive diagnosis of cervical cancer, es-

Table 4. Missed invasive carcinoma with various diagnostic techniques.

Method	Rate	Authors
Cytology	2.7%	Knutzen and Sherwood 1977
Colposcopy	2.0%	Knutzen and Sherwood 1977
Cone biopsy	0.7–4%	Silbar and Woodruff 1966; Villasanta and Durkan 1966; Crapanzano 1972; White et al. 1976
Target biopsy	0–1%	Ortiz et al. 1969; Crapanzano 1972; White et al. 1976; Hovadhanakul et al. 1976; Knutzen and Sherwood 1977; Deppe et al. 1978
	18%	Cecchini et al. 1978
Satisfactory colposcopy	0%	Townsend et al. 1970
Unsatisfactory colposcopy	88%	Townsend et al. 1970
	100%	Hollyock and Chanen 1972; Chanen and Hollyock 1974; Dolan et al. 1975

188

pecially of its intraepithelial variants (Table 1). Undirected biopsies are of less accurate diagnostic value than cytology (Chao et al. 1969).

2. *Cone biopsy*. The fear of overlooking invasive cancer by punch biopsy and having subsequent inadequate treatment by simple hysterectomy is the major motivation behind conization; although this technique is not infallible in excluding the invasion (Table 4). The overall rate of diagnostic error for conization is 3.5% (Ferguson and Demick 1960; Anderson and Linton 1967; Sabatelle et al. 1969; Chao et al. 1969).

The benefit of precise histologic diagnosis, however, is challenged by the various adverse effects of the technique such as hemorrhage, cervical stenosis and uterine perforation. The incidence of hemorrhage is approximately 10% (Chao et al. 1969; Villasanta and Durkan 1966; Nishimura et al. 1978). Cervical stenosis is found in 7% of the cases (Hester and Read 1960), and uterine perforation occurs in about 1% of all conizations (Davis et al. 1972; Hester and Read 1960). Although stenosis can be prevented by sounding the endocervical canal and late hemorrhage does not occur with synthetic absorbable sutures (Nelson et al. 1979), diagnostic conization should be limited to precisely defined indications. Two groups of patients are at higher risks for complications of cone biopsy: young women (Claman and Lee 1974), and pregnant

patients, due to eversion of the squamo-columnar junction and increased vascularity of the cervix. Boutselis (1972) observed an overall complication rate for conization of 21%, with abnormal bleeding accounting for half, and subsequent abortion or premature labor making up the other half. Blood transfusions because of massive hemorrhage are required in 6% to 11% (Daskal and Pitkin 1968; Rogers and Williams 1967). Cone biopsy during pregnancy is associated with a considerable risk of an inadvertent operative interruption of the pregnancy (Bottomy and Boyd 1961; Boutselis and Ullery 1964), intrauterine infection (Rogers and Williams 1967), and termination of pregnancy by abortion or premature labor (Dean et al. 1962; Ferguson and Brown 1960). The average fetal loss is approximately 5–15% (Chao et al. 1969; Daskal and Pitkin 1968; Davis et al. 1972; Villasanta and Durkan 1966).

In a combined total of 149 cone biopsies during pregnancy, no invasive carcinoma was noted (Rogers and Williams 1967; Daskal and Pitkin 1968), suggesting that the high fetal loss must be considered avoidable. With the onset of pregnancy, the amount of residual tumor left after conization remarkably increases (Boutselis 1972), thereby increasing the rate of diagnostic error. Conization on the basis of a single abnormal Pap smear cannot be recommended.

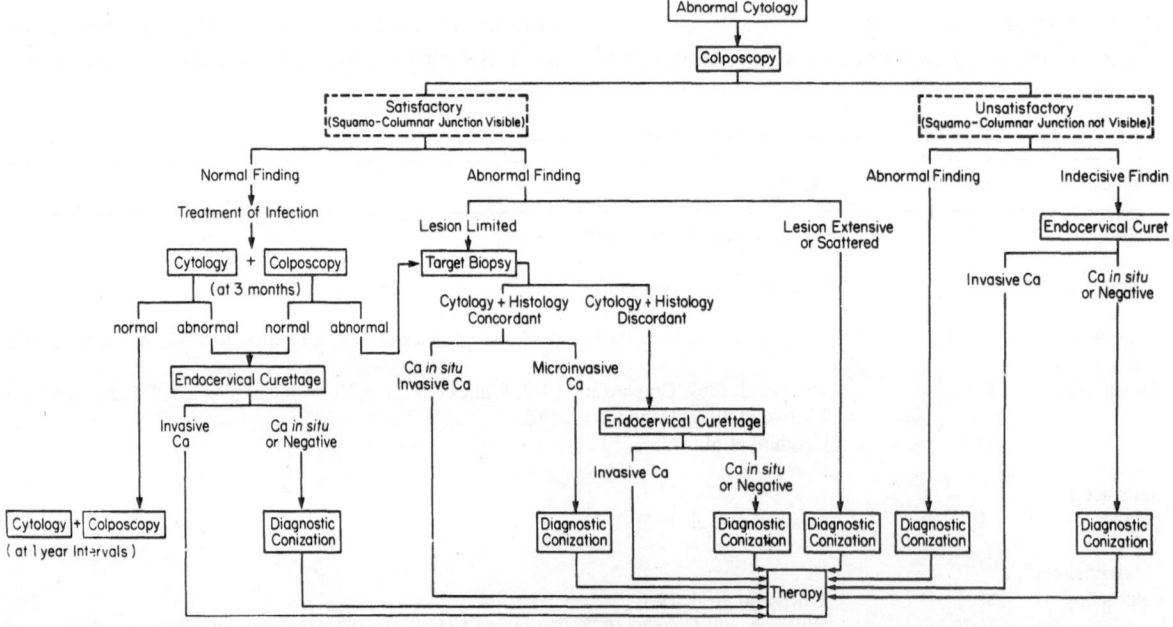

Figure 1. Suggested role of colposcopy in the evaluation of abnormal cytology.

II.B.2. Follow-up of abnormal cytology with colposcopy

The histologic condition reflected by a suspicious smear usually includes mild to severe dysplasia, carcinoma *in situ*, and less frequently, early invasive carcinoma. The 45% frequency of unnecessary conizations for inflammatory atypia (Stucin et al. 1972) suggests the need of an accurate but less radical diagnostic technique to evaluate a case of abnormal cytology.

II.B.2.a. Colposcopic classification.

Colposcopy classifies patients with abnormal cytology into three major groups (Figure 1).

1. Patients with normal colposcopical findings: The squamo-columnar junction is fully visible, and no focal suspect lesion is detected colposcopically. Follow-up consists of repeat cytology and colposcopy; diagnostic conization is indicated only if follow-up cytology is either positive or repeatedly suspicious.

2. Patients with abnormal colposcopical findings: The final diagnosis is based on the histology of the colposcopically directed punch biopsy (target biopsy). Cone biopsy is indicated only in a few patients.

3. Patients with unsatisfactory colposcopical findings: If the squamo-columnar junction is not fully visible, colposcopy fails to exclude a lesion inside the endocervical canal. Positive or repeatedly suspicious cytology is therefore followed by endocervical curettage and/or diagnostic conization.

II.B.2.b. Cervical biopsy.

1. *Target biopsy* (colposcopically directed punch biopsy). Several patients with doubtful or positive cytology show no obvious target lesion on examination with the unaided eye. The main benefit of colposcopy is to identify and localize lesions not visible by gross inspection. Results of colposcopic and colpomicroscopic studies indicate that CIN is significantly limited to the T-zone on the ectocervix

in young women and extends into the lower end of the endocervical canal in older women (Coppleson et al. 1978; Chanen and Hollyock 1974; Tovell et al. 1976). In young women of childbearing age where conization should be avoided, the lesion is usually clearly visible during colposcopy and easily accessible for a target biopsy.

Satisfactory colposcopy for a target biopsy includes that the lesion: (a) is entirely visible, (b) does not extend into the endocervical canal, and (c) covers less than 25% of the portio. There are three main arguments in favor of colposcopically directed punch biopsy instead of cone biopsy:

1. Target biopsies have the same diagnostic accuracy as cone biopsies but have fewer risks (Table 2). A comparison of cone biopsy and directed punch biopsy in the same patient shows a high correlation in the histological findings of both methods (Beller and Khatamee 1966; Ortiz and Odell 1970; Savage 1975). Excluding cases of unsatisfactory colposcopy, the diagnostic error rate is below 1% (Stafl and Mattingly 1973; Knutzen and Sherwood 1977), otherwise the percentage of missed invasion dramatically increases (Table 4). Complications of punch biopsy occur in fewer than 0.1% of cases as contrasted with the 10% rate of serious hemorrhage and 1% additional complications attributable to conization (Burke and Mathews 1977).

2. In case of small focal lesions, the directed biopsy is probably more accurate than routine examination of the cone. Without thorough sectioning of the cone specimen, isolated areas of carcinoma *in situ* or micro-invasive cancer can easily be missed (Krumholz and Knapp 1972).

3. Avoiding unnecessary conizations of the cervix can reduce the laboratory, hospital and physician expenses of diagnosing early cervical cancer by more than 85% (Stafl and Mattingly 1973). Colposcopically directed biopsy is a suitable method in approximately 80 to 94% of the patients (Crapanzano 1972; Krumholz and Knapp 1972; Ortiz and

Table 5. Avoidance of diagnostic conization by colposcopically directed biopsy.

Rate	Authors
45–75%	Chanen and Hollyock 1974; Trombetta 1975; Cruikshank et al. 1976; White et al. 1976; Yajima et al. 1978
80–90%	Donohue and Meriwether 1972; Krumholz and Knapp 1972; Ostergard and Gondos 1973; Dolan et al. 1975; Odell 1976; Swan 1976; Kohan et al. 1977; Selim et al. 1977; Pang et al. 1977
>90%	Stafl and Mattingly 1973

Odell 1970). By target biopsies, diagnostic cervical conization can be avoided in 50–90% of the cases with abnormal Pap smears (Table 5).

Colposcopy with target biopsy allows an adequate management of the pregnant patient with an abnormal Pap smear. The exact diagnosis of a cervical lesion during pregnancy is difficult due to inflammation, decidual reaction, and hyperactive epithelial changes (Bottomy and Boyd 1961). Exclusion of invasive carcinoma is essential in preventing an unsuspected invasive lesion from being untreated during the duration of pregnancy, and in determining the method of delivery. Vaginal delivery in case of invasive cancer lowers the maternal 5-year survival rate (Gusberg et al. 1970; Boutselis 1972) but is not contraindicated in the presence of intraepithelial neoplasia (Sall et al. 1969; Boutselis 1972).

In the pregnant woman, colposcopy is especially suitable due to the physiologic eversion of the cervix which affords an excellent colposcopic visualization of the entire squamo-columnar junction as the most likely origin of malignant transformation. Benedet et al. (1977) found an exact agreement between colposcopic appearance and histology in 89% of their pregnant patients. Expert colposcopists maintain that there is no need to take biopsies if there are no colposcopic features of microinvasive or invasive carcinoma (DePetrillo et al. 1975; Talebian et al. 1976). The carefully selected patient (e.g., the cytologic smear does not suggest invasive carcinoma and the satisfactory colposcopic finding is compatible with an early cervical lesion) (Figure 2), may be followed through pregnancy without conization and re-evaluated and treated postpartum (Trombetta 1976; Selim et al. 1977; Nelson et al. 1979; Dudan et al. 1973). The very low incidence of invasive cancer in pregnancy makes inadequate diagnosis most unlikely (Ortiz and Newton 1971). Postponement of definitive surgical treatment until after the puerperium does not usually lead to an advancement of the disease (Jones et al. 1965; Stafl and Mattingly 1973). Successful management of the pregnant patient requires expertise with the colposcopic technique, strict adherence to the indications for immediate conization, and adequate follow-up.

2. *Cone biopsy under colposcopic guidance.* Including colposcopy in the diagnostic procedure,

there are only the following indications for cone biopsy in the management of patients with abnormal smears: (a) cases considered as inappropriate candidates, e.g., those deemed unreliable in routine follow-up; (b) cases with repeated abnormal smears in the absence of a colposcopic lesion; (c) cases where the abnormal T-zone extends up into the endocervix beyond the visual limitations of the colposcope so that an endocervical lesion with the possibility of invasion must be suspected (unsatisfactory colposcopy); (d) cases where the lesions are colposcopically too extensive (e.g., more than 25% of the cervix is involved) or too diffuse for meaningful biopsy; (e) cases with indecisive colposcopic findings and negative cervical curettage; (f) cases with positive endocervical curettage suggestive of any abnormality except invasive cancer, and (g) cases diagnosed by target biopsy as microinvasive carcinoma in order to perform the depth of invasion. If cone biopsy is the elected diagnostic procedure, pre-operative colposcopic evaluation will improve the procedure as conization itself does not guarantee the complete removal of the cervical lesion (Trombetta 1975). Determining the extent of the lesion by colposcopy achieves a cone biopsy that is conservative enough to allow accurate histological diagnosis and radical enough to act as definitive treatment if required. Reduction in the size of the cone reduces the high morbidity of this procedure in pregnancy and avoids the possible complication of cervical incompetence in women of childbearing age.

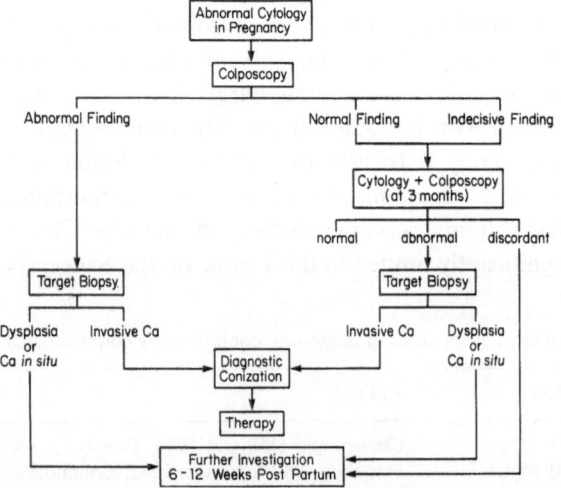

Figure 2. Suggested role of colposcopy in the evaluation of abnormal cytology in pregnancy.

II.B.2.c. Endocervical curettage (ECC)

One important limitation of colposcopy is the incomplete visualization of a neoplastic process extending into the endocervical canal. To solve this dilemma, endocervical curettage (ECC) was introduced by Younge (1958), but has not become an established part of colposcopic examination following abnormal cervical cytology. Some authors recommend it as a routine procedure during colposcopic follow-up (Ortiz et al. 1969; Dolan et al. 1975; Townsend et al. 1970; Nelson et al. 1979; Kolstad 1966; White et al. 1976; Ostergard and Gondos 1973).

The combination of colposcopy, target biopsy and ECC can rule out the presence of invasive carcinoma in 85% of patients with abnormal cervical cytology (Ostergard and Gondos 1973). However, the rate of missed invasive lesions is not increased by the omission of ECC (Swan 1979), and the procedure has definite drawbacks. In a few cases where occult invasion is diagnosed and conization is avoided, curettage specimens are frequently insufficient for adequate pathological interpretation, especially in menopausal patients (Urcuyo et al. 1977; Shingleton et al. 1977). Determining the presence and/or depth of invasion is often difficult, and requires conization after ECC. Histologic interpretation of the cone may be hampered after a recent curettage (Chanen and Hollyock 1974; Urcuyo et al. 1977). ECC should not be performed routinely as the procedure is of minimal value in unsatisfactory colposcopy.

In cases with discrepancies between Pap smear and colposcopy, an endocervical lesion must be suspected (Ronk et al. 1977; Urcuyo et al. 1977), and ECC becomes mandatory (Townsend et al. 1970). Negative curettings in inconclusive cases do not rule out the possibility of endocervical carcinoma and must be followed by cone biopsy and fractional curettage.

III. CONCLUDING REMARKS

CIN is usually asymptomatic, first becoming evident in routine Pap smears. Cytology is undoubtedly the most practical method for cervical cancer screening. However, even with the most experienced cytologists and optimal laboratory facilities, the false-negative rate of a single smear reaches 10–30%. The effectiveness of colposcopy lies in its ability to detect small areas of malignant epithelium which are not represented in cervical cytology. It further detects areas of dysplasia and may clarify the interpretation of the atypical smear. Ideally, every woman should have a colposcopic examination at as regular intervals as a Pap smear. However, the combination of routine cytology and routine colposcopy in a mass screening program is not practical for several reasons: colposcopy is expensive and relatively time consuming, the number of experienced colposcopists is limited, and the improvement of diagnosis by the combined use of the two methods does not seem statistically significant to recommend its routine use on a large scale. The practical compromise adopted is a two-level screening program that improves the detection rate of serious abnormalities from the 80–90% range to the 90–95% range: After routine screening by exfoliative cytology (first level), colposcopy is used for the interpretation and management of the abnormal smear (second level).

Colposcopy as an intermediate diagnostic step between cytology and histology refines the evaluation and management of patients with early cervical neoplasia, defining the site and the type of biopsy as well as the need for ECC. The use of target biopsy will lead to diagnostic accuracy, decreased morbidity, and lower hospitalization costs. The questionable 'blind' four quadrant biopsy with a diagnostic error rate of over 20% can be abandoned. The need for diagnostic conization of the cervix as an accurate, but risky method, can be avoided in young women with benign lesions, in older women with endocervical invasive carcinoma, and particularly in pregnant patients. Thus, the number of diagnostic conizations can drop by 85-95%. Colposcopy also saves many unnecessary biopsies from cervices that appear suspicious during naked eye inspection. Therefore, the additional time and expenses required appear justified. The combination of cytology, colposcopy with target biopsy, and ECC is successful only in experienced hands. This modality of diagnostic procedure is not available to every practicing gynecologist, until combined colposcopy training is integrated in all obstetrics/gynecology residency

192

programs. Colposcopy training centers with experienced personnel are needed most, so that an increasing number of gynecologists can apply this diagnostic tool in their own practices.

REFERENCES

Akerele FA: The use of colposcopy in the evaluation of abnormal Papanicolaou smears in a large group practice. MD, State Med J 36: 55, 1977.

Allahverdian V, Valaitis J, Kalis O, Pearlman S: Cytology and colposcopy in the diagnosis and management of outpatients with cervical intraepithelial neoplasia. J Reprod Med 24: 1, 1980.

American Society for Colposcopy and Colpomimicroscopy: Glossary of Colposcopic Terms. International Symposium Florida 1973. J Reprod Med 16: 212, 1976.

Anderson SG, Linton EB: The diagnostic accuracy of cervical biopsy and cervical conization. Am J Obstet Gynec 99: 113, 1967.

Beller FK, Khatamee M: Evaluation of punch biopsy of the cervix under direct colposcopic observation (target punch biopsy) Obstet Gynec 28: 622, 1966.

Benedet JL, Boyes DA, Nichols TM, Millner A: Colposcopic evaluation of patients with abnormal cervical cytology. Br J Obstet Gynaecol 83: 177, 1976.

Benedet JL, Boyes DA, Nichols TM, Millner A: The role of colposcopy in the evaluation of abnormal vaginal vault smears. Gynecol Oncol 5: 338, 1977.

Benedet JL, Boyes DA, Nichols TM, Millner A: Colposcopic evaluation of pregnant patients with abnormal cervical smears. Br J Obstet Gynecol 84: 517, 1977.

Boelter WC, Newman RL: The correlation between colposcopic grading directed punch biopsy, and conization. Am J Obstet Gynecol 122: 945, 1975.

Bottomy JR, Boyd RA: The clinicians dilemma: Conization for evaluation of carcinoma in situ of the cervix in pregnancy. Southern Med J 54: 584, 1961.

Boutselis JG: Intraepithelial carcinoma of the cervix associated with pregnancy. Obstet Gynecol 40: 657, 1972.

Boutselis FG, Ullery JC: Intraepithelial carcinoma of the cervix in pregnancy. Am J Obstet Gynec 90: 593, 1964.

Burke L, Mathews BE: Colposcopy in clinical practice. Philadelphia: F.A. Davis Company, 1977.

Cecchini S, Bonardi L, Cipparone G, Ottaviano M, Pierohi G: Contribution of cytology, colposcopy, target biopsy and conization to the early diagnosis of precancerous and cancerous lesions of the cervix uteri. Tumori 64: 389, 1978.

Chanen W, Hollyock VE: Colposcopy and the conservative management of cervical dysplasia and carcinoma in situ. Obstet Gynecol 43: 527, 1974.

Chao S, McCaffrey RM, Todd WD, Moore JG: Conization in evaluation and management of cervical neoplasm. Am J Obstet Gynecol 103: 574, 1969.

Christopherson WM: Present role of cytology in cancer detection and diagnosis. Prog Clin Cancer 4: 185, 1970.

Claman AD, Lee N: Factors that relate to complications of cone biopsy. Am J Obstet Gynec 120: 124, 1974.

Coppleson M: The value of colposcopy in the detection of preclinical carcinoma of the cervix. J Obstet Gynecol Br Emp 67: 11, 1960.

Coppleson LW, Brown B: 1974. Estimation of the screening error rate from observed detection rates in repeated cervical cytology. Am J Obstet Gynecol 119: 953, 1974.

Coppleson M, Pixley E, Reid B: Colposcopy, a Scientific and Practical Approach to the Cervix and Vagina in Health and Disease. Springfield, Illinois: Charles C. Thomas, 1978.

Crapanzano JT: Office diagnosis in patients with abnormal cervicovaginal cytosmears; correlation of colposcopic biopsy and cytologic findings. Am J Obstet Gynecol 113: 967, 1972.

Cruikshank D, Kaminsky DB, Ekbladh LEV: Colposcopic evaluation of cervical intraepithelial neoplasia. J Reprod Med 17: 327, 1976.

Daskal JL, Pitkin RM: Cone biopsy of the cervix during pregnancy. Obstet Gynecol 32: 1, 1968.

Davis RM, Cooke JK, Kirk RF: Cervical conization. Obstet Gynecol 40: 23, 1972.

Dean RE, Isbell NP, Woodard DE: Cervical carcinoma in situ in pregnancy. Obstet Gynec 20: 633, 1962.

Denzler U: The effectiveness of cytology in the prevention of cancer of the uterine cervix. Geburtsh Frauenheilk 38: 1028, 1978.

DePetrillo A, Townsend D, Morrow CP, Lickrish GM, DiSaia PJ, Roy M: Colposcopic evaluation of the abnormal Papanicolaou test in pregnancy. Am J Obstet Gynecol 121: 441, 1975.

Deppe G, Marin AC, Shapiro WJ, Koffler D, Cohen JC: Colposcopy in the detection and management of patients with cervical intraepithelial neoplasia. Mt Sinai J Med (NY) 45: 75, 1978.

Dolan TE, Boyce J, Rosen Y, Lu T: Cytology, colposcopy and direct biopsy: What are the limitations? Gynecol Oncol 3: 314, 1975.

Donohue LR, Meriwether W: Colposcopy as a diagnostic tool in the investigation of cervical neoplasias. Am J Obstet Gynecol 113: 107, 1972.

Dudan RC, Yon JL, Ford JN & Averette, H.E.: Carcinoma of the cervix and pregnancy. Gynecol Oncol 1: 283, 1973.

Dunn L.J. (1979). Cervical cytologic evaluation. And what to do when findings are abnormal. Postgrad Med 65: 187.

Feldman MJ, Kent DR, Linzey EM, Goldstein AJ: The making of a colposcopist. A safe and sensible approach. J Reprod Med 16: 73, 1976.

Ferguson JH, Demick PE: Diagnostic conization of the cervix. N Eng J Med 262: 13, 1960.

Ferguson JH, Brown GC: Cervical conization during pregnancy. Surg Gynec Obstet 111: 603, 1960.

Fritsches HG, Busch WE: The importance of complementary cytology and colposcopy in a detection program. Acta Cytol 21: 10, 1977.

Griffiths CT, Younge PA: The clinical diagnosis of early cervical cancer. Obstet Gynecol Surv 24: 967, 1967.

Gronrovs MP, Hautera O, Jarvi S, Kangos and I Rauramo: Cytology and colposcopy in mass screening for cervical cancer. Acta Cytol 1: 37, 1967.

Gusberg SB, Frich GC, Corseadens: Gynecologic Cancer, 4th edition. Baltimore: The Williams & Wilkins Co, 330 pp, 1970.

Herbeck G, Menken FC: Colposcopy in the management of early cervical neoplasia. End scopy 9: 232, 1977.

Herbeck G: Current experiences in screening and early diagnosis of cervical neoplasia. Fortschr Med 11: 481, 1979.

Hester LL, Read RA: An evaluation of cervical conization. Am J Obstet Gynecol 80: 715, 1960.

Hill EC: Pre-clinical carcinoma, colposcopy, and the negative smear. Am J Obstet Gynecol 95: 308, 1966.

Hinselmann H: Verbesserung der Inspektionsmoeglichkeit von Vulva, Vagina und Portio. Muench Med Wschr 77: 1733, 1925.

Hollyock VE, Chanen W: The use of the colposcope in the selection of patients for cervical cone biopsy. Am J Obstet Gynecol 114: 185, 1972.

Hovadhanakul P, Mehra U, Teragno K, Taylor H, Cavanagh D: Comparison of colposcopy directed biopsies and cold knife conization in patients with abnormal cytology. Surgery Gynecol & Obst 142: 333, 1976.

Hulka BS: Cytologic and histologic outcome following an atypical cervical smear. Am J Obstet Gynecol 101: 190, 1968.

Jones EG, Varga A, Leff JG, Schwinn CP, Slate WG, Wargin JT, Bullock WK: Efficiency of multiple biopsy for cancer detection during pregnancy. Obstet Gynec 26: 70, 1965.

Kanka J, Svoboda B, Stolz J: The advantages of combining colposcopy and cytology in the prevention of uterine cervix cancer. Acta Univ Carol Medica 20: 279, 1974.

Kern G, Rissmann E, Hund G: Die Leistungsfaehigkeit der Kolposkopie bei der Fruehdiagnostik des Collumcarcinoms Archiv fur Gynaekologie 199: 526, 1964.

Kern G, Aslami A, Kern E: Folgen der Zervixkonisation Geburtshilfe Frauenheilkd 27: 879, 1967.

Kioko GM: Cervical cysplasia in a large, predominantly black practice as diagnosed by colposcopy in patients with normal and class II Papanicolaou smears. J Reprod Med 22: 222, 1979.

Kirkup W, Singer A, Hill AS: The accuracy of colposcopically directed biopsy in patients with suspected intraepithelial neoplasia of the cervix. Br J Obstet Gynec 87: 1, 1980.

Knutzen VK, Sherwood AGB: Colposcopy and selective biopsy in patients with abnormal cervical cytology. Afr Med J 52: 478, 1977.

Kohan S, Beckman M, Bigelow B, Carp M, Douglas GW: Colposcopy and the management of cervical intraepithelial neoplasia. Gynecol Oncol 5: 27, 1977.

Kolstad P: Carcinoma of the cervix, Stage O: Diagnosis and treatment. Am J Obstet Gynecol 96: 1098, 1966.

Kolstad P: Diagnosis and management of precancerous lesions of the cervix uteri. Internat gynaecol obstet 8: 551, 1970.

Krumholz BA, Knapp RC: Colposcopic selection of biopsy sites. Obstet Gynecol 39: 22, 1972.

Krumholz BA, Talebian IF: Colposcopy clinic: an evaluation of 500 new patients. J Reprod Med 16: 31, 1976.

Lang WR: The respective roles of cytology and colposcopy in obstetrics and gynecologic practice. J Reprod Med 16: 249, 1976.

Maisel FJ, Nelson HB, Ott RE, Morgenstern NL, van Ravenswaay TR: Papanicolaou smear, biopsy and conization of the cervix. Am J Obstet Gynecol 86: 931, 1963.

Martin P: How preventable is invasive cervical cancer. Am J Obstet Gynecol 113: 541, 1972.

Naujoks H, Koepf F, Leber I: Preoperative evaluation by colposcopy and cytology in cervical intraepithelial neoplasia (CIN). Geburtshilfe Frauenheilkd 39: 372, 1979.

Navratil E: Colposcopy. Dysplasia, Carcinoma in situ and Micro-invasive Carcinoma of the Cervix Uteri. Compiled by Gray LA. Springfield: Charles C. Thomas, p 228, 1964.

Navratil E: Is there a place for the colposcope in an established cytologic screening program for uterine cancer? Acta Cytol 9: 391, 1965.

Nelson, JH, Averette HE, Richart RM: Detection, diagnostic evaluation and treatment of dysplasia, carcinoma in situ and early invasive cervical carcinoma. CA 29: 174, 1979.

Nishimura A, Tsukamota N, Sugimori H, Hamasaki Y, Matsuyama T, Masamichi K, Kashimura T, Taki J: Evaluation of the colposcopically directed biopsy and the cone biopsy. Gynecol Oncol 6: 229, 1978.

Nyirjesy I: Atypical or suspicious cervical smears. JAMA 222: 691, 1972.

Odell LD: The use of the colposcope in the detection and management of patients with early cervical neoplasia. J Reprod Med 16: 235, 1976.

Olson AW, Nichols EE: Colposcopic examination in a combined approach for early diagnosis and prevention of carcinoma of the cervix. Obstet Gynecol 15: 372, 1960.

Ortiz R, Odell LD: Observation of the use of the colposcope for cervical neoplasia. J Reprod Med 4: 45, 1970.

Ortiz R, Newton M, Langlois PL: Colposcopic diagnosis of carcinoma of the cervix. Obstet Gynecol 34: 303, 1969.

Ortiz R, Newton M: Colposcopy in the management of abnormal cervical smears in pregnancy. Am J Obstet Gynecol 109: 46, 1971.

Ostergard DR, Gondos B: Outpatient therapy of preinvasive cervical neoplasia: selection of patients with the use of colposcopy. Am J Obstet Gynecol 115: 783, 1973.

Pang JC, Chir B, Hsu C, Kwan-Chan KM: Cytology and colposcopy in the diagnosis of cervical neoplasia. Gynecol Oncol 5: 134, 1977.

Pedersen E, Hoeg K, Kolstad P: Mass screening for cancer for the uterine cervix in Ostfold County, Norway. Acta Obstet Gynecol Scand 50: 69, 1971.

Richart RM: Evaluation of the true false negative rate in cytology. Am J Obstet Gynecol 89: 723, 1964.

Richart RM: Natural history of cervical intraepithelial neoplasia, Mod Treat 5: 748, 1968.

Rogers RS, Williams JH: The impact of the suspicious Papanicolaou smear on pregnancy. Am J Obstet Gynecol 98: 488, 1967.

Ronk DA, Jimerson GK, Merrill JA: Evaluation of abnormal cervical cytology. Obstet Gynec 49: 581, 1977.

Sabatelle R, Sedlis A, Sall S, Tchertkoff V: Cervical biopsy versus conization. Cancer 23: 663, 1969.

Sall S, Weingold AS, Stone M: Cancer of the cervix in pregnancy. Bull NY Acad Med 45: 328, 1969.

Satoh S: A comparison of presurgical and postsurgical diagnosis of cervical lesions. Acta Obstet Gynaecol Jpn 30: 1285, 1978.

Savage EW: Correlation of colposcopically directed biopsy and conization with histologic diagnosis of cervical lesions. J Reprod Med 15: 211, 1975.

Selim MA, So-Bosita JL, Blair OM, Little BA: Cervical biopsy versus conization. Obstet Gynec 41: 177, 1973.

Selim MA, Vasquez H, Masri R: Indications for and experience with colposcopy in the management of neoplasia of cervix. Surg Gynecol Obstet 145: 529, 1977.

Shingleton HM, Partridge EE, Austin JM: The significance of age in the colposcopic evaluation of women with atypical Papanicolaou smears. Obstet Gynecol 49: 61, 1977.

Shulman JJ, Hontz A, Sedlis A: The Pap smear: Take two. Am J Obstet Gynecol 121: 1024, 1975.

Silbar EL, Woodruff JD: Evaluation of biopsy, cone, and hysterectomy sequence in intraepithelial carcinoma of the cervix. Obstet Gynecol 27: 89, 1966.

Singleton WP, Rutledge F: To cone or not cone the cervix. Obstet Gynecol 31: 430, 1968.

Soule EH, Dahlin DC: Cytodetection of preclinical carcinoma of the cervix: 12 years experience with initial screening and repeat cervical smears. Mayo Clin Proc 35: 508, 1960.

Stafl A, Mattingly RF: Colposcopic diagnosis of cervical neoplasia. Obstet Gynecol 41: 168, 1973.

194

Stafl A, Friedrich EG Jr, Mattingly RF: Detection of cervical neoplasia, reducing the risk of error. Clin Obstet Gynecol 16: 238, 1973.

Stafl A, Mattingly RF: Angiogenesis of cervical neoplasia. Am J Obstet Gynecol 121: 845, 1975.

Stucin M, Kovacic J, Bonta S, Raiker S: Management of the suspicious cytologic cervical smear to the final diagnosis and therapy. Gynecol Oncol 1: 90, 1972.

Swan RW: Colposcopic evaluation of the female lower genital tract. J Miss State Med Assoc 17: 181, 1976.

Swan RS: Evaluation of colposcopic accuracy without endocervical curettage. Obstet Gynecol 53: 680, 1979.

Talebian F, Krumholz BA, Shayan A, Mann LI: Colposcopic evaluation of patients with abnormal cytologic smears during pregnancy. Obstet Gynecol 47: 693, 1976.

Talebian F, Shayan A, Burton A, Krumholz A, Palladino VS, Mann LI: Colposcopic evaluation of the patient with abnormal cervical cytology. Obstet Gynecol 49: 670, 1977.

Tovell H, Banogan P, Nash A: Cytology and colposcopy in the diagnosis and management of preclinical carcinoma of the cervix uteri learning experience. Am J Obstet Gynecol 124: 924, 1976.

Townsend D, Ostergard DR, Mishell DR Jr, Hirose FM: Abnormal Papanicolaou smears. Evaluation by colposcopy, biopsies, and endocervical curettage. Am J Obstet Gynecol 108: 429, 1970.

Tredway DR, Townsend DE, Hovland DN, Upton RT: Colposcopy and cryotherapy in cervical intraepithelial neoplasia. Am J Obstet Gynecol 114: 1020, 1972.

Trombetta GC: Colposcopy: a prerequisite for cone biopsy. J Reprod Med 14: 86, 1975.

Trombetta GC: Colposcopic evaluation of cervical neoplasia in pregnancy. J Reprod Med 16: 243, 1976.

Urcuyo R, Rome RM, Nelson JH: Some observations on the value of endocervical curettage performed as an integral part of colposcopic examination of patients with abnormal cervical cytology. Am J Obstet Gynecol 128: 787, 1977.

Van Nagell JR, Parker JC, Hicks LP, Conrad RP, England C: Diagnostic and therapeutic efficacy of cervical conization. Am J Obstet Gynecol 124: 134, 1976.

Villasanta U, Durkan JP: Indications and complications of cold conization of the cervix. Obstet Gynecol 27: 717, 1966.

White AJ, Saidi MH, Weinberg PC: Management of cervical neoplasia with colposcopy. J Reprod Med 16: 315, 1976.

Wied GL, Legoretta G, Mohr D, Rauzy A: Cytology of invasive cervical carcinoma and carcinoma in situ. Ann NY Acad Sci 97: 759, 1962.

Younge PA: Problems concerning the diagnosis and treatment of carcinoma in situ of the uterine cervix. Am J Roentegenol Radium Ther Nucl Med 79: 479, 1958.

Younglove RH, Newman RL: Atypical cervical cytology and colposcopic directed biopsy. Int J Gynaecol Obstet 15: 548, 1978.

27. OUTPATIENT DIAGNOSIS AND SELECTION OF TREATMENT OF CERVICAL INTRAEPITHELIAL NEOPLASIA USING COLPOSCOPY

K.D. Hatch, H.M. Shingleton and Hazel Gore

I. OUTPATIENT DIAGNOSIS OF CERVICAL NEOPLASIA USING COLPOSCOPY

Patients with abnormal Pap smears can be effectively evaluated as outpatients with careful correlation of cervical cytology, colposcopically directed biopsies, and interpretation of endocervical curettage (ECC) material (Stafl 1973; Ostergard 1973). Proper therapy can then be selected. Patients with invasive carcinoma can move directly to radiotherapy or radical surgery without a diagnostic conization. Patients with adequately evaluated cervical intraepithelial neoplasia (CIN) can have appropriate therapy selected. Diagnostic conization can be reserved for those patients who have an unsatisfactory colposcopic exam; noncorrelation of cytologic, histologic, and colposcopic data; findings consistent with microinvasion; or findings consistent with but not diagnostic of invasion. Approximately 85% of patients can be adequately evaluated as outpatients saving millions of medical care dollars (Austin 1978). This chapter will describe the use of cytology, colposcopy, directed cervical biopsies, and endocervical curettage to diagnose cervical neoplasia and choose appropriate therapy.

II. DIAGNOSTIC TECHNIQUES

II.A. Colposcopic examination

After discussing the colposcopic exam with the patient, a standard speculum is introduced to expose the cervix. A cytologic smear is performed and excess leukorrhea is removed with a swab. The cervix is examined first with the naked eye to determine if a grossly visible lesion is present. The colposcope is then brought into focus and the cervix is examined beginning at low power (6 ×) and proceeding to higher magnifications (16 ×) (25 ×). The original squamous epithelium can be identified on the exocervix by its characteristic dense submucosal fine capillary network (Figure 1). The columnar epithelium should then be identified by its typical vilous character and the entire squamo-columnar junction visualized (Figure 2). The space between the original squamous epithelium and the squamo-columnar junction is the transformation zone (T-zone). The old T-zone is identified by nabothian cysts and their characteristic stretched, dilated and often bizarre blood vessels (Figure 3). The active T-zone borders the columnar epithelium (Figure 2) and contains metaplastic squamous cells. The T-zone contains the majority of neoplastic changes. It should be examined for friability, surface contour irregularity, abnormal vascular pat-

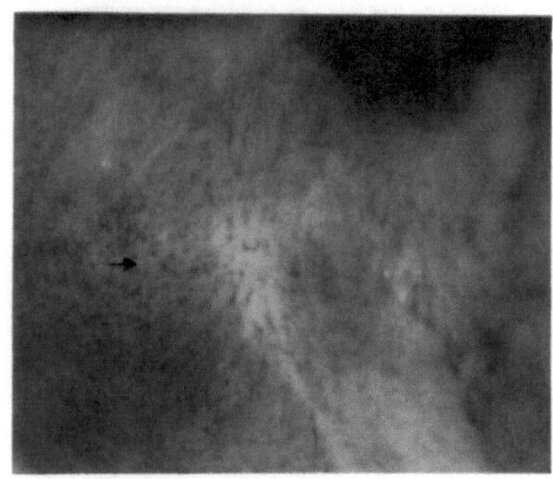

Figure 1. View of submucosal capillary vascular network in the original squamous epithelium (arrow). The cervical os is at 0, × 15.

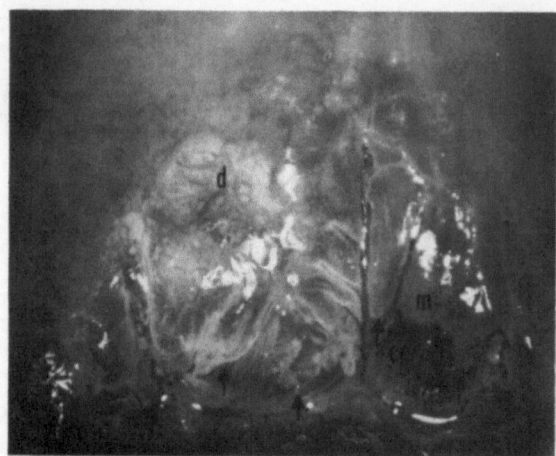

Figure 2. View of a patient with an abnormal T-zone. Arrows show the squamo-columnar junction. Cervical ridges with columnar epithelium at CE. Squamous metaplasia at M. CIN I at D. A fine mosaic and punctation pattern is present and the external border is not distinct, × 9.6.

tern, and surface color abnormalities and opacities. Any of these characteristics may indicate if an invasive lesion is present (Figure 4). Use of the green filter increases the contrast between blood vessels and the surrounding stroma and epithelium. A 3% acetic acid solution should then be placed on the cervix for 30 seconds to one minute and the cervix again examined. Areas of dysplasia become more opaque reflecting the fact that their nuclei are larger and more chromatin-dense than the surrounding metaplastic or mature squamous epithelial cells. These areas of opacity are termed acetowhite lesions as they become apparent after the application of acetic acid. They should be examined for thickness, surface contour, vascular pattern, distance between vascular markings, and clarity of demarcation. The higher grade CIN lesions are thicker with irregular surface contour and have a prominent vascular pattern with increased distance between vascular markings (Figure 5). (Coppelson 1967). Conversely, the thinner lesions whose borders are not well defined with no vascular pattern and smooth surface contour are likely to be only mildly to moderately dysplastic (Figure 6). The vascular patterns looked for in the acetowhite lesions are punctation – a collection of capillaries seen end on; and mosaic – a network of stromal vessels between islands of white epithelium forming a mosaic-like pattern (Figure 5) (Kolstad 1972.

There are several other important observations to be made and recorded: (1) Is the lesion entirely seen and can the entire transformation zone be seen? If the lesion extends into the canal, or the T-zone cannot be fully visualized within the canal, the colposcopic evaluation is *unsatisfactory* and the colposcopist will have to rely on the endocervical curettings to direct further therapy. If the curettings contain dysplastic elements, then a diagnostic con-

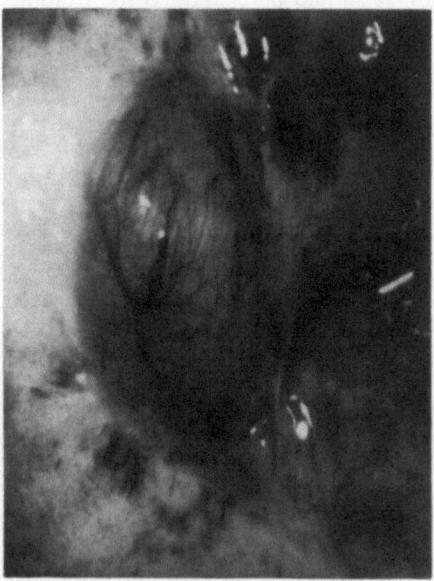

Figure 3. View of normally branching vessels pushed to the surface by a nabothian cyst. Such findings indicate this is the old T-zone, × 15.

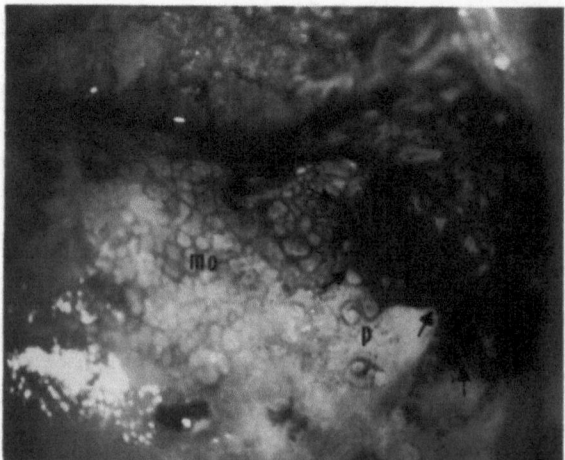

Figure 4. View of a patient with a predominantly mosaic pattern (MO) with some punctation (P). Loss of surface epithelium, friability and irregular contour at arrows suggests an invasive lesion. A cone is mandatory for diagnosis if the directed biopsies do not reveal invasion or reveal just MIV, × 9.6.

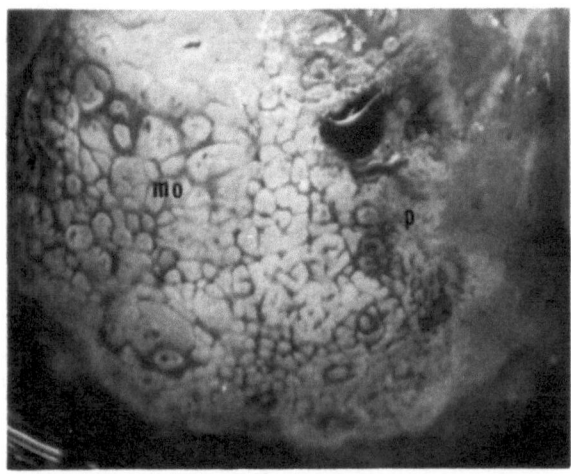

Figure 5. View of a patient with CIN III. The edge of the lesion is prominent, the intercapillary distance in the mosaic pattern is wide and irregular (MO), punctation is present (P) and the lesion is intensely acetowhite, × 9.6.

ization is indicated. The cone, could also be therapeutic. (2) Does the lesion suggest microinvasion (MIV) or invasion? If the colposcopic impression suggests MIV or invasion, then a diagnostic cone is mandatory providing colposcopic biopsies were not diagnostic of invasion themselves. A cervical biopsy of MIV also indicates a diagnostic cone as mandatory. (3) How large is the lesion and is it too distorted from obstetric scarring to accept a rigid cryoprobe? If the lesion is entirely seen and the entire transformation zone can be visualized, the exam is *satisfactory*. The size of the lesion and concern over applicability of the cryoprobe then becomes important if the colposcopist plans to treat the lesion with cryosurgery. The decision whether to treat with cryosurgery requires great care in interpretation of colposcopic findings, ECC material, cervical biopsy, and cytology. Mild to moderate dysplasia lesions respond well to cryotherapy (Kaufman 1978); however, CIS lesions are not so easily eradicated (Ostergard 1980).

II.B. Biopsy techniques

After evaluation of the cervix, an endocervical curettage is performed by scraping the endocervix with a small curette, allowing the dislodged fragments to catch in the mucous and clot, then pulling this coagulum from the cervical os with a uterine dressing forceps or ring forceps. This is placed on a

piece of paper towel or other suitable receptacle and placed in 10% formalin. It is processed routinely with hematoxylin and eosin staining (Gore 1976). Three colposcopically directed biopsies of the lesion are taken and placed on a piece of dry paper towel, oriented with the stroma side down, and placed in 10% formalin. Bleeding is controlled after the biopsy by ferric subsulfate solution (Monsel's solution) or silver nitrate cautery.

II.C. Interpretation of biopsy and ECC material

The colposcopic impression, ECC material, cervical biopsies, and cytology are carefully evaluated during a conference with the colposcopist and pathologist. Each must be aware of the other's findings and active communication is mandatory. The ECC is interpreted as unsatisfactory, negative, mild to moderate dysplasia, severe dysplasia to CIS, suspect invasive carcinoma, or invasive carcinoma (Gore 1976). It is important not to report curettings that are unsatisfactory as negative as it may lead to clinician into a false sense of security. An evaluation of the amount of dysplasia in the curettings is helpful when the ECC is positive (Shingleton 1976). One or two isolated fragments in the entire specimen that otherwise contains adequate endocervical material may indicate contamination of the specimen by a loosened fragment from the exocervical lesion. Conversely, several fragments of dysplasia

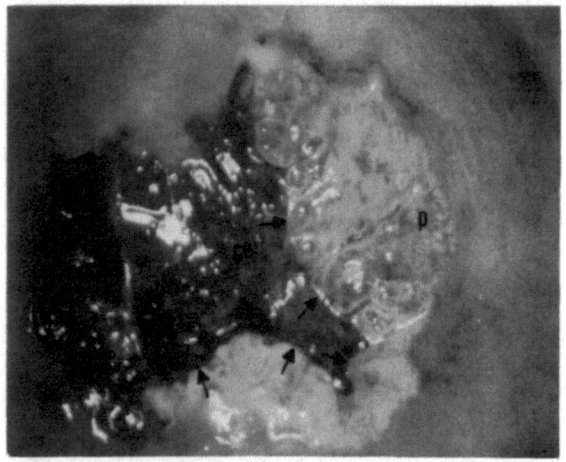

Figure 6. View of a patient with CIN II lesion. The edges of the lesion are easily seen but not raised, a fine punctation pattern is present at P, the surface contour is smooth and has no ulceration. The squamo-columnar junction is easily seen (arrows) and columnar epithelium is normal (CE), × 9.6.

scattered throughout the specimen and found in different levels indicates a true positive ECC necessitating a cone. When the ECC contains fragments of dysplasia worse than that seen on the cervical biopsies, the ECC is considered positive and a cone is required. When the ECC suggests invasive carcinoma, conization is mandatory for definitive diagnosis.

Cervical biopsies are interpreted as negative, unsatisfactory, CIN I, II or III, MIV, or invasion. Unsatisfactory biopsies must be repeated or conization performed if the cytology remains abnormal. Patients with cervical biopsies suggesting MIV must undergo a diagnostic conization to insure that there is no area of frank invasion. Patients with a diagnosis of invasive carcinoma may proceed to planned therapy without an intervening conization. Patients with a biopsy of CIN must have careful correlation of cytology, cervical biopsies, ECC material, and colposcopic examination before treatment is selected. If there is significant non-correlation (greater than 1 degree of severity difference) between the cytology and histology, re-evaluation with colposcopy or conization is indicated. If the information correlates well (no greater than 1 degree of severity difference), then treatment will be based on the patient's wishes concerning future childbearing, the size and appearance of a lesion, and the severity of the lesion (Figure 6).

II.D. Practical application of colposcopy

From 1970 to 1979, 2,588 patients with abnormal cervical cytology were evaluated. No neoplasia was found in 639 patients and they were treated medically for cervicitis. Cryosurgery was selected as treatment for 968 patients with a 20% persistent disease rate in CIN III and a 10% persistent disease rate in CIN I and II (Hatch 1980). A cone or hysterectomy was performed in 981 patients allowing the opportunity to correlate the findings from the Colposcopy Clinic with those of the final specimen (Table 1). Exact correlation was obtained in 66% of the patients and correlation within 1 degree of severity was found in 95%. One patient with CIN I and II, and 9 patients with CIN III on

Table 1. Correlation of outpatient diagnosis with cone or hysterectomy diagnosis.

Outpatient diagnosis	Cone hysterectomy diagnosis					
	Invasive	MIV	CIN III	CIN I & II	Neg.	Total
Invasive	70	2	6	0	0	78
Microinvasive	5	10	26	0	0	41
CIN III	9	31	464	90	33	627
CIN I & II	1	2	83	107	42	235
Total	85	45	579	197	75	981

Heavy lines indicate exact correlation; the lighter lines indicate correlation within 1 degree of severity.

their outpatient evaluation had invasive carcinoma when they were coned. Each of the 10 had an indication for conization from their outpatient evaluation and after the cone were treated with appropriate therapy. Examination of the patients with MIV reveals why this diagnosis can only be made from a cone or hysterectomy specimen. Only 10 of 41 patients thought to have MIV on outpatient evaluation had the diagnosis confirmed by cone or hysterectomy. Five had invasive carcinoma instead and 26 had CIN III. All of the patients with MIV on outpatient evaluation had conization performed prior to definitive therapy. Seventy-five patients had negative findings on cone or hysterectomy after having CIN on their outpatient evaluation. It is assumed these patients had their entire lesion removed by the biopsies or the lesion was small enough that routine sectioning of the specimen failed to disclose the lesion.

III. CONCLUDING REMARKS

Colposcopy is a cost efficient means of evaluating patients with abnormal cervical cytology. It should not replace the Pap smear as a screening technique, however, since it requires specialized training, consumes more time and requires an investment in medical equipment greater than that for a Pap smear. The two techniques should be used together to provide the most cost-efficient medical care.

REFERENCES

Austin JM, Charles ED, Shingleton HM: Colposcopy or cervical conization? An economic comparison. S Med J 71: 580, 1978.

Coppleson M, Reid BL: Preclinical carcinoma of the cervix uteri. Its nature, origin and management. Oxford: Pergamon, 1967.

Gore H, Shingleton HM, Austin JM: A classification of endocervical curettage. Gynecol Oncol 4: 53, 1976.

Hatch KD, Shingleton HM, Austin JM, Soong SJ, Bradley DH: Cryosurgery of cervical intraepithelial neoplasia-Report of 968 patients. Obstet and Gynecol (in press).

Kaufman RH, Irwin JF: The cryosurgical therapy of cervical intraepithelial neoplasia. Am J Obstet Gynecol 131: 381, 1978.

Kolstad P, Stafl A: Atlas of colposcopy. Oslo: Universitetsforlaget, 1972.

Ostergard DR: Cryosurgical treatment of cervical intraepithelial neoplasia. Obstet Gynecol 56: 231, 1980.

Ostergard DR, Gondos B: Outpatient therapy of preinvasive cervical neoplasia: Selection of patients with the use of colposcopy. Am J Obstet Gynecol 115: 783, 1973.

Shingleton HM, Gore H, Austin JM: Outpatient evaluation of patients with atypical Papanicolaou smear: Contribution of endocervical curettage. Am J Obstet Gynecol 126: 122, 1976.

Stafl A, Mattingly RF: Colposcopic diagnosis of cervical neoplasia. Obstet Gynecol 41: 168, 1973.

28. ADENOCARCINOMA OF THE CERVIX: HISTOPATHOLOGIC AND CLINICAL FEATURES

H.M. Shingleton, Hazel Gore and J.H. Wilters

Adenocarcinoma comprises between 4–10% of all cervical carcinomas and in recent years, the incidence, both in absolute numbers and relative to squamous cell carcinoma, seems to be increasing (Shingleton et al. 1981; Morley and Seski 1976; Davis and Moon 1975). Whether this is related in some way to widespread use of oral contraceptive pills is speculative (Czernobilsky et al. 1974; Hanjani and Sonder 1980). Availability of a large number of patients with adenocarcinoma of the cervix in a short time period prompted a study of this tumor with regard to histopathologic classification, radiocurability, routes and frequency of metastasis, recurrence and survival.

I. CLASSIFICATION OF ADENOCARCINOMA OF THE CERVIX

Various classifications of adenocarcinoma of the cervix have been proposed. In an effort to determine whether histologic patterns are of prognostic significance, tissue from patients treated between 1970–1980 was reviewed and all patterns present in each tumor were recorded. From this, a classification (Table 1) was devised, sometimes combining one or more of the initial patterns for simplification. In several aspects, this is similar to the classification proposed by the World Health Organization (WHO) (Table 1).

I.A. Endocervical pattern

In both series, the endocervical aspect was the most common type of pattern. In the WHO classification, this is subdivided according to differentiation with a separate subdivision of mucinous adenocarcinoma for that variant with prominent mucin. The classification derived from our review considers a more restricted endocervical pattern without demonstrable mucin in H and E sections while listing separately mucinous patterns. These include mucin in individual cells (Figure 1), more abundant mucin development with mucin in glands (or clefts), and a myxoma pattern (Figures 2a and b). In this, there is extension of mucin into the stroma similar to the better known myxoma peritonei.

*Table 1.*Classification of adenocarcinoma of the cervix.

UAB classification	WHO classification
Adenocarcinoma or adenosquamous carcinoma	Adenocarcinoma, endocervical type
Endocervical (no mucin)	Well differentiated
Mucinous tumors	Moderately differentiated
Papillary	Poorly differentiated
Hobnail/clear cell (mesometanephric)	Mucinous adenocarcinoma
Adenoid cystic/microglandular	Adenocarcinoma *in situ*
Adenocanthoma	Endometrioid adenocarcinoma
	Clear cell (mesonephroid) adenocarcinoma
Collision tumors	Adenoid cystic carcinoma
Adenocarcinoma and CIN surface element	Adenosquamous carcinoma
Adenocarcinoma and squamous cell carcinoma	Undifferentiated carcinoma

Hafez, E.S.E., Smith, J.P. (eds.), Carcinoma of the Cervix: Biology and Diagnosis. ISBN-13: 978-94-009-7487-6
© 1982, Martinus Nijhoff Publishers, The Hague/Boston/London.

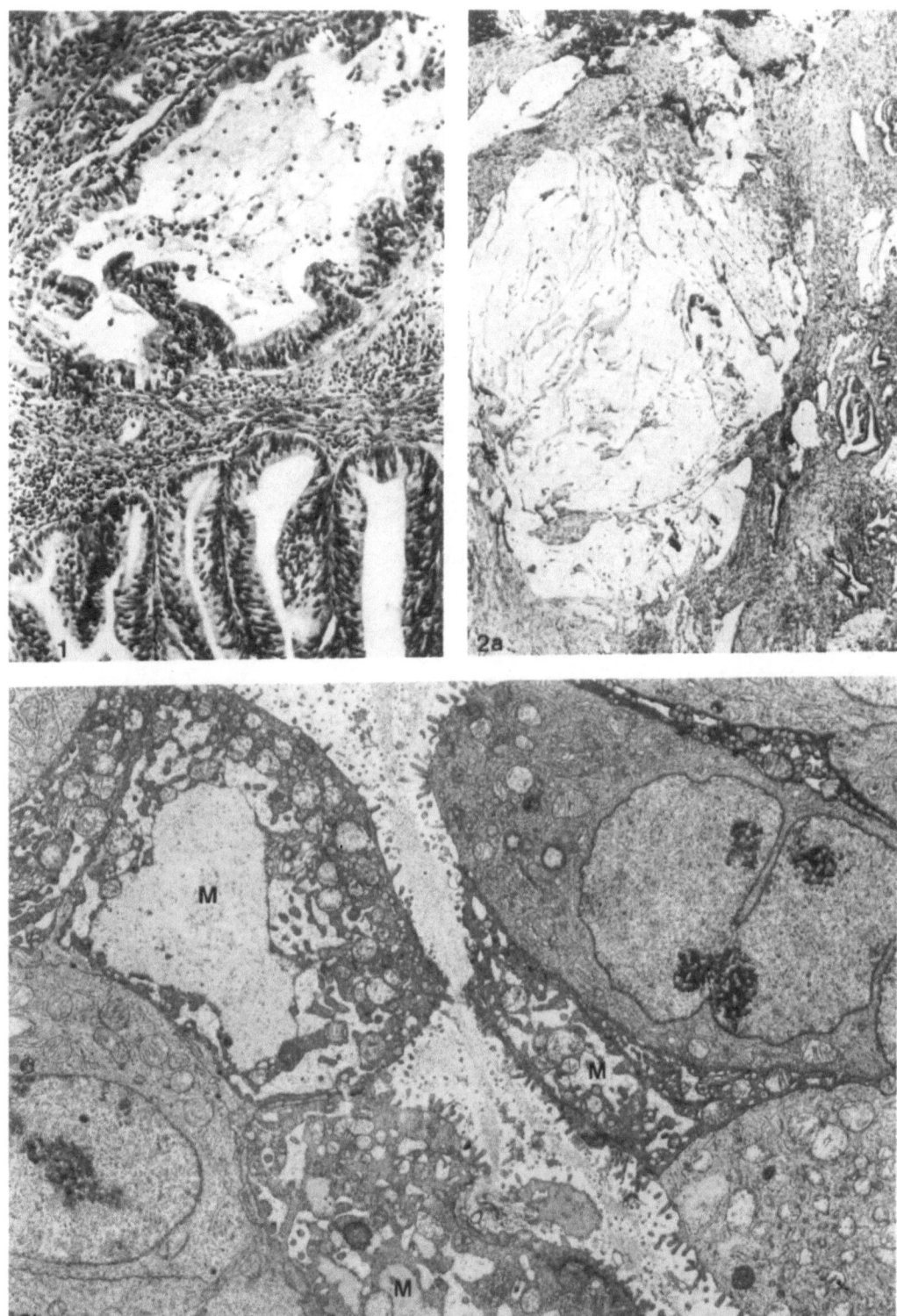

Figure 1. In this well-differentiated tumor, individual cells contain mucin and there is mucin in one gland space, H & E × 116.8.
Figure 2a. Mucin has accumulated in the stroma, producing a 'myxoma cervicis' pattern similar to that of myxoma peritonei. Whether such cervical tumors extend to involve the peritoneum is unclear, H & E × 41.6.
Figure 2b. Within this electron photomicrograph of a mucin producing tumor similar to that in Figure 2a are cells containing aggregates and pools of mucin (M) and some cells without mucin. (In this figure the non-mucin containing cells are in the upper right and lower left, with nuclei and zones of cytoplasm without mucin. The nuclei of the mucin containing cells are not present in this level of section.) × 5200.

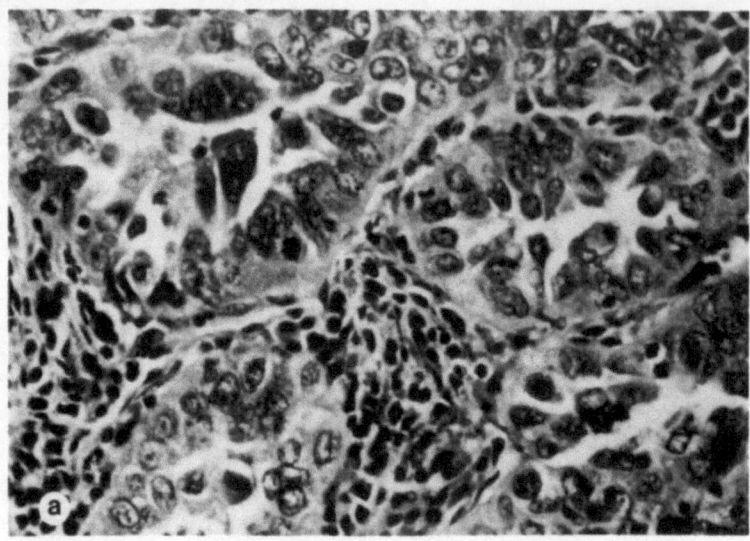

Figure 3a. There is a most distinctive hobnail pattern epithelial lining these crowded malignant glands, H & E × 424.

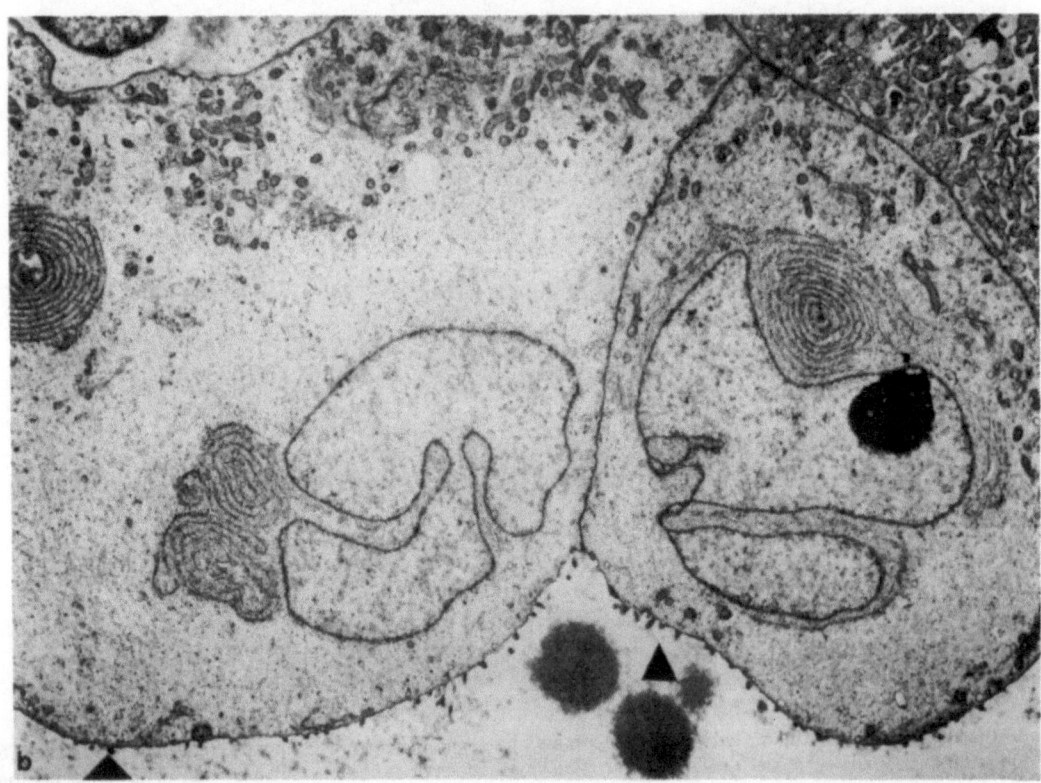

Figure 3b. In this electron micrograph from the specimen illustrated in Figure 3a, the cell nuclei have bizarre shapes but fine nuclear chromatin distribution. Within one cell nucleus (right) is large single nucleolus. The cytoplasm adjacent to the nuclei is devoid of organelles other than concentric laminations of the endoplasmic reticulum and at the periphery of the cytoplasm are numerous mitochondria. Blunt malformed microvilli project into the lumen at the cell surfaces (arrows), × 4080.

The papillary pattern was usually a secondary pattern, most commonly associated with the endocervical type. The WHO classification also includes an adenocarcinoma *in situ*. This has been described by Friedell and McKay (1953) essentially as single malignant appearing glands or surface glandular epithelium without clearcut invasion. This is a difficult diagnosis to make with certainty and no example was found in the review series. This may have been due to a tendency to interpret focal areas of neoplastic glands as being superficially invasive.

I.B. Endometrioid pattern

Endometrioid adenocarcinoma is identical to or closely resembles adenocarcinoma of the endometrium. The diagnosis depends on exclusion of corpus cancer; tumors with an endometrial appearance would have been included in this group only if there were absolute proof of lack of involvement of the endometrial cavity by the malignant process. At times, this is indistinguishable from the endocervical pattern, and, indeed, this is not an uncommon problem in the evaluation of curettings in an attempt to establish the primary site of an adenocarcinoma. The rigid criteria established in this study related to the desire to have as pure a group as possible for treatment and survival results; with less rigid criteria, especially in studies in which clinical information is lacking or incomplete, such a group would be large.

I.C. Clear cell pattern

A variety of terms has been applied to the group of tumors loosely termed clear cell carcinoma. A hobnail pattern (Figures 3a and b) resembling mesonephric derivatives and a clear cell pattern (Figures 4a and b) resembling metanephric derivatives are included in this group, sometimes termed mesonephroid (as in the WHO classification, although clear cell tumors are 'metanephroid'), or mesometanephric (or mesometanephroid). Although these tumors seem to recapitulate derivaties of the mesonephros and metanephros, sometimes direct continuity may be established with endocervical epithelium indicating that such a pattern may also be found in a paramesonephric derivative. The term mesometanephric (or perhaps more correctly mesometanephroid) is only descriptive and does not imply cell of origin.

I.D. Adenoid cystic pattern

The adenoid cystic pattern is cribriform and superficially similar to that found in salivary gland tumors. It is commonly focal and may occur with or without the basaloid cells described in cervical tumors (Baggish and Woodruff 1966; Moss and Collins 1964; Daroca and Dhurandhar 1980). Ultrastructural studies of the microglandular pattern indicate that many of these tumors are different from adenoid cystic tumors of the head and neck in that the spaces are gland lumina (Figure 5).

Table 2. Histologic patterns in 137 adenocarcinomas.

Pattern	Adenocarcinoma ($N = 92$)			Adenosquamous ($N = 45$)		
	Pure	Mixed with second pattern	Mixed with several patterns	Pure	Mixed with second pattern	Mixed with several patterns
Endocervical	30	17	3	18	1	0
Papillary	0	22	4	0	1	4
Mucinous	11	9	2	4	6	5
Adenoid cystic	3	5	1	7	3	2
Hobnail/clear	2	4	2	1	0	0
Adenoacanthoma	0	1	0	–	–	–
Probable malignant squamous element	0	11	4	–	–	–

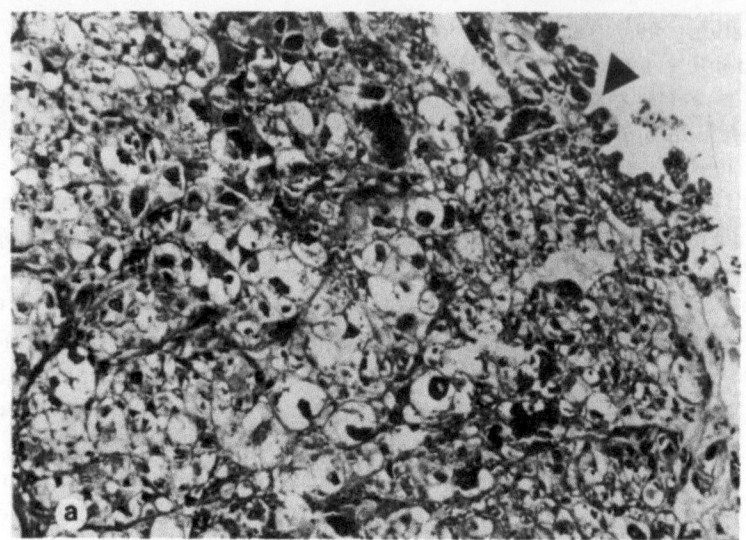

Figure 4a. Adenocarcinoma of clear cell pattern with hobnail pattern epithelium lining a gland space (arrow), H & E × 252.

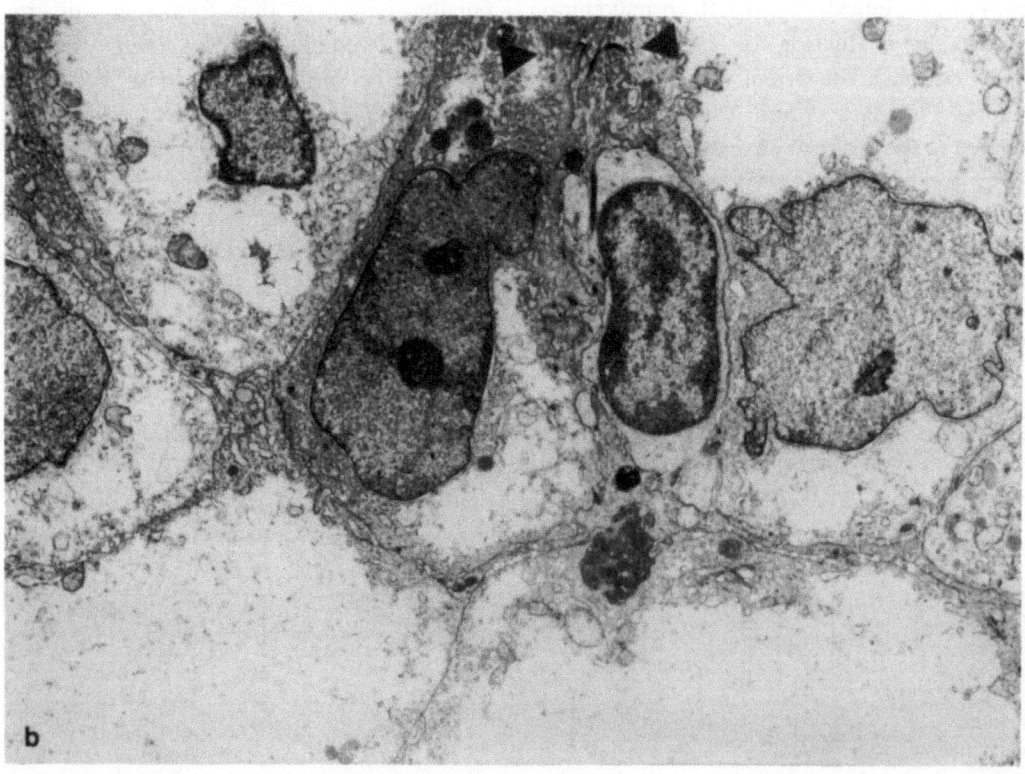

Figure 4b. The pattern in Figure 4a may be correlated with this electron micrograph where the large irregular nuclei are surrounded by clear areas of cytoplasm containing granular material. The arrows indicate well formed desmosomes with associated filaments suggesting that these are malignant squamous cells distended by pools of glycogen, × 4080.

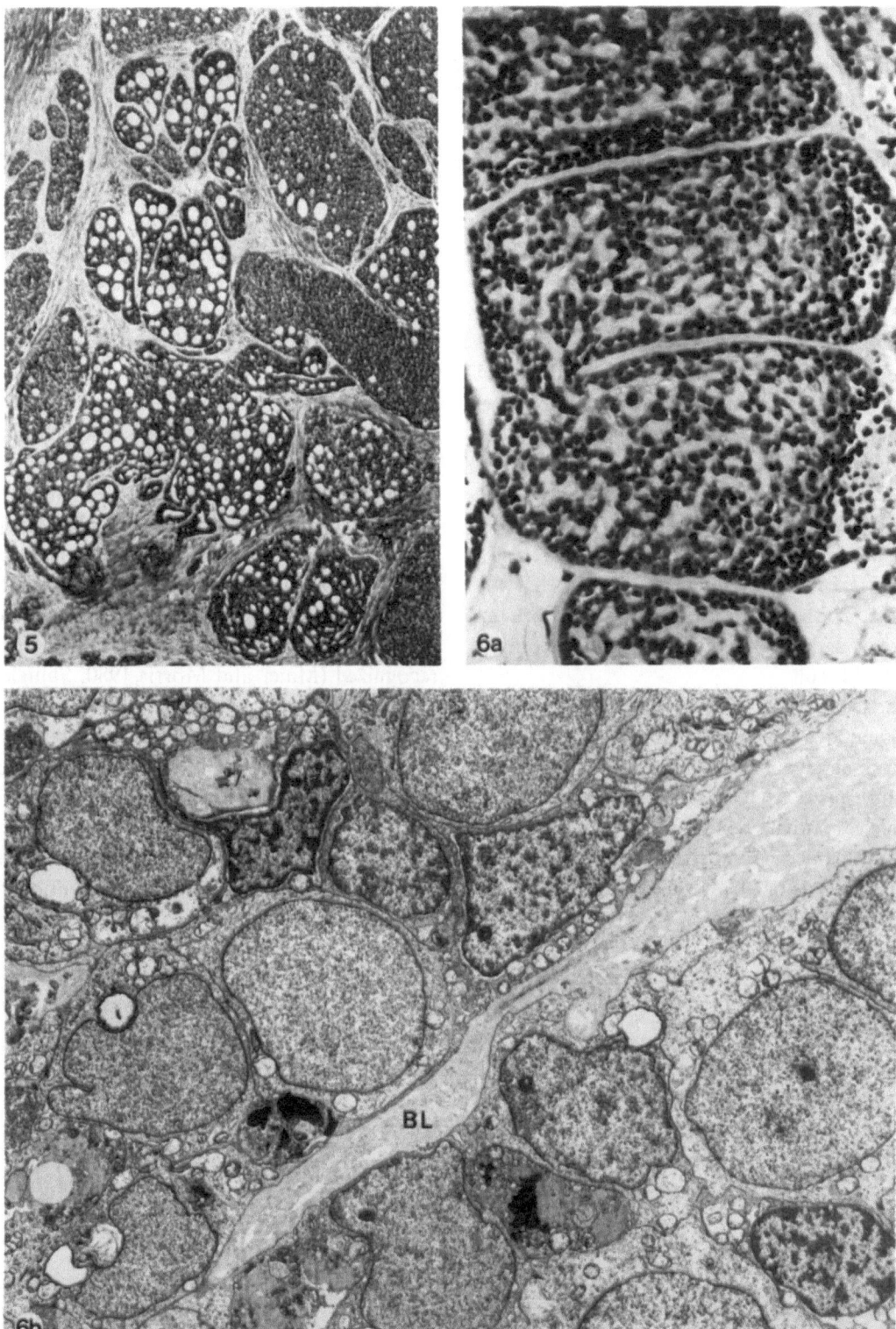

Figure 5. Within this almost pure example of the basaloid type of adenoid cystic tumor are large groups of fairly regular cells, sometimes in solid sheets and sometimes containing small rounded spaces, H & E × 41.6.

Figure 6a. Also included in the adenoid cystic group is the cylindroma pattern similar to that of adenoid cystic tumors elsewhere in the body. Stromal cylinders traverse the tumor and on cross section simulate gland spaces, H & E × 300.8.

Figure 6b. Within this photomicrograph of the cylindroma shown in Figure 6a, the spaces between groups of tumor cells contain extracellular collections of laminated basal membrane-like material (BL). This electron microscopic appearance is identical to that described in adenoid cystic tumors of the head and neck, × 4320.

Since this is in marked contrast to the cylindromatous pattern (Figures 6 a and b) similar to that found in adenoid cystic tumors of the head and neck and perhaps included in the cylindroma group (Tchertkoff and Sedlis 1962), it is more appropriate to accept adenoid cystic as a pattern rather than a specific tumor (Shingleton et al. 1977).

I.E. Adenocarcinoma with squamous elements

Adenosquamous carcinomas have an intimate admixture of adenocarcinoma and squamous cell carcinoma, frequently associated with other patterns (Figure 7). (Table 2). Identification of the malignant squamous cell element may be virtually impossible. In most tumors where probable malignant squamous cells were postulated from H and E sections, definite malignant squamous cells were identified at the ultrastructural level. With experience, diagnosis of adenosquamous becomes a little less difficult.

Adenoacanthoma, an adenocarcinoma with benign squamous elements, usually occurring as small, well-defined metaplastic nodules (Figure 8) is rare and must be distinguished from adenosquamous carcinoma. Such tumors would undoubtedly be included in other classifications as endocervical or endometrioid adenocarcinoma qualified by the degree of differentiation of the adenocarcinomatous element.

I.F. Other patterns

Undifferentiated tumor (WHO classification) seems to be an attempt to find a place for 'all the other tumors'. If the tumors are so undifferentiated to preclude their assignment to one of the other diagnostic categories, it might be questioned whether they are really adenocarcinomas. It may well be proper to delete from consideration tumors with this degree of dedifferentiation unless ultrastructural studies can determine the true tumor type.

Of special interest are those tumors considered as collision tumors where malignant glandular and squamous elements seem to have developed separately within the same general area. Collision of adenocarcinoma and squamous cell carcinoma or adjacent growth of these two tumors without a close admixture where malignant glandular and squamous elements are actually growing as a unit, has long been recognized. less recognized is the presence of a cervical intraepithelial neoplastic surface (or cleft-involving) element, including moderate dysplasia to carcinoma *in situ* association with adenocarcinoma (Figure 9). this combination is seen more frequently than has otherwise been recognized (Maier and Morris 1980; Shingleton et al. 1980).

A 'glassy cell carcinoma' as described by Glucksmann and Cherry (1956), and further reported by Littman et al. (1976), was not encountered in this series. A few of the tumors had focal areas which contained 'glassy cells' and which otherwise met some of the diagnostic criteria, but invariably other areas had well-differentiated adenocarcinoma (or squamous cell carcinoma), excluding them from the classic group. The criteria for diagnosing this lesion are unclear. If differentiation of either element of an 'adenosquamous' carcinoma is not allowable, then it is somewhat difficult to understand how a diagnosis of adenosquamous carcinoma can be made without ultrastructural studies.

Table 3. Lesion size related to lesion type; adenocarcinoma and matched controls.[a]

	Stage I							
	Exophytic		Ulcerative		Endophytic		Polypoid	
	Adeno.	Squam.	Adeno.	Squam.	Adeno.	Squam.	Adeno.	Squam.
1 cm or less	1	4	7	2	19	8	1	0
2 cm	7	9	9	13	2	1	2	0
3 cm or more	15	13	1	3	3	0	3	1
	23	26	17	18	24	9	6	1

[a]Sixteen patients with squamous cell lesions did not have information for this comparison.

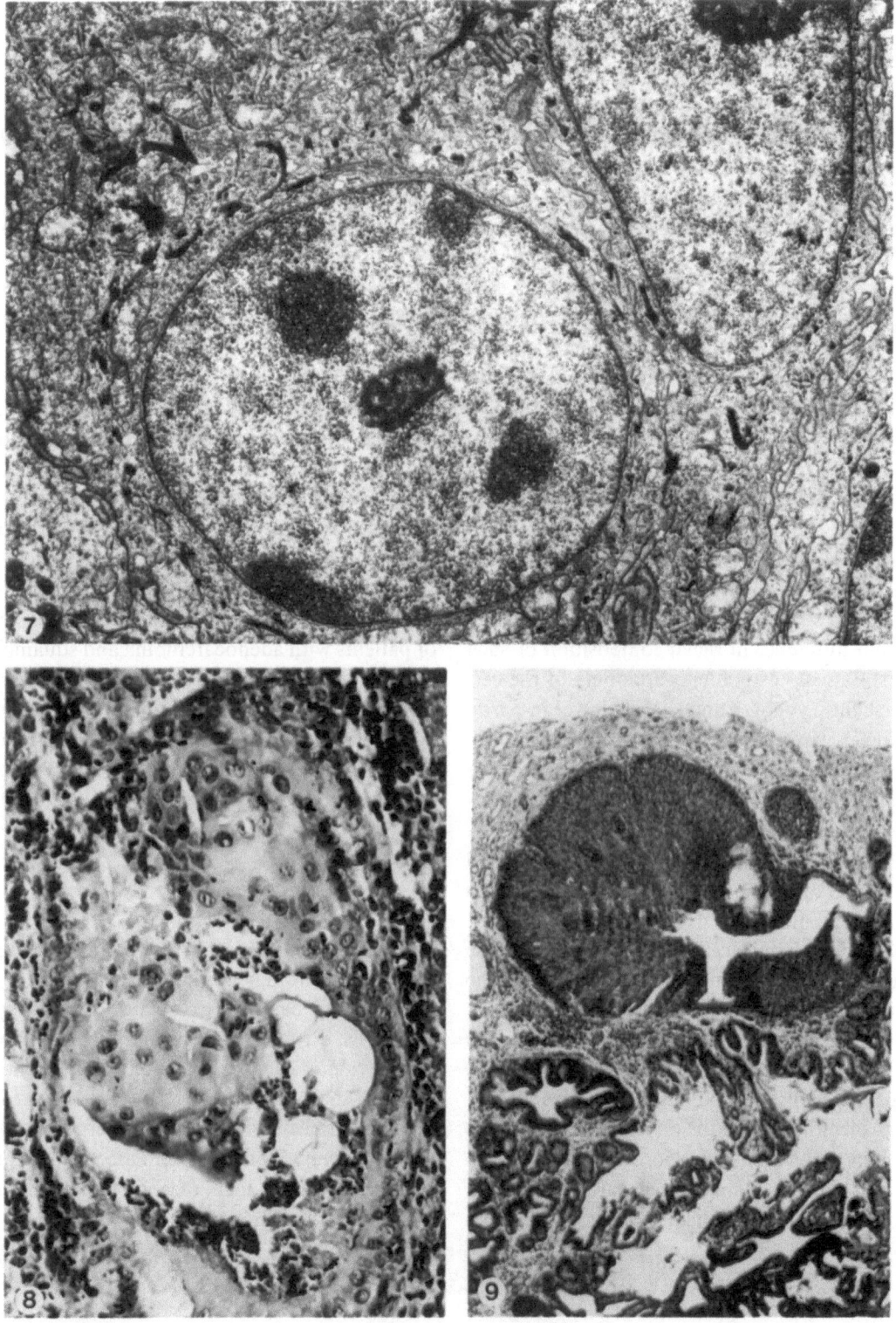

Figure 7. This electron photomicrograph from a solid area in the tumor contains two malignant cells with bundles of dense tonofibrils in the perinuclear area, features of squamous cells. The nuclei contain coarse chromatin aggregates, × 10,400.

Figure 8. Focus of histologically benign squamous metaplasia within an adenocarcinoma, the pattern of adenoacanthoma, H & E × 300.8.

Figure 9. Carcinoma *in situ* within a cleft adjacent to but apparently separate from a well-differentiated adenocarcinoma of the endocervical type with a papillary focus at the lower right. This is one of the 'surface' CIN with associated adenocarcinoma group, H & E × 69.6.

Some adenocarcinomas have as many as four patterns and almost half have at least two patterns (Table 2). The adenosquamous tumors often have other patterns within them (other than the adenocarcinoma and squamous components). Those patients who were considered to have a 'probable' malignant squamous element within their tumors (Table 3) were ultimately placed in the adenosquamous category. Many of these patients had material available for transmission electron microscopic studies and invariably a squamous component was identified in their tumors by this method.

II. CLINICAL FEATURES AND TREATMENT RESULTS

In comparing patients with adenocarcinoma of the cervix (including adenosquamous carcinoma) to patients with squamous cell carcinoma, there is no significant difference in racial composition of such patients. Patients with adenocarcinoma of the cervix are slightly younger and slightly lower in parity than those with squamous cell carcinoma. The mean age of adenocarcinoma patients compared to the adenosquamous carcinoma patients is not significantly different.

The clinical type of lesion has been compared with the size of lesion in a group of patients with stage I carcinoma of the cervix or both adenocarcinoma and squamous cell carcinoma types (Table 3). Since an adenocarcinoma is derived from the endocervix, it might be predicted that such a tumor would most likely be endophytic or polypoid. In actuality, the majority are exophytic or ulcerative, perhaps reflecting the common presence of endocervical epithelium on the cervical portio. Adenocarcinoma, however, is more frequently endophytic than is squamous cell carcinoma when compared with the matched controls. The distribution of size of lesion within each of the clinical categories is very similar when comparing adenocarcinoma and squamous cell carcinoma.

Less differentiated lesions are generally associated with higher numbers of metastases in pelvic nodes. When the size of lesion is correlated with nodal metastases, larger lesions are associated with more metastases (Burghardt and Pickel 1978). In the Alabama series, among stage I cervical carcinomas, there was no statistical difference between the number of metastases to lymph nodes associated with adenocarcinoma and squamous cell carcinoma, nor were adenosquamous lesions associated with higher numbers of node metastases than were 'pure' adenocarcinomas. The presence of poor stromal response did not correlate with lymph node metastases, differing from a previous report (Gusberg et al. 1971).

The preliminary survival data in this series (three years) suggests that there is no difference in survival of patients with adenocarcinoma and squamous cell carcinoma, nor was there a difference in survival when cervical adenocarcinoma was compared to adenosquamous carcinoma. Increasing tumor volume, may be correlated with decreased survival and disease-free rates (Shingleton et al. 1981).

III. CONCLUDING REMARKS

Adenocarcinoma of the cervix often presents a mixture of histologic tumor patterns, none of which in this study has been correlated specifically with prognosis. Prognosis is primarily determined by tumor volume, degree of histologic differentiation, and to some extent by the type of treatment selected. Transmission electron microscopy is helpful in studying poorly differentiated tumors and for categorization of such tumors as squamous cell carcinoma or adenocarcinoma.

REFERENCES

Baggish MS, Woodruff JD: Adenoid-basal carcinoma of the cervix. Obstet Gynecol 28: 213, 1966.

Burghardt E, Pickel H: Local spread and lymph node involvement in cervical cancer. Obstet Gynecol 52: 138, 1978.

Czernobilsky B, Kessler I, Lanat M: Cervical adenocarcinoma in a woman on long term contraceptives. Obstet Gynecol 43: 517, 1974.

Daroca PJ, Dhurandhar HN: Basaloid carcinoma of the uterine cervix. Am J Surg Path 4: 235, 1980.

Davis JR, Moon LB: Increased incidence of adenocarcinoma of the uterine cervix. Obstet Gynecol 45: 79, 1975.

Friedell GH, McKay DG: Adenocarcinoma in situ of the endocervix. Cancer 6: 887, 1953.

Glucksmann A, Cherry CP: Incidence, history and response to radiation of mixed carcinomas (adenoacanthomas) of the uterine cervix. Cancer 9: 971, 1956.

Gusberg SB, Yannopoulos K, Cohen CJ: Virulence indices and lymph nodes in cancer of the cervix. Am J Roentgenol Radium Ther Nucl Med 111: 2, 1971.

Hanjani P, Sonder H: Association of adenocarcinoma of the endocervix and oral contraception. (Abstract). In Hafez E, Smith J (eds): Proceedings of the International Symposium on Carcinoma of the Cervix, 1980.

Littman P, Clement PB, Henriksen B, Wang CC, Robboy SJ, Taft PD, Ulfelder H, Scully RE: Glassy cell carcinoma of the cervix. Cancer 37: 2238, 1976.

Maier RC, Norris HS: Coexistence of cervical intraepithelial neoplasia with primary adenocarcinoma of the endocervix. Obstet Gynecol 56: 361, 1980.

Morley GW, Seski JC: Radical pelvic surgery versus radiation therapy for Stage I carcinoma of the cervix (exclusive of microinvasion). Am J Obstet Gynecol 126: 785, 1976.

Moss LD, Collins DN: Squamous and adenoid cystic basal cell carcinoma of the cervix uteri. Am J Obstet Gynecol 88: 86, 1964.

Shingleton HM, Lawrence WD, Gore H: Cervical carcinoma with adenoid cystic pattern. Cancer 40: 1112, 1977.

Shingleton HM, Gore H, Soong SJ, Bradley D: Adenocarcinoma of the cervix. 1. Clinical evaluation and pathologic features. Am J Obstet Gynecol (in press) 1981.

Tchertkoff V, Sedlis A: Cylindroma of the cervix. Am J Obstet Gynecol 84: 749, 1962.

29. DISTINCTION BETWEEN CERVICAL AND ENDOMETRIAL ADENOCARCINOMA WITH IMMUNOPEROXIDASE STAINING OF CARCINOEMBRYONIC ANTIGEN

M. KORHONEN, T. WAHLSTROM, J. LINDGREN and M. SEPPALA

Adenocarcinoma of the uterine cervix comprises about 5–10% of all cervical cancer, however, according to the literature, its incidence is increasing (Tasker and Collins 1974), as is the incidence of endometrial carcinoma. Adenocarcinoma of the cervix is epidemiologically different from squamous cell carcinoma; the patients tend to be older (Abad et al. 1969), and more often unmarried, nulliparous and hypertensive. Unlike the squamous cell carcinoma, adenocarcinoma does not seem more likely to develop in urban population (Korhonen 1980). The prognosis of cervical adenocarcinoma is slightly less favorable than that of squamous cell carcinoma (Korhonen, to be published).

Adenocarcinoma of the endometrium is usually found in patients in their fifties or older. Not only is it relative more common in unmarried and nulliparous women, it is also associated with obesity, diabetes and hypertension. Because endometrial adenocarcinoma is the most common malignant tumor of the female genital tract, every adenocarcinoma of the uterus is likely to be labeled as endometrial. Accurate differential diagnosis is crucial because cervical adenocarcinomas should be treated differently from endometrial adenocarcinomas.

Two main difficulties involved in the diagnosis of adenocarcinoma of the uterine cervix are its detection and its differentiation from endometrial adenocarcinoma.

I. DETECTION OF CERVICAL ADENOCARCINOMA

Cervical adenocarcinoma is more difficult to diagnose than squamous cell adenocarcinoma of the cervix. According to one series (Korhonen 1978), the symptoms and the length of the symptomatic period are identical and there is no difference in the distribution of cases to clinical stages. Moreover, in 29% of cases of cervical adenocarcinoma, no tumor was clinically visible. The corresponding figure for squamous cell carcinoma is 2% (Graham et al. 1962). Because of its intracervical localization, adenocarcinoma of the cervix is easily missed in clinical examination as well as in colposcopy.

Although detection rates up to 97% have been reported (Reagan and Ng 1973), the cytologic diagnosis of cervical adenocarcinoma is less accurate than that of squamous cell carcinoma. Table 1 shows the results of cytology in the series of Korhonen (1978). The rate of false-negative cytology was 14% for all, and 31% for stage I adenocarcinomas of the cervix. The detection rate of squamous cell carcinomas reported from the same hospital was 98.7% (Timonen and Purola 1962). A relatively low detection rate for adenocarcinoma of the cervix may be attributed to sampling errors, probably due to the intracervical localization of the tumor. The sampling technique used was a combination of cervical scrape and endocervical swab with a cotton-tipped stick; the combination proved to be better than use of cervical scrape alone. The key to the good results

Table 1. Accuracy of cytology in the detection of cervical adenocarcinoma (Korhonen 1978).

| Clinical stage | No. of cases | Cytologic diagnosis | | |
		Negative (%)	Suspicious (%)	Positive (%)
I	48	31	17	52
II	33	3	21	77
III	28	–	11	89
IV	3	–	–	100

reported by Reagan and Ng (1973) may be the sampling technique using endocervical aspiration. In a minority of cases the smears contained well-differentiated cells of cervical adenocarcinoma which, in the presence of autolysis, usually had been misinterpreted as normal or reactive endocervical cells.

II. METHODS AVAILABLE FOR DISTINCTION BETWEEN ENDOMETRIAL AND CERVICAL ADENOCARCINOMA

II.A. Clinical methods

Histologic verification of adenocarcinoma of the cervix is often based on the material obtained by curettage. Fractional curettage is the most commonly used clinical method to differentiate between cervical and endometrial adenocarcinoma. Comparing results of fractional curettage to the localization of tumor in surgical specimens, fractional curettage gave the correct result in only 11 out of 29 cases, when tumor tissue was present in the removed uterus (Korhonen 1978). Usually the fractional curettage indicated more extensive tumor than was found in the surgical specimen. Hysterography has been recommended by many authors (Norman 1950; Schwartz et al. 1975), but it too has given inconclusive results in the hands of others (Joelson et al. 1971). Hysteroscopy was then recommended, which seems to be a very accurate method, perhaps the best available.

II.B. Histopathology and histochemistry

Histologically, it is not possible to reach definite conclusions about the origin of an adenocarcinoma of the uterus. Although these tumors often repeat the differentiation type of the cells at their site of origin, they may show any of the differentiation patterns of the Mullerian epithelium or a combination thereof. The so-called endometrioid adenocarcinomas of the cervix account for about 15% of cervical adenocarcinomas (Anderson and Frazer 1976). Cervical adenocarcinomas vary greatly in histology and the pattern may vary even from one section to another in the same tumor (Hepler et al. 1952).

Table 2 summarizes Sorvari's (1969) study of mucosubstances of uterine adenocarcinomas. He found all 59 cervical adenocarcinomas and 97% of endometrial adenocarcinomas to be positive for mucin. In cervical adenocarcinomas, the amount of mucin was usually larger and was found in the cytoplasm. In endometrial carcinomas, the mucin was usually localized in the apical border of the cell and little or no mucin was seen in the cytoplasm. Sorvari also found qualitative differences between the chemical composition of mucins of the two carcinomas, but no mucin pattern was specific to either of them.

The presence of mucosubstances is characterized by great variability; some cells may be strongly positive for mucin and the adjacent cell may be negative. Clear cell adenocarcinomas of the cervix are usually mucin negative (Korhonen 1978). Mucin stainings may be helpful but the variability and the ambiguous interpretation of stainings are the limiting factors.

II.C. Cytology

Reagan and Ng (1973) compared the cytologic presentation of cervical and endometrial adenocarcinoma. The cells originating in cervical adenocarcinoma were more numerous; they were larger, often columnar in shape, and when stained with EA-65, they usually had a granular and acidophilic cytoplasm. The cells from endometrial adenocarcinomas were few in number; they were smaller, roundish, and the cytoplasm was finely vacuolated and basophilic. The nuclei of cervical adenocarcinoma were larger; hyperchromasia was more pronounced, and multiple nucleoli and macronuc-

Table 2. Mucosubstances in uterine adenocarcinoma (Sovari 1969).

	Cervical adenoca. 59 cases	Endometrial adenoca. 105 cases
Mucin positive	100%	97%
Distribution of mucin		
endometrial type (apical border)	21%	80%
cervical type (cytoplasm)	66%	10%
not determined	13%	10%

leoli were more common than in nuclei of endometrial adenocarcinoma.

While these features may give a hint about the localication of an adenocarcinoma, the contribution of cytology to the differential diagnosis of uterine adenocarcinomas remains to be evaluated.

III. CARCINOEMBRYONIC ANTIGEN (CEA)

Carcinoembryonic antigen was first described in carcinomas of the gastrointestinal tract and in fetal gut, liver and pancreas (Gold and Freedman 1965). It is a glycoprotein, has a molecular weight of about 200,000 and contains 60–70% carbohydrate and 30–40% protein. CEA has since been detected in several types of tumors, including carcinomas of the stomach, pancreas, breast, uterus, ovary and bladder. It is, however, strictly specific for neither malignant nor embryonic tissue; it is also found in nonneoplastic diseases such as ulcerative colitis and hepatic cirrhosis and also in very small amounts in normal tissues. Circulating CEA can be measured in plasma by using RIA. Elevated concentrations of CEA (2.5 ng/ml or more) are often found in patients with aforementioned and other diseases. Sixty percent of patients with cervical, 50% with ovarian, and 30% with endometrial carcinoma have an elevated CEA level (van Nagell et al. 1978). In addition, elevated CEA levels have been found significantly more often (29%) in patients with cervical intraepithelial neoplasia than in healthy volunteers (11%); but compared to levels in patients with benign gynecologic diseases, no significant difference existed (van Nagell et al. 1976).

In cancer patients, the circulating CEA is usually elevated, particularly if metastases are present, and the increase seems to have some correlation to the total tumor burden. At one time it was hoped that CEA might be used as a diagnostic tumor marker. Unfortunately it was not found to be sufficiently specific. Eleven percent of unselected healthy persons and as many as 19% of those who smoke have an elevated CEA level (Fuks et al. 1975). Nevertheless, plasma CEA determinations were helpful in the management of certain cancer patients. High CEA levels may suggest the presence of metastases. After a CEA-positive tumor is treated surgically, the CEA rapidly drops within the normal range. A failure of CEA level to decrease is usually associated with incomplete removal of the tumor. Reappearance of elevated plasma CEA may indicate a recurrence and it often precedes a clinically detectable recurrent tumor by months or years (Fuks et al. 1975).

A fascinating new application of CEA is the use of 131 I-labeled CEA antibody for the radioimmunodetection of neoplasms (Goldenberg et al. 1980).

IV. IMMUNOPEROXIDASE STAINING OF TISSUE CEA

The advent of immunoperoxidase histochemistry has allowed a new convenient method for the visualization of antigens by light microscopy. The great advantage over the immunofluorescence method is the permanency of the sections. Immunoperoxidase staining allows detection of many types of antigens, enzymes, viral antigens, hormones, immunoglobulins, etc. (DeLellis et al. 1979). In addition, this method has been used successfully to detect CEA in tissues. Because the antigenicity of CEA is stable and not destroyed by paraffin embedding of the tissue, this method is applicable to routine histologic specimens. Several modifications of immunoperoxidase staining are available (Primus et al. 1978). The staining is positive if the tissue contains 3–5 μg of CEA per gram of tissue (Goldenberg et al. 1976).

With the use of this method, CEA was detected in adenocarcinomas of the stomach, colon, pancreas, lung and ovary; in squamous cell carcinomas of the lung and cervix; and in transitional cell carcinoma of the bladder (Goldenberg et al. 1976). Benign tumors usually show negative staining although positive reactions are seen in the adenomas of the colon (Goldenberg et al. 1976), especially in the areas which show morphologic atypia (Isaacson and Le Vann 1976) and in serous cystadenoma of the ovary (Goldenberg et al. 1976). Intraepithelial neoplasias of the cervix show a positive staining in 26-60% depending on the severity of the lesion and squamous cell carcinomas of the cervix in 66% of the cases (Lindgren et al. 1979).

V. CEA STAINING IN THE DIFFERENTIAL DIAGNOSIS OF CERVICAL AND ENDOMETRIAL ADENOCARCINOMA

A study was undertaken to determine the value of CEA staining in distinguishing cervical from endometrial adenocarcinoma (Wahlstrom et al. 1979). Deparaffinized and rehydrated sections were treated with 0.5% hydrogen peroxide in absolute methanol to destroy the endogenous peroxidase activity of the tissue. Exposure of sections to normal sheep serum was followed by application of rabbit anti-CEA serum, sheep anti-rabbit IgG serum and rabbit anti peroxidase serum. After incubation with peroxidase, the latter enzyme was detected histochemically with the use of diaminobenzidine and hydrogen peroxide. Adjacent control sections were stained similarly except that the CEA antiserum was absorbed with purified CEA and sections from colorectal carcinoma were used as a positive control. An example of CEA-positive adenocarcinoma of the uterine cervix is presented in Figure 1. The details of the staining procedure as well as the preparation of antisera and the absorbtion of antisera for nonspecific antigens and the antigens related to CEA (NCA, NCA-2, CELIA) have been published earlier (Lindgren et al. 1979).

Specimens from 163 cases of cervical adenocarcinoma and 137 cases of endometrial adenocarcinoma were stained for CEA. The results are shown in Table 3. Cervical adenocarcinomas were positive in 80% of cases. Pure cervical adenocarcinomas were positive in 80%, cervical adenocarcinomas with squamous elements were positive in 100% of cases and clear cell adenocarcinomas of the cervix were always CEA-negative.

Only 8% of endometrial adenocarcinomas showed a positive staining reaction for CEA and all of these adenocarcinomas with squamous elements.

The incidence of adenocarcinoma of the endometrium is over 20 times that of adenocarcinoma of the cervix. Hence, more than 2/3 of all CEA-

Table 3. Tissue CEA in uterine adenocarcinomas.

Histologic type of adenocarcinoma	Cervical adenocarcinoma		Endometrial adenocarcinoma	
	CEA + all cases	%	CEA + all cases	%
Adenosquamous carcinoma or adenoacanthoma	45/45	100	11/11	100
Clear cell adenocarcinoma	0/11	0	0/4	0
Other adenocarcinomas	86/107	80	0/122	0

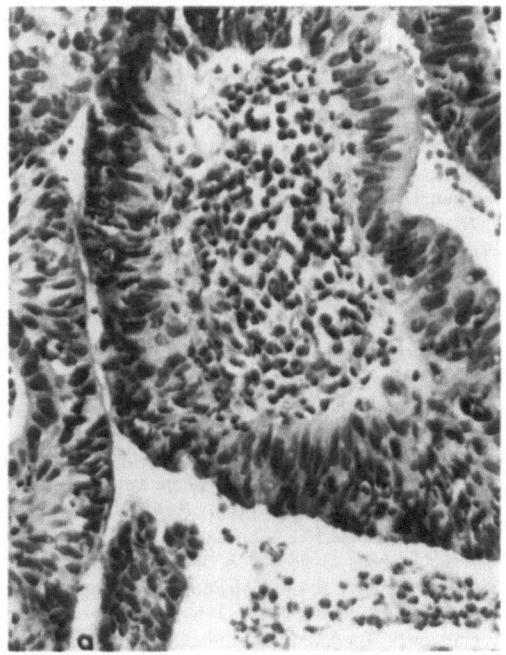 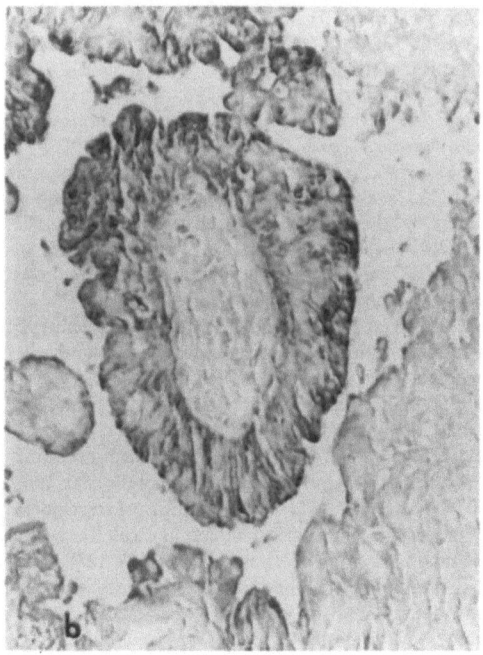

Figure 1. Immunoperoxidase staining of CEA in cervical adenocarcinoma. (a) Hematoxylin and eosin staining, (b) staining with anti-CEA serum, showing CEA in the cytoplasm.

positive adenocarcinomas of the uterus can be estimated to be endometrial and less than 1/3 of them cervical. Nevertheless, the immunoperoxidase staining of CEA can be a useful diagnostic method when combined with a careful histologic examination. The CEA staining has no diagnostic value in case of adenosquamous carcinomas or adenoacanthomas, because these are tumors with squamous elements also CEA-positive regardless of their origin. Clear cell adenocarcinomas, however, are CEA-negative in both cervix and in endometrium. After these histologic types have been excluded, all adenocarcinomas with positive CEA staining are cervical and 99% of CEA-negative adenocarcinomas are endometrial.

Adenosquamous carcinomas, adenoacanthomas and clear cell adenocarcinomas comprise 35% of

adenocarcinomas of the cervix (Korhonen 1978). In the group of endometrial adenocarcinomas studied, 8% contained squamous elements. According to the literature, about 7% of endometrial carcinomas are adenosquamous (Ng 1968) and the percentage of adenoacanthomas varies from 0.8–43.7% (Charles 1965). The CEA staining is, when applicable, a valuable method in the differential diagnosis of cervical and endometrial adenocarcinoma. A crucial limitation is the lack of applicability to a significant proportion of cases.

The interpretation of CEA staining is unambiguous, and commercial CEA antibodies are available. The immunoperoxidase method is simple, inexpensive, suitable for a routine laboratory and has many other applications in diagnostic pathology (De Lellis et al. 1979).

REFERENCES

Abad RS, Kurohara SS, Graham JB: Clinical significance of adenocarcinoma of the cervix. Amer J Obstet Gynecol 104: 517, 1969.

Anderson MC, Frazer AC: Adenocarcinoma of the uterine cervix; a clinical and pathological appraisal. Brit J Obstet Gynecol 83: 320, 1976.

Charles D: Endometrial adenoacanthoma. A clinicopathological study of 55 cases. Cancer 18: 737, 1965.

DeLellis RA, Sternberger LA, Mann RM, Banks PM, Nakane PK: Immunoperoxidase techniques in diagnostic pathology. Report of a workshop sponsored by National Cancer Institute. Am J Clin Path 71: 483, 1979.

Fuks A, Banjo C, Shuster J, Freedman SO, Gold P: Carcinoembryonic antigen (CEA): Molecular biology and clinical significance. Biochem Biophys Acta 417: 123, 1975.

Gold P, Freedman SO: Specific carcinoembryonic antigens of the human digestive system. J Exp Med 122: 467, 1965.

Goldenberg DM, Sharkey RM, Primus FJ: Carcinoembryonic antigen in histopathology; Immunoperoxidase staining of conventional tissue sections. J Nat Cancer Inst 57: 11, 1976.

Goldenberg DM, Sharkey RM, Primus FJ: Immunocytochemical detection of carcinoembryonic antigen in conventional histopathology specimens. Cancer 42: 1546, 1978.

Goldenberg DM, Kim EE, DeLand FH, Bennett S, Primus FJ: Radioimmunodetection of cancer with radioactive antibodies to carcinoembryonic antigen. Cancer Res 40: 2984, 1980.

Graham JB, Sotto LS, Paloucek FP: Carcinoma of the cervix. Philadelphia: Saunders, 1962.

Hepler TK, Dockerty MB, Randall LM: Primary adenocarcinoma of the cervix. Amer J Obstet Gynecol 63: 800, 1952.

Isaacson P, LeVann HP: The demonstration of carcinoembryonic antigen in colorectal carcinoma and colonic polyps using an immunoperoxidase technique. Cancer 38: 1348, 1976.

Joelsson L, Levine RU, Moberger G: Hysteroscopy as an adjunct in determining the extent of carcinoma of the endometrium. Amer J Obstet Gynecol 111: 696, 1971.

Korhonen MO: Adenocarcinoma of the uterine cervix. An evaluation of the available diagnostic methods. Acta Path Microbiol Scand Sect A, Suppl 264: 1, 1978.

Korhonen MO: Epidemiological differences between adenocarcinoma and squamous cell carcinoma of the uterine cervix. Gynecol Oncol 10: 312, 1980.

Korhonen MO, Nieminen U: Adenocarcinoma of the uterine cervix: Results of treatment and prognosis compared to squamous cell carcinoma (to be published).

Lindgren J, Wahlstrom T, Seppala M: Tissue CEA in premalignant epithelial lesions and epidermoid carcinoma of the uterine cervix; Prognostic significance. Int J Cancer 23: 448, 1979.

van Nagell JR, Donaldson ES, Wood EG, Goldenberg DM: The clinical significance of carcinoembryonic antigen in the plasma and tumors of patients with gynecologic malignancies. Cancer 42: 1527, 1970.

van Nagell JR, Meeker WR, Parker JC Jr, Kashmiri R, McCollum V: Carcinoembryonic antigen in intraepithelial neoplasia of the cervix. Amer J Obstet Gynecol 126: 105, 1976.

Ng ABP: Mixed carcinoma of the endometrium. Amer J Obstet Gynecol 102: 506, 1968.

Norman O: Hysterography in cancer of the corpus of the uterus. Acta Radiol (Stockh) Suppl 89: 1, 1950.

Primus FJ, Sharkey RM, Hansen HJ, Goldenberg DM: Immunoperoxidase detection of carcinoembryonic antigen. Cancer 42: 1540, 1978.

Reagan JW, Ng ABP: The cells of uterine adenocarcinoma. Monographs in clinical cytology 1. Basel: Karger, 1973.

Schwartz PE, Kohorn EI, Knowlton AH, Morris J: Routine use of hysterography in endometrial carcinoma and postmenopausal bleeding. Obstet Gynecol 45: 378, 1975.

Sovari TE: A histochemical study of epithelial mucosubstances in endometrial and cervical adenocarcinomas. Acta Path Microbiol Scand Suppl 207: 1, 1969.

Tasker JT, Collins JA: Adenocarcinoma of the uterine cervix. Amer J Obstet Gynecol 118: 344, 1974.

Timonen S, Purola E: Early diagnosis of uterine carcinoma. Ann Chir Gynaec Fenn 51: 405, 1962.

Wahlstrom T, Lindgren J, Korhonen M, Seppala M: Distinction between endocervical and endometrial adenocarcinoma with immunoperoxidase staining of carcinoembryonic antigen in routine histological tissue specimens. Lancet 2: 1159, 1979.

30. LYMPHOGRAPHY, ANGIOGRAPHY AND PHLEBOGRAPHY IN THE STAGING AND FOLLOW-UP OF CERVICAL CARCINOMA

A. ONNIS, L. LABI and S. VALENTE

The vascular structures of the pelvis represent an artero-phlebo-lymphatic rete. The three interrelated components of this system are important for onco-logic diagnosis, either for their thin branches at the pelvis viscera level, or for the complex structure of the largest vessels, which enable recognition of a presence of pathologic expansive process (Dos Santos 1968; Farinas 1941; Montanari 1974). Using an appropriate contrast media (such as oil contrast medium), it is possible to obtain complete radiologic evidence of each vascular system.

The complete visualization at the same moment of the single vascular components of each artero-phlebo-lymphatic district is rarely possible, since particular techniques are needed. Some vascular structures cannot be visualized radiologically. In fact, in direct lymphoadenography, the lymphatic collectors coming from the genito-uro-digestive visceral structures of the pelvis are not shown. In these cases, radiologic evidence of the visceral lymphatic rete lacks, contrary to what is obtainable for the arterious and venous districts. This does not mean that lymphatic vessels, radiologically recognizable, are not able to provide information on pathology provess, in particular in the pelvic visceral area.

In the evaluation of lymphoadenographic semeiology, it is necessary to distinguish the behavior of the lymphatic collectors from that of the lymphonodes. The latter can provide direct information on neoplastic processes in the areas of their corresponding lymphatic drainage, the replacement of the lymphonodal tissue by the neoplastic one. The picture is radiologically represented by partial or total filling defect, up to the missed visualization of the node site of metastasis.

Concerning the lymphatic system, a relationship exists among the different vascular structures and components of the artero-phlebo-lymphatic rete.

Contrastographic techniques are needed in onco-logic gynecology to investigate these structures to provide a unitary evaluation of the radiologic contribution to the multiple clinical problems.

I. RADIOLOGIC ANATOMY AND PELVIC ANGIO-GRAPHIC TECHNIQUES

The examination of the structural and dynamic aspects of the arterious and venous components of the pelvic vascular rete enable a drawing of the main lines of angiographic semeiology. The radiographic anatomy does not correspond to the classic anatomy, as noticed in almost all the vasal districts angiographically investigated. The contrasto-graphic visualization of vasal structures is strictly related to the functional conditions.

I.A. Pelvic arterious radiographic anatomy

The pelvic arterious vascularization does not show the same radiographic pictures because the visualiz-ation of some branches is not constant, e.g. the ovarian arteries are visualized in one-third of the cases are not often bilaterally.

The course of the arteries, which is quite constant in the parietal sector, is variable in the visceral sector, in relation to the viscera topographic and functional situation. For example, the parametrial tracts of the uterine arteries, almost rectilinear in the nullipara, become tortuous with the increase of parity. They meet at the marginal tract level which runs along the uterine axis. The consequent angio-graphic aspect, defined as *uterine arterious forceps*, implicates the viscerum thickness. The intramural branches of the uterine arteries become detached from the marginal tracts perpendicularly; angiographically, it displays a double hayrack-like appearance due to this tortuous vessel, which tends to meet on the median plane, without reaching it.

The visualization on the radiogram varies, not only in relation to the spatial disposition of the uterine body, but in relation to the selectivity of the angiographic technique. The uterus functional state makes the intramural branches more evident during the premenstrual period, less evident in the intermenstrual period, and absent in senile age. The marked visualization of hypertrophic intramural branches under physiologic conditions is present only during pregnancy and puerperium. It is also accompanied by small arteries and capillaries; this shows all the uterine parenchima.

I.B. Techniques of pelvic arteriography

The following are radiographic techniques for the investigation of the pelvic arteries: (a) *inferior translumbar aortography*, by puncture of the aorta at the second lumbar vertebra's body level (Dos Santos 1968); (b) *iliac retrograde arteriography*, by puncture of the femoral artery at the inguinal level and injection under pressure of the contrast medium (Farinas 1941); (c) *aortic transfemoral catheterism* (Seldinger 1953) allows the injection of a contrast medium into the aorta through a catheter introduced into the femoral artery at the inguinal level; (d) *selective catheterism of the hypogastric artery and its branches* allows the injection of radiopaque liquid to a predetermined vascular sector (Onnis et al. 1967, 1974). Under radioscopic control, it is possible, using the Odman's precurved catheters, to reach the hypogastric artery and the uterine or pudenda artery.

A recent modification allows a bilateral investigation through the femoral artery of one side only. This technique is useful for those cases of neoplasia that involve a modification of the vascular system.

I.C. Pelvic venous radiographic anatomy

The pelvic venous flow is more complex than the arterious flow. The venous visceral system is connected by plexi, so the blood flow has various possible directions. Each pelvic organ drains through a main flow and many collaterals. The bladder drains prevalently into the hypogastric vein; the uterus drains through the uterus vein into the hypogastric and contemporaneously through the ovarian veins into the inferior cava and left renal vein. The connection between the ovarian and uterine venous area forms an entir system. The ovarian veins basically run parallel to the corresponding arteries. They are widely anastomosed with the lumbar plexus, the retroperitoneal, ureteral veins, and lateral abdominal wall. The uterine venous system joins the marginal vein which runs along the lateral edge of the uterine body cervix and superior part of the vagina. The caliber of all these venous ways essentially depends on the volume of the arterious flow, and obstacle to the venous drainage.

If the arterious flow exceeds the capacity of the venous bed, a progressive dilatation of the ovarian and/or uterine plexi occurs. Similar modifications can be due to a difficult venous drainage with a normal arterious flow. Such an occurrence can be induced by increased venous pressure, by sectorial strictures and compressions of the venous walls. Flogistic processes, and their adherential outcome, viscera dislocations, presence of masses compressing the thin venous walls, are the most frequent causes.

I.D. Pelvic phlebographic techniques

Many radiologic techniques visualize the parietal venous sector only: (a) *indirect parietal phlebography* by injection of contrast medium into the pelvic bony tissue: only the drainage's way coming from the bonds themselves are visualized; (b) *direct parietal phlebography* is performed by the saphenae and femoral catheterisms at the inguinal level, and translumbar way; (c) *visceral phlebography* is performed by injection of a contrast medium into the uterine wall thickness.

The confluence of venous rete towards the uterine and ovarian veins forms an inconstant picture even under normal conditions; the ovarian or uterine venous drainage or the omolateral one are often visualized. The transuterine phlebography is not only relatively dangerous but also traumatic, and often has only a partial diagnostic value.

I.E. Pelvic lymphatic radiographic anatomy

The lymphatic flow is related to the venous flow; the lymphatic system is formed by vessels and lymphatic stations. The radiologic evidence of the pelvic lymphatic system shows results and pictures in different periods. In fact, the lymphatic vessels are first visualized, while the nodes require a longer time to reach a complete penetration of contrast. The radiologic images allow a study of the pelvic lymphatic collectors.

The *external iliac collectors* follow the inguinal collectors and are disposed around the external iliac blood vessels forming three chains. Such classic disposition is present in 35% of the cases; the chains are often four or more. The numerous transversal and oblique anastomosis often make a clear distinction of the lymphatic chains impossible. The *common iliac collectors* follow the external iliac ones and are disposed in three chains with many variants. The *lumbo-aortic collectors* follow the latter; the right collector passes laterally to the inferior cava, the left one laterally to the aorta.

The *hypogastric* or *internal iliac collectors* become opaque in 40% of the cases for progression against the stream of the contrast medium, beginning from the internal chain of the common iliac collectors. Such visualization is often unilateral but prevalently left. The topographic and morphologic studies of lymphographic pictures in the nodes require a subsequent radiological stage (*late images*). The lymphographic investigation visualizes the *inguinal* nodes in some gynecological cancers, especially in cervical cancer.

The *external iliac nodes* are disposed in the internal, medial and external chains. The internal chain is formed by three groups: an inferior (internal retrocrural), a middle (obturator node) and a superior. The middle chain is formed by three groups: an inferior (visible in 40% of the cases), a middle (visible in 50% of the cases) and a superior (visible in 65% of the cases). The external chain, sited between the artery and the psoas muscle, is always formed by three groups: an inferior (visible constantly), a middle (visible in 35% of the cases), a superior (visible in 45% of the cases).

The common iliac nodes are divided into three groups: (1) and internal group or and/of the promontory (visible in 90% of the cases); (2) a middle retrovascular group, that is posteriorly to the common iliac vessels, and (3) an external group (almost completely visible), laterally to the common iliac artery.

The hypogastric nodes are visualized for progression against the stream of the contrast medium from the common iliac nodes and only in 10% of the cases bilaterally. The lumbo-aortic nodes are numerous and closely arranged. They are often disposed in two chains: at the right and left side of the aorta.

The number of nodes visible in the radiograms is variable, even under physiologic conditions; their symmetric disposition and dimension are constant. Visualization also depends on the functional characteristics: in each chain some nodes receive the lymph directly from the drained organs, others only from the nodes. Moreover, for the numerous anastomotic vesswls, the former are always included in the lymphatic circulation, the latter can also be excluded in some functional moments and therefore not visible.

I.F. Pelvic lymphographic techniques

The introduction of the contrast medium by previous catheterism of the back of the feet lymphatic collectors is conducted by automatic systems and exact modalities of pressure and quantity until the column reaches the last lumbar vertebrate. The hydrosoluble contrast media presents poor results due to its fast reabsorption and irregular progression. Moreover, they cause pain. The oil contrast media gives a regular constant and homogeneous contrast of the lymphatic vessels. They accumulate in the nodes and remain there for a long time. The radiographic investigation is usually conducted as follows: (a) once the infusion is ended, to visualize the lymphatic collectors by three projections: antero-posterior, right and left oblique anterior; and (b) after 24 hours to study the nodes by the time imbued by contrast medium.

The inconveniences are rare, and are represented by allergic phenomena to iodine, local anaesthetics, feverish reactions due to the spreading of contrast medium in the tissues, pulmonary micro-embolism. It is necessary to avoid inconveniences when infecting the contrast medium, which quantity must be defined during radiological control.

218

II. PELVIC ANGIOGRAPHIC PATHOLOGY IN GYNE-COLOGICAL ONCOLOGY

II.A. Arteriographic pathology

The visceral arteries are more abundant than the parietal arteries. They present more evident aspects of *dislocation* when undergoing exstrinsic compression. The vesical arteries can be displaced to cover medial pelvic expansive processes, or displaced controlaterally from those at lateral pelvic site. The passage from the parametrial tracts to the marginal ones of the uterine arteries of both sides represents the *uterine arterious forceps*. The stiffness and angle-shot of the arterious branches, at their origin, can often imply of the expansive processes sited at the bifurcations level.

II.B. Radiological pictures

The picture is represented by the long-term out-come of a previous radiant treatment. The arteries appear thinning, stretched and stiffed. Following the radiant treatment, a picture of diffuse hyper-emia is noticed. In the presence of pelvic metastasis, the metastatic foci can lead to a localized, dense and delicate arterious malformation. When the process is of neoplastic nature, thin neoformed small ar-teries exist and are disposed of in a disorderly way forming a fine reticulum.

A myometrial expansive process dilates, leng-thens, compresses, moves the arterious branches, often displacing them to surround the tumoral mass, making them tortuous and disposed in a disorderly way (Figure 1).

II.C. Phlebographic pathology

Phlebography is useful to determine functional or anatomic variations of the pelvic veins. The func-tional variations consist of: (1) *slackening* of the venous flow with prolonged stanching of contrast

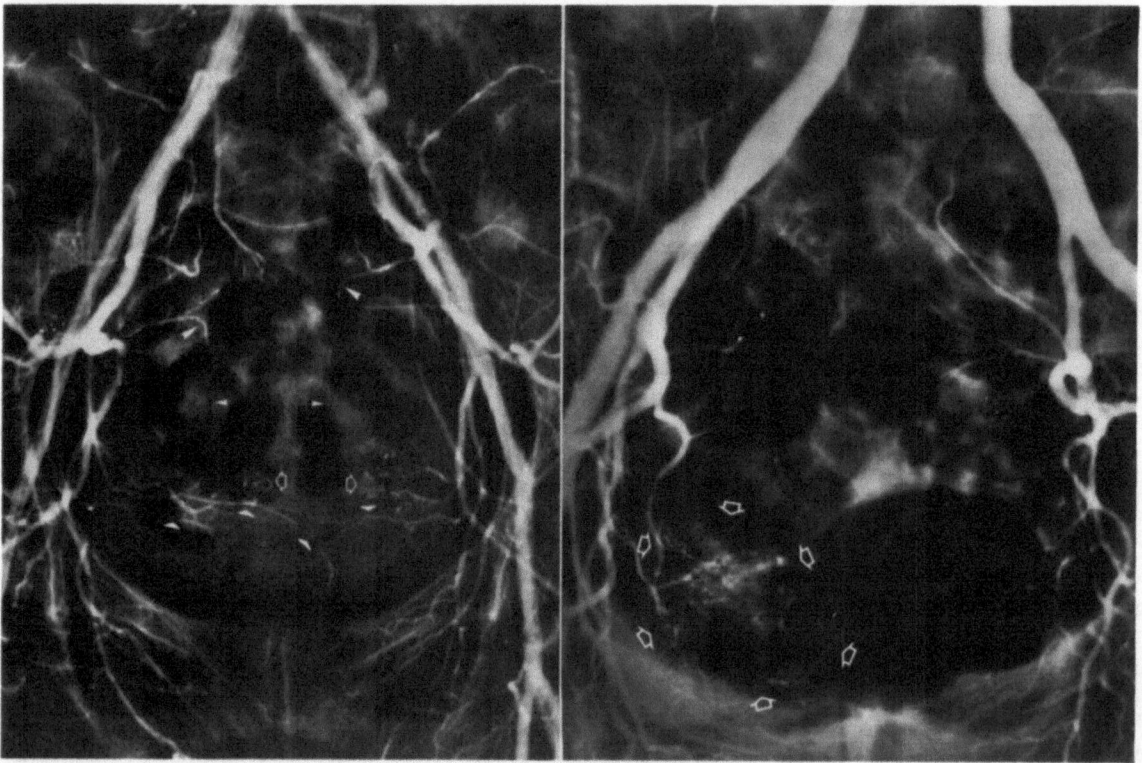

Figure 1. Left: Pelvic arteriography in a patient who underwent endocavitary (radium or transcutaneous ^{60}Co) radiotherapy two years before the angiographic examination. Visceral arteries uniformly thinner and stretched, the lateral sacral (long arrows) and the vesical arteries (triangular arrows) are evident. The uterine aa. (empty arrows) present irregular caliber and rigid aspect. Right: Relapse of cervical carcinoma with invasion of the right parametrium. Dense vascular neoformation, sustained by uterine, obturator and vesical aa.: it furnishes blood to an irregularly roundish are of 4 cm of diameter, which is projected over the pubis.

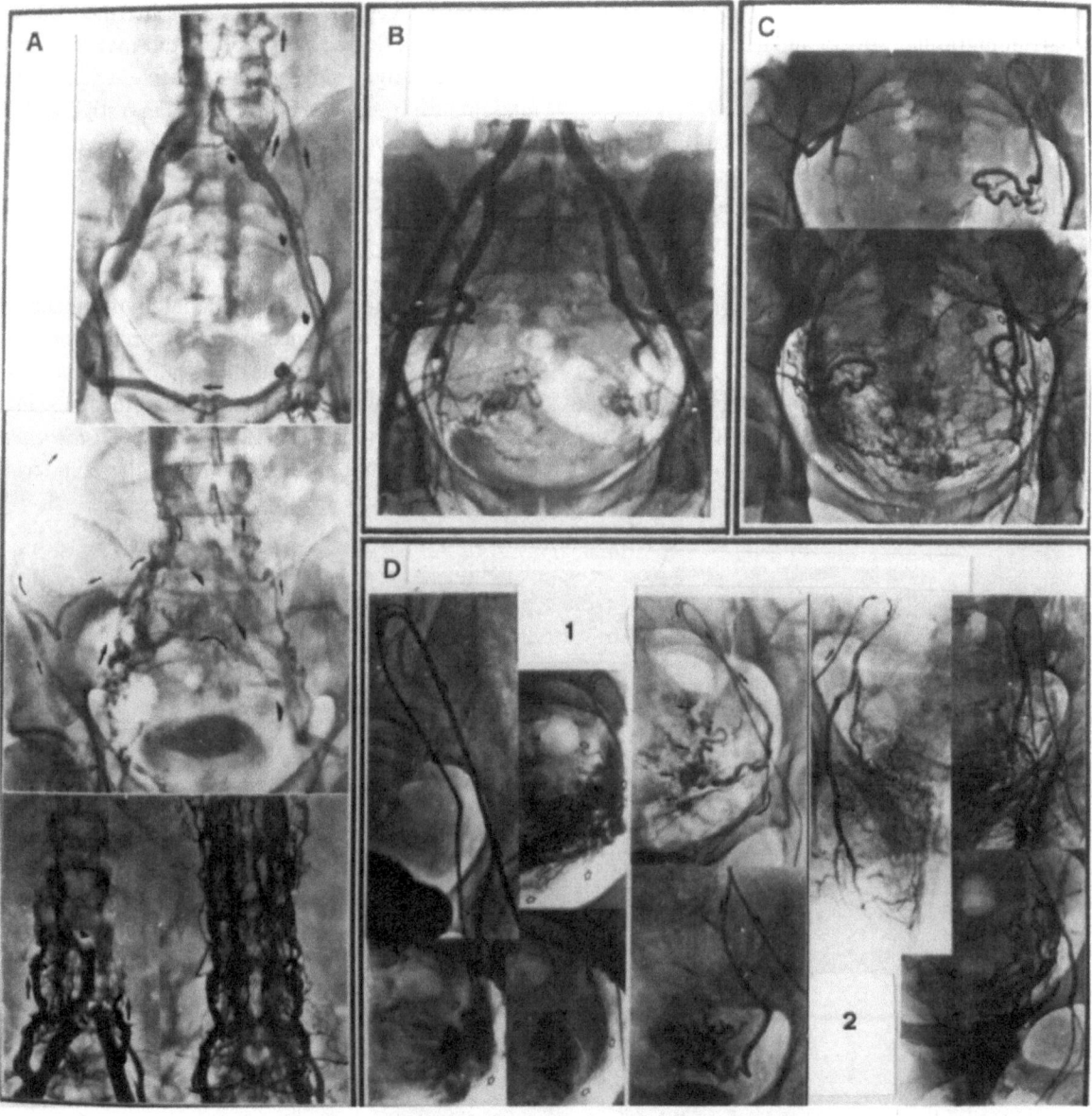

Figure 2. (A) Pelvic phlebography; (B) pelvic arteriography; (C) hypogastricography; (D) selective catheterisms; (1) uterine aa.; (2) vesical and pudenda aa.

medium; (2) *reflux* of contrast medium injected under pressure in the collateral veins; and (3) *current inversion* in the large vessels and collateral venous circles with phlebographic visualization of branches outside the hypogastric area.

These pictures can vary with the position assumed by the patient during the examination e.g., in dorsal decubitus, the sacral branches are mainly visualized, in an upright position, mainly of the other braches.

The anatomic variations consist of: (1) *caliber*

increase, more evident in the ovarian veins; the uterine veins seldom dilate due to its larger tributary area; (2) *number increase* which can be noticed particularly in the ovarian vein and in the ovarian parametrial plexi; (3) *varicose aspects*, when the caliber and number increase is not sufficient to support an overcharge, the venous walls subside; (4)*compression, dislocation* and *traction*: the ovarian veins are the most susceptible of dislocations; (5) *obstructions* occur in some cases of cervical carcinoma with involvement of the parametrial area;

such an occlusion can be followed by a uterine parenchimographic effect; and (b) *direct involvement of the venous walls* due to neoplastic infiltration or to thrombosis.

The parietal involvement appears as radiographic aspects of multiple filling defects which quickly evolves toward a true occlusion which leads to formation of collateral circles or to current inversion (Figure 2).

II.D. Lymphographic pathology

The diagnostic investigation of the pelvic lymphatic system can be indicated by *preoperative examination* in different stages of cervical carcinoma other than the vulva, vagina, ovary and uterine body. Therefore, the degree of lymphonodal invalvement, and indications for surgical treatment and the modalities of radiant therapy can be investigated by *postoperative control of the lymphoadenectomy radicality*.

II.E. Radiological pictures

Indications diagnosing lymphonodal involvement of a genital malignant cancer present variable significance; in fact, there are signs of presumption and certainty. The lymphatic vessels can present the following pathologic modifications (Figure 3): (a) *Dislocation* from their normal site; (b) *reflux* in the collateral

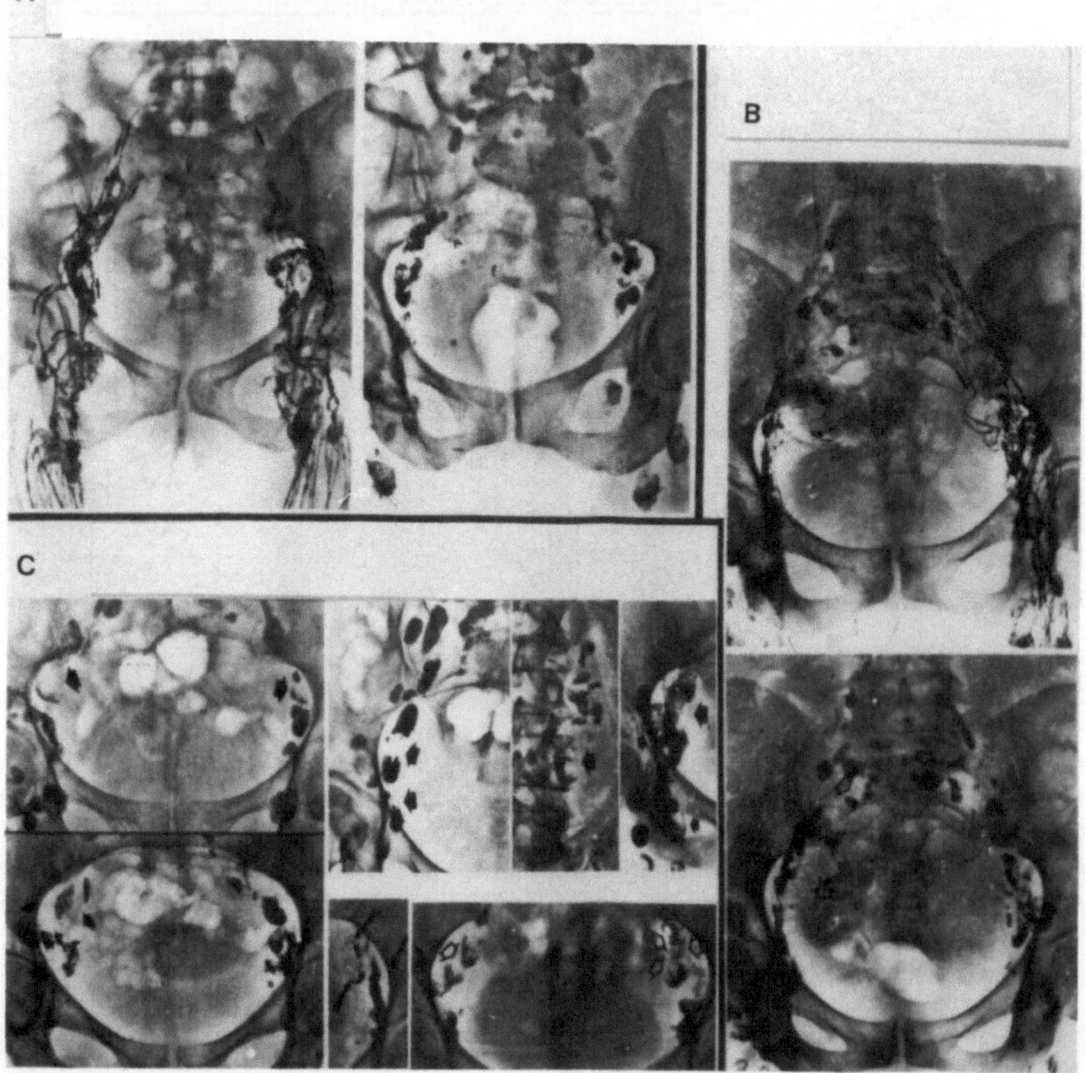

Figure 3. (A) Normal lymphography; (B) collateral vessels and suspect lymphographic picture; (C) lymphonodal metastasis.

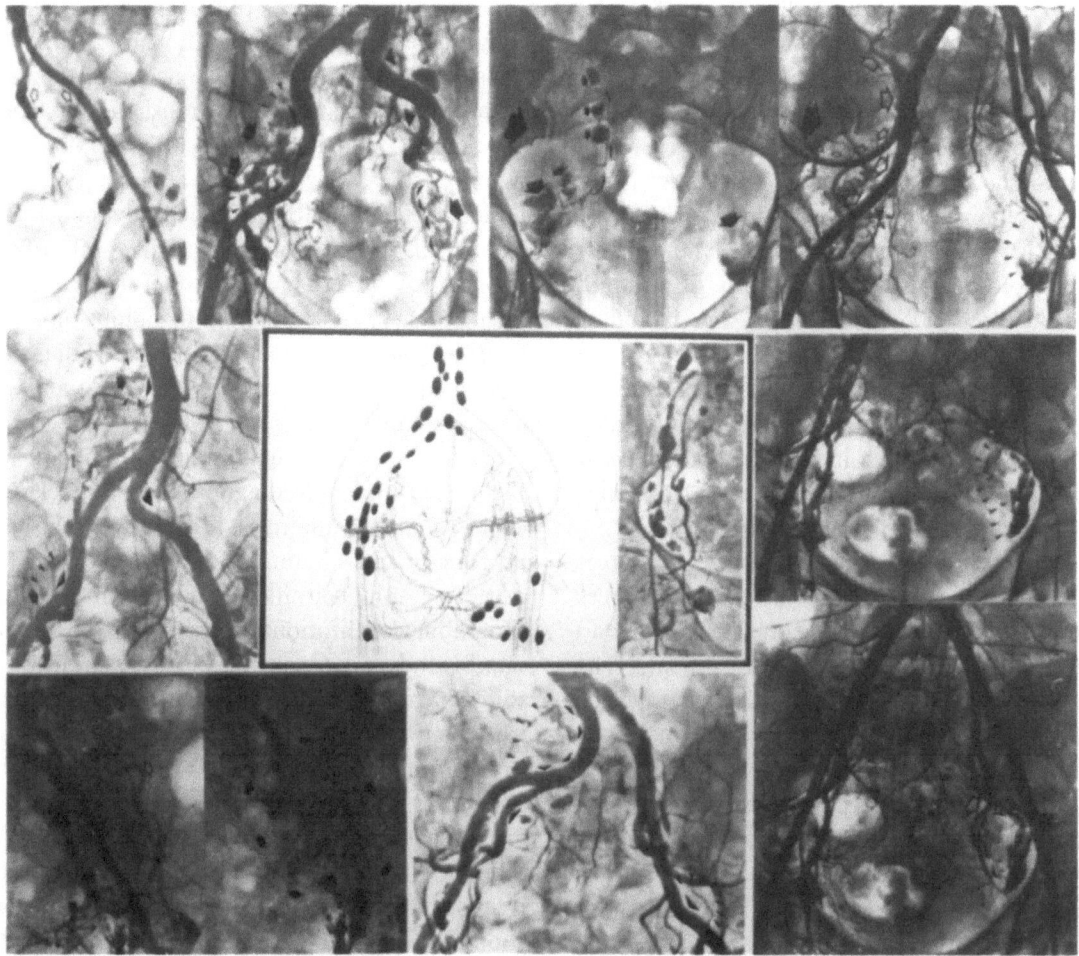

Figure 4. Some pictures of lympho-arteriographic association.

and anastomotic vessels; (c) *progression stop* of contrast medium often associated to both the anastomotic vessels visualization and the upward lymphatic stasis; (d) *caliber variations* which can include total, sectorial or bead-like dilatations, strictures, increased tortuosity; (e) *spread out*, which indicates an obstacle in the lymphatic vessel course, but can also represent a falsification due to exaggerate pressure infusion of contrast medium; (f) *lymphatic stasis* (24 hours after the use of extrafluid Lipiodol); such a picture has a different value depending on the level of its finding: it is pathognomonic only if it is present in abnormal or anastomotic collateral vessels already visible in precocious radiograms and not in the main lymphatic vessels (external iliac, common iliac, lumbo-aortic, hypogastric).

Lymph nodes present the following pathological aspect: *volume increase*: such a picture can be due to both neoplastic involvement or hyperplasia following inflammations. The picture of lymphonodal image enlargement with lacunar aspect is suspicious.

III. CONCLUDING REMARKS

The necessity of an integration between clinico-laboratory investigation and angiography, for the staging of gynecological cancers, is universally admitted (Figure 4).

Groin-pelvic lymphography in cervical carcinoma is considered an unchangeable tool of diagnosis in the exploration of the lymphatic system tributary of cervix uteri. The use of the radioactive isotope 32P carried out by oily contrast medium, permits the control of micrometastasis, and in some cases to avoid the selective dissection of nodes radiologically excluded by the lymphatic circulation. The number of false positive is acceptable as that basic error of many other diagnostic techniques and in particular of those with contrastographic method: 6% of false positive and 15% of false negative (Onnis 1974). False negatives are mainly due to micrometastasis because of limitations of many radiological methods (e.g. scheletric and thoracic, and those of other districts), also including the scintiscan.

The statistical analysis of the series demonstrates how a positive or suspicious lymphography permits the 'N' stadiation, which indicates a systematic or selective management of the lymphonodal chains, both of surgical or radiological type.

The nodes prolonged opacification is of great value both for the radiotherapy by external sources and for a widely demolisher surgery, in order to make controls after the different treatments. The nodes persistent opacification also permit the follow-up of morphological aspect and control the eventual presence of micrometastasis, which could slip to the action of a radiotherapy by external source, or isotopes carried by contrast medium (radiant lymphography).

The arteriographic semeiology is rich in direct or indirect signs of the neoplasia in its diffusion and invasivity. The existence of rich and large neoformed circles in any pelvic district is typical of a productive process in the expansion stage and must be precisely defined in its limits and spatial dimen-

sions. For this purpose, phlebography, lymphography and scintiscan investigation is used by endovasal infusion MAAI[131]. Concerning the technique, the transcutaneous-transfemoral aortic catheterism (Seldinger 1953), permits helpful information on the pelvic and genital circulation, with minimal traumatism for the patient. By the selective catheterism (transcutaneous-transfemoral) of the hypogastric arteries, or of the uterine or internal pudenda artery, it is possible to obtain more detailed and precise information for a better diagnosis – particularly on the uterine, parametrial and vulvovaginal circulation.

Results of this investigation are particularly useful for the differential diagnosis between sclerosal pelvic situations (due to radiotherapy or surgery) and persistencies or tumoral relapses.

Arteriography permits the individualization and topographic localization of persistencies or tumoral relapses and a consequent selective surgical and radiotherapeutic treatment. The images are particularly significant and reliable in case of selective arteriography of the hypogastric artery, or of its collaterals.

Investigation of the venous pelvic district, either within the parietal or visceral circulation, often gives radiological pictures of difficult interpretation. It also permits useful informations on the site and extension of productive processes; integrating, in this way, the arteriographic and lymphographic reports.

REFERENCES

Dos Santos: Attualità in Oncologia Ginecologica, aggiornamenti diagnostici e terapeutici. Padova: Cedam, 1968.

Farinas PL: New technique for the angiographic examination of the abdominal aorta and its branches. Am J Roentgenol Rad Ther and Nuclear Med 46: 641, 1941.

Montanari GD, Grella P, Viozzi A: Risultati a distanza della terapia endolinfatica con radionuclidi nel carcinoma del collo dell'utero. Clin Exp Obst Gyn, I supp: 54, 1974.

Onnis A, Marsiletti GC, De Salvia D, Bevilacqua L: Percutaneous selective catheterization of the hypogastric artery and its branches. Am J Obst Gyn 98: 966, 1967.

Onnis A: Intralymphatic isotope therapy with P32 in the treatment of female genital cancer. Clin Exp Obst Gyn I: 53, 1974.

Seldinger SI: Catheter replacement of the needle in percutaneous arteriography. Acta Radiol 39: 368, 1953.

Vecchietti G, Onnis A, Bresadola S, Romagnolo A, Colombini C: Studies and clinical possibilities of intralymphatic isotopic therapy in malignant diseases of the female reproductive system. Opening lecture for International Symposium on the preparation and bio-medical application of labeled molecules. The Centers of Radiation Chemistry and Radio-Elements of C.N.R. and EURATOM, Venice 23 August, 1964.

Vecchietti G, Onnis A, Bresadola S, Romagnolo A, Colombini C: Studies and clinical possibilities of intralymphatic isotopic therapy in malignant diseases of the female reproductive system. Acta Isotopica 5: 121, 1965.

Vecchietti G, Onnis A: La radioisotopoterapia in oncologia ginecologica. Padova: Cedam, 1967.

31. CONCLUDING REMARKS: FUTURE RESEARCH

E.S.E. HAFEZ

Recent advances on the epidemiology (Table 1), cytology ultrastructure (Table 2), etiology (Table 3), and diagnosis (Table 4), of carcinoma of the cervix have been reported, summarized and discussed (cf. Hafez and Smith 1980).

I. EPIDEMIOLOGY

Extensive attempts have been made to evaluate the annual trends and mortality rate from carcinoma of the cervix in various parts of the world. In the U.S.A. the annual trends in cancer incidence and mortality have been evaluated by the Surveillance, Epidemiology, and End Results (SEER) program of the National Cancer Institute based on data from 11 population-based cancer registries. *In situ* carcinoma is most common in the U.S.A. among women in age groups ranging from 20 to 40, showing nearly continuous declines among all age groups after 40. There is continuous increase in incidence of invasive carcinoma as age increases, with the highest rates among women of 55 years of age. In the U.S.A. during 1969–1971, *in situ* carcinoma of the cervix was the second most frequently occurring cancer among white females (exceeded only by breast cancer) and was the most frequent among black females. Breast cancer rates surpassed those of *in situ* cervical cancer among black women. Thus, in the late 1970s, incidence rates for *in situ* cervical carcinoma became the second highest among all U.S. females. Invasive carcinoma of the cervix rated the fifth highest incidence of all cancers in white females between 1969–1971 and was third highest among black females. A reduction in invasive carcinoma is attributed to the efforts of mass screening programs and their ability to detect earlier stage disease among previously unscreened populations. In several developed countries there is increased acceptance by women of the Papanicolaou (Pap) smear as part of routine health care procedure and improved health care delivery to all socioeconomic strata.

The incidence of carcinoma of the cervix seems to be associated with low income and limited education,

and in the United States with Black and Hispanic populations. Pap smears are more frequent in affluent, better educated, white population. Thus, those more in need of screening are less likely to receive it. Within high risk communities, older women are least likely to have Pap smears.

Carcinoma of the cervix is the most common form of cancer in the developing countries of the Americas. In Central American countries the highest incidence is in younger women, contrasting to the incidence in the U.S. and European countries. The common finding in European and American countries of an inverse relationship between cervix and breast cancers does not apply in Jamaica in that both types are common and both cancers show a similar age specific pattern.

In most countries of the Middle East conservative Muslim mode of life, male circumcision, sexual conservatism, and ritual hygiene probably operate in reducing incidence of carcinoma whereas aesthetic factors and complacency in seeking medical advice operate in delaying diagnosis.

The incidence of cervical carcinoma in Jewish patients is relatively low compared to non-Jewish women. In Jewish populations, the number of cases of cervical carcinoma equals to or exceeds the number of either endometrial or ovarian tumors.

Mortality rates for carcinoma of the cervix are higher in most Latin American and Caribbean countries than in the U.S. and Canada. Black and white women in the U.S.A. have longest median survival (ten years or more) when carcinoma is diagnosed among women 35 years or younger. Among 35–44 years of age, women's median survival was 10 years for white women and 7.2 years for black.

The prognosis in endocervical glandular neoplasms is related to the clinical stage, degree of

Hafez, E.S.E., Smith, J.P. (eds.), Carcinoma of the Cervix: Biology and Diagnosis. ISBN-13: 978-94-009-7487-6
© 1982, Martinus Nijhoff Publishers, The Hague/Boston/London.

differentiation, tumor type, and nuclear DNA findings. Patients with pure endocervical adenocarcinoma have better prognosis than those with mixed carcinomas.

I.A. Screening programs

Several screening modalities have been used for detection of cervical carcinoma which requires utilization to reach women of high risk in urban populations: e.g. (a) utilization of selected neighborhood health clinics or 'standing' clinics that conduct daily screening services for their community; (b) initiation of mobile 'outreach' clinics in YMCA facilities, churches and other community programs; and (c) operation of clinics at selected places of employment to facilitate accessibility for working women. The Pan American Health Organization (PAHO) has initiated in 1965 an interesting screening program in Chile. The screening coordinated by the Ministry of Public Health, is nationwide in scope and includes a network of 12 regional cytology laboratories throughout the country. In 1976, PAHO and the U.S. National Cancer Institute (NCI) have launched effective cancer control programs in Latin America known as the 'Latin American Cancer Research Information Project' (LACRIP) (Litvak 1976). LACRIP was designed to gather information on cancer related activities in Latin America and to assist Latin American investigators, clinicians and administrators in the development of better approaches to the prevention, diagnosis and treatment of cancer. This most successful project now includes the active participation of 48 recognized centers in Latin American and 12 in the U.S.; their collaborative research activities include a significant number of clinical and epidemiologic studies on cervical neoplasia.

II. ETIOLOGY

II.A. Viruses

There is considerable evidence suggesting a close relationship between herpes simplex virus type 2 (HSV-2) and cervical neoplasia. Extensive research has been undertaken to identify and characterize markers of HSV-2, including virus specific antigens,

in cervical tumors and tumor-derived cells. Several attempts have been made to demonstrate the expression of HSV-2 specified antigens within the cancer cells in the absence of an infectious virus (Dressman et al. 1980). The technique employed for the detection of these antigens has entailed the use of hyperimmune rabbit or hamster antisera to HSV with immunofluorescence (IF) staining. VP 143 of HSV-2 was prepared in rabbits using protein purification and immunization procedures (Curtney and Benyesh-Melnick 1974). These and other studies indicate that: (a) expression of nucleolar antigen may have a diagnostic role in cervical cancer; and (b) HSV-2 fingerprints implicate the virus as a factor in this cancer.

VP 143 was readily localized within nuclei of squamous epithelial cells of patients with herpes cervicitis. Staining for VP 143 was also seen in cervical cells of certain patients with carcinoma *in situ* and a few patients with invasive squamous cell carcinoma. However, the staining was perinuclear within the cytoplasm in a pattern similar to that noted in HSV-2-transformed cells. These results provide further evidence for a role of HSV-2 in human cervical carcinoma.

II.B. Immunological factors

Immunologic factors are of utmost importance in squamous cell carcinoma of the uterine cervix. The peripheral blood lymphocytes of these patients express specific immunological sensitivity by tumor-associated antigen. Cell-mediated immunity was evaluated in patients with this malignancy at this time of initial clinical diagnosis, prior to treatment. The tube Leukocyte Adherence Inhibition Assay (LAI assay) is capable of identifying patients with squamous cell carcinoma of the cervix and to discriminate between patients with cervical squamous neoplasia, other types of tumors and the normal state (Chen et al. 1975; Chiang et al. 1976; Halliday and Miller 1972; Halliday et al. 1974).

II.C. Sexually transmitted disease

Repeated exposure of the uterine cervix to the male partner's asymptomatic urogenital infection can lead to precancerous or cancerous lesions. Dahlberg (1976) performed bacteriologic cultures of prostatic fluid and/or semen as well as cytologic examinations of prostatic excretions. Contraceptive methods excluded use of the condom. Precancerous lesions of the cervix reversed to normal with: (a) antibacterial treatment of males; (b) change of contraceptive method; and (c) change of partner.

II.D. Effect of oral contraceptive and IUDs

The effects of oral contraceptives on the occurrence of cervical neoplasia are controversial. Women at higher risk for cervical lesions may tend to choose OCs more often than other contraceptive methods. Women selecting OC have a higher screening rate and might be sexually more active. The diaphragm might have a protective effect against cervical carcinogenesis. Sexual behavior accounts for some, but not all of the apparently higher risk of cervical neoplasia among OC users. There is no apparent association between the use of OCs and the incidence of invasive carcinoma.

Cervical carcinogenesis may be hormone-dependent as judged by: (a) the histological sensitivity of the cervix to hormonal influences; (b) the decreasing incidence of cervical cancer after menopause; and (c) the results of animal experiments with estrogens and progesterones. Oral contraceptives caused atypical squamous epithelium, increased squamous metaphasia, basal cell and glandular hyperplasia of the cervix that could be misdiagnosed as malignant, but proved to be benign by using light and electron microscopy.

Prolonged usage of an IUD is often associated with exfoliation of atypical cells that might be mistaken to represent carcinoma. The occurrence of dysplasia of varying severity increases with IUD use. The time required to progress from mild to moderate dysplasia decreases with IUD use. However, the life-table rate of progression from dysplasia to carcinoma *in situ* is unaffected by IUD users. There is no evidence that IUDs accelerate the development of cervical carcinoma or the progression of dysplasia to cancer. However, there are no controlled studies on sizeable population to evaluate the effect of IUDs on cervical atypias. As with OC studies IUD users and non-users were not necessarily matched regarding factors associated with increased risk of cervical carcinogenesis, i.e. age, sexual behavior parity, and socioeconomic status. Controlled long-term follow-up for different types of medicated IUDs are needed.

II.E. Genetic aspects

Several structural aberrations were observed in the chromosomes of patients, e.g. deletions and marked variability in size and shape of homologous chromosomes. The consistently observed chromosomal abnormalities in different stages of carcinoma of the cervix confirm the diagnostic value of the presence of such aberrations in cases of equivocal diagnosis. Thus, the presence of an abnormal clone of cells with chromosomal aberrations may indicate the presence of malignancy.

III. BIOLOGY

III.A. Histochemistry

There are remarkable variations in the ability of cells to produce and to store glycogen. Poorly differentiated cancer cells lack glycogen whereas well-differentiated cancer cells may store these inclusions. This phenomenon is probably related to the degree of cellular maturation and is a reflection of the altered genetic makeup of these cells.

Heat stable alkaline phosphatase (ALP), usually found in the placenta or in certain types of cancers is found in normal diploid reserve cells from which most cervical cancers seem to originate. ALP isoenzyme patterns change during the course of carcinogenesis and seem to resemble the so-called 'enzyme deviation'.

III.B. Ultrastructure

Transmission and scanning electron microscopy have been used to study the fine structure of tumor patterns in cervical carcinoma. Emphasis was placed on: (a) the classification of poorly differentiated tumors, especially adenocarcinomas with questionable elements of squamous cell; (b) the relation of pathologic patterns of adenocarcinomas with radiation or surgical curability, i.e. identification of good or poor prognosis patterns; (c) the significance of the adenoid cystic pattern, a rare and unusual tissue type; (d) the significance of adenosquamous carcinoma; and (e) the changes in patterns of adenocarcinoma that recur following irradiation therapy.

Squamous lesions of cervical intraepithelial neoplasia (CIN) are characterized by a progressive diminution in ultrastructural squamous characteristics concomitant with increasing severity of the lesion. Neoplastic basal cells in all three grades of CIN may be similar, exhibiting high nucleo-cytoplasmic ratio (NCR), irregular convoluted nuclei, and numerous surface microvilli with normal to decreased desmosomes. In CIN grade I–II, or mild-moderate dysplasia, midlevel cells show enlarged convoluted nuclei with decreased amount of glycogen and increased number of ribosomes. In CIN III, or severe dysplasia-carcinoma *in situ* the nucleo-cytoplasmic ratio is increased and nuclei often show shallow invaginations with multiple nucleoli and coarsely clumped chromatin. The apical microvilli of cells increase to a great extent with few poorly formed desmosomes. Glycogen is absent and tono-filaments are greatly decreased or absent.

Ultrastructural characteristics of invasive squamous cell carcinoma of the cervix vary with the degree of differentiation. In well-differentiated squamous lesions the surface microvilli tonofilaments are abundant whereas glycogen may aggregate into pools. Nuclei are enlarged and pleomorphic with bizarre nuclear invaginations and irregular chromatin clumps. Cells may form partial or complete basal laminae. In poorly differentiated squamous tumors the desmosomes are poorly developed, and the tonofilaments, and glycogen are decreased.

In well-differentiated carcinoma, cell surfaces are characterized by well-developed microvillous projections. Desmosomes are numerous and well formed. In poorly differentiated carcinoma, the desmosomes are less numerous and sometimes poorly formed. The basement membrane separating the malignant cell nests from the stroma is often missing or incomplete. The nuclei of cells of well-differentiated cancer are pleomorphic and usually enlarged. The well-developed elongated microvillous pattern noted in well-differentiated carcinomas is associated with an increase in the surface area that facilitates active metabolic exchange.

It would appear that the cancer squamous cells lose their ability to produce microridges which characterize the squamous epithelium. The normal superficial or intermediate squamous cells are characterized by the presence of microridges, covering the total cell surface. When applying SEM to routine cervical smear preparations, the characteristic features of normal ectocervical squamous epithelium and microridges covering the cell surface are noted whereas more rounded cells appear to be covered by short microvilli. Cell surface ultrastructure characteristics – like microridges and microvilli – cannot be utilized for the discrimination of normal and early neoplastic cells, at least not as easily as previously reported. Cell surface labelling techniques have been applied altering functional properties of cell surface organization in the search for an early marker of irreversible neoplastic transformation.

IV. CELL GROWTH, TYPES AND GRADING

IV.A. Cell growth

Uncontrolled growth, invasion, and the forming of metastasis are processes of great academic and clinical significance. Each of these processes result from an alteration in the behavior of individual cells giving rise to such phenomena as loss of contact inhibition, decreased mutual adhesiveness or escape of immunological surveillance. Alterations in behavior of cells may be associated with specific modifications in cell surface organization.

Microinvasive carcinoma of the cervix represents a transition from dysplasia or carcinoma *in situ* and frank invasion. By histological criteria, microinvasion is clearly invasive but lacks the malignant potential of invasive cancer and is therefore amenable to conservative therapy. Microinvasion can arise from the surface epithelium of the ectocervix or from within endocervical glands and may be focal or multifocal. Lesions begin as nonconfluent projections penetrating into the stroma as finger-like or bulky, broad downgrowths that incite a local stromal reaction with edema fibrosis and inflammatory cell infiltration. Distinctive cellular changes occur in these microinvasive foci which reflect differentiation and maturation toward kertin production. Isolated droplets of neoplastic cells are often found scattered in the stroma around microinvasive projections.

Deeper, more advanced microinvasion may exhibit finger-like or bulky downgrowth, but these foci tend to coalesce and anastomose forming a confluent growth pattern. Although lymphatic or blood vascular permeation can occur with any degree of stromal invasion, it is more commonly noted with advanced confluent microinvasion. Regional lymph node metastases are rarely seen with microinvasive lesions less than 3 mm in depth but do occur with large volume confluent microinvasion with advanced stromal invasion and vascular infiltration.

IV.B. Types

Microinvasive carcinoma makes up an ever increasing proportion of stage I invasive cervix cancer.

In microinvasive carcinoma, the upper limitation of the depth of invasion has been variously stated to be 1, 2, 3, 4 and 5 mm. 'Hyperkeratotic dysplasia' of the cervix, involves cervical dysplasia with a granular layer and a keratotic surface. This type is mostly noted in patients less than 50 years of age who exhibit severe dysplasia or carcinoma *in situ*. 'Mucoepidermoid tumor' refers to growths that are composed of epidermoid cells and contain variable amounts of mucin. While these two characteristics are consistently present, other features of these tumors may be quite variable. Hellweg (1957) expanded the concept to include mucoepidermoid carcinomas (MEC) of the cervix. Cervical MECs should be differentiated from both adenosquamous carcinoma and adenocancroid. Both of these tumor types are composed of squamous and glandular differentiation products and both may produce mucin. The essential difference lies in the relative predominancy of one of the three diagnostic elements, i.e. squamous differentiation products, glandular differentiation products and mucin.

The frequency of lymph node metastases at the pelvic wall is higher in younger patients than in elderly women. In patients with cervical squamous cell carcinoma there is verifiable correlation between tumor grading, tumor growth, tumor location, tumor spread and age of patients.

Neoplasms of the vagina that arise following apparent successful treatment of cervical carcinoma are becoming recognized as a distinctive entity. A second primary neoplasm in the vagina that occurs following cervical carcinoma could represent a separate neoplasm, a 'field' response to a common carcinogen or be due to radiation carcinogenicity that results from previous treatment.

IV.C. Grading

Since there are varying degrees of malignancy in groups of a given stage, it is important to determine their grade or degree of malignancy according to the histological and nuclear grade as well as to the stromal reaction. Staging is determined clinically and estimates the extent of disease and size of the tumor, whereas histological type and grading provide its microscopic characteristics. Glandular neoplasms of the endocervix show remarkable morphologic variations; some are pure adenocarcinomas whereas other have both a glandular and squamous component (mixed adenosquamous carcinomas) (Glucksman and Cherry 1956; Reagan and Ng 1973).

Considering tumor localization and tumor growth, most carcinomas located at the portio are of the purely exophytic type whereas most endocervical tumors are of the endophytic type. Of the exophytic growing tumors, 25% are well differentiated, whereas this type of cell differentiation is found in only 11% of the endophytic tumors. Poorly differentiated cancers have a higher incidence of lymph and blood vessel invasion.

In advancing grades of CIN the decrease in the number of pseudopodia per basal cell is a significant progressive phenomenon. The absence of apparent differences in pseudopodia at either end of the disease continuum reflects the necessary and arbitrary categorization of histological grades. The modification of stromal-basal cell interactions resultant from this dedifferentiation, may account in part for the pathogenesis of CIN. An important feature of microinvasive carcinoma is the tendency for the invading cells to mature. Such maturation is common and might explain why most invasive squamous cancers are of the large cell non-keratinizing or of the keratinizing type. A heavy infiltrate of lymphocytes alone or in combination with plasma cells often surround the invasive foci. Histologically there is usually extensive carcinoma *in situ* associated with finger- or tongue-like projections into the stroma. Invasive foci are usually isolated, but at times may be confluent. Until major advances are provided in the area of early diagnosis and treatment with predictable promise for cure, attention must be directed to the study of the natural history of the disease, its histologic patterns, cell type, nuclear grade, and stromal reactions.

V. DIAGNOSIS

Diagnosis of carcinoma of the cervix is based on cervico-vaginal cytology, colposcopy, colposcopic biopsy and histopathologic evaluation. The principal factor for the success of colposcopy in diagnosis of cervical neoplasia is the expertise of the examiner. One of the most important benefits of colposcopy is a significant decrease in the frequency of diagnostic conizations. The correlation between the result in colposcopic directed biopsy and in the definite surgery specimen demonstrate that only in 0.3% of cases, more significant changes are noted in operative specimens than in colposcopically directed biopsies. The results demonstrate that organized training programs in colposcopy and careful quality control can significantly increase the accuracy of cervical cancer detection and decrease its cost.

Cone biopsy, an essential diagnostic and therapeutic method in a cervical pathology may cause a few complications, which include heavy bleeding, perforation and infection (early-appearing complications) and stenosis or cervical incompetence (late-appearing complications). The most common complication is bleeding, the frequency of which may vary from 4–20% of cases. Post-cone bleeding occurs in most cases due to the softening of the suture employed, thus explaining its retarded occurrence.

Squamous carcinoma with invasion no greater than 5 mm from the surface rarely results in lymph node metastases and rarely, if ever, produces death from disease (Christopherson et al. 1976; Leman et al. 1976; Roche and Norris 1975). Others have allowed a depth of invasion of 5 mm but limited the lesion to those with less than 10 mm of lateral spread (Lohe 1978). The diagnosis of microinvasive carcinoma requires that the minimal tissue be a cone, since a biopsy adjacent to a large clinical carcinoma may only show superficial invasion. Microinvasive carcinoma is usually asymptomatic and the diagnosis results from cytologic screening. The technique of Feulgen microspectrophotometry was used to study pure adenocarcinomas and mixed carcinomas. The nuclear DNA findings are correlated with the clinicopathologic characteristics in an attempt to better define the morphogenesis and prognostic factors of these neoplasma. The technique is used to measure the stem cell modal values (Fu et al. 1980).

Differential diagnosis between cervical and endometrial adenocarcinoma is a common clinical problem. Fractional curettage, which is the most commonly used clinical method, gives inaccurate results in most cervical tumors (Korhonen 1978). Histologically, adenocarcinomas of the cervix are variable and may show any of the differentiation patterns of the Mullerian epithelium. In a few patients with cervical adenocarcinomas epithelial differentiation pattern is similar to that usually noted in endometrial adenocarcinomas and it is not possible to distinguish histologically between these two neoplasmas. However, there are differences between cervical and endometrial adenocarcinoma in the amount, localization and chemical composition of histochemically stainable mucin (Sorvari 1969). Histochemical demonstration of carcinoembryonic antigen (CEA) using immunoperoxidase technique may be a valuable technique for the distinction between cervical and endometrial adenocarcinoma.

The diagnosis of carcinoma of the cervix during pregnancy has presented several problems. The availability of cytologic screening coupled with the increased use of colposcopically guided cervical biopsy have made the diagnosis more frequently discovered during pregnancy (0.6 to 1.25%). Extensive conization is usually avoided completely during the first trimester and very seldom utilized later. Since the widespread utilization of colposcopy examination of abnormal cervical cytology smears, the need to perform diagnostic conizations had decreased over 90%. Pregnancy must not modify the approach to adequate diagnostic techniques.

Arteriography facilitates the individualization and topographic localization of tumoral relapses and a consequent selective surgical and radiotherapeutic treatment. The images are particularly significant and reliable in case of selective arteriography of the hypogastric artery, or of its collaterals. The diagnostic information supplied by phlebography does not appear relevant in comparison with the arteriographic and lymphographic technique.

VI. ANIMAL MODELS AND EXPERIMENTAL CARCINOGENESIS

The histogenesis of various types of squamous cell cancers of the cervix was studied in two model systems of the mouse and analogous lesions to the various histological grades of cervical cancer. When coal-tar hydrocarbon, i.e. benzopyrene, was applied to the mouse cervix, the animals developed frank invasive cancer of the cervix in 6–8 weeks. All lesions were of the keratinizing type of cancer. They were preceded by dysplasia and then microinvasive cancer prior to frank invasion. The animals which developed cancer had dysplasia earlier in the induction period.

Epidermal cell differentiation is a continuous process with increasing irreversibility and increasing loss of proliferative potency. Reversal of this differentiation is noted in animal models when epithelia were treated with specific substances known as promoters (Boutwell 1974). In the course of promoter use in tissue culture systems, inhibition of cellular differentiation with specific anatomic and biochemical alterations have been measured (Diamond et al. 1978; O'Brien 1976). Preinvasive cervical neoplasia can be considered an epithelial tissue under the influence of an unknown promoter substance whose effects result in dedifferentiation. A cell line designated SKG-1 was established from human uterine epidermoid cancer of a 40 year old female. The material obtained by radical hysterectomy, was finely minced, stirred slowly in a 0.25% trypsin solution for 30 min and centrifuged at 900 rpm for 10 min. The sediment, suspended in the culture medium (Ham's F-12 with 20% calf serum) was cultured into Petri dishes at 37° C in humidified 5% CO_2 and 95% air. Future research is needed to establish new animal models for experimental carcinogenesis in vitro and in vivo.

REFERENCES

Boutwell RK: Function and mechanism of promoters of carcinogenesis. CRC Crit Rev Toxicol 2: 419, 1974.

Chen SS, Koffler C, Cohen CJ: Cellular Hypersensitivity in Patients with Squamous Cell Carcinoma of the Cervix. Am J Obstet Gynecol 121: 91, 1975.

Chiang WT, Wei PY, Alexander ER: Circulatory and Cellular Immune Responses to Squamous Cell Carcinoma of the Uterine Cervix. Am J Obstet Gynec 126: 116, 1976.

Christopherson MM, Gray LA, Parker JE: Microinvasive carcinoma of the uterine cervix. Cancer 38: 629, 1976.

Courtney RJ, Benyesh-Melnick M: Isolation and characterization of a large molecular weight polypeptide of herpes simplex virus type I. Virology 62: 539, 1974.

Dahlberg B: A symptomatic vacteriospermia. Urology 8: 563, 1976.

Diamond L, O'Brien T, Rovena G: Tumor promoters inhibit terminal cell differentiation culture. In Slaga JJ, Sivak A, Boutwell RK (eds): Carcinogenesis, Vol. 2, Mechanisms of Tumor Promotion and Cocarcinogenesis. New York: Raven Press, 1978.

Disaia PF, Nallick RH, Townsend DE: Antibody Cytotoxicity Studies in Ovarian and Cervical Malignancies. Obst Gynecol 42: 644, 1973.

Dressman GR, Burek J, Adams E, Kaufman RH, Melnick JL, Posell KL, Purifoy DJM: Expression of Herpes-virus-induced Antigens in Human Cervical Cancer. Nature 283: 591, 1980.

Fu YS, Temmin L, Olaizola Y, Regan JW: Nuclear DNA characteristics of microinvasive squamous carcinoma of the uterine cervix. In Fenoglio CM, Wolff MW (eds): Process in Surgical Pathology, Vol. 1, 1980.

Hafez ESE, Smith JP: Carcinoma of the Cervix: Biology, Etiology & Diagnosis. Proc of Intern Sympos Kiawah Island, SC, U.S.A., September, 1980, p 65.

Halliday WJ, Miller S: Leukocyte adherence Inhibition: A simple test for Cell-Mediated Immunity and Serum Blocking Factors. International J Cancer 9: 477, 1972.

Halliday WJ, Malluish AE, Isbister WH: Detection of anti-Tumor Cell- Mediated Immunity and Serum Blocking Factors in Cancer Patients by the Leukocyte Adherence Inhibition Test. Br J Cancer 29: 31, 1974.

Glucksman A, Cherry CP: Incidence, histology and response to radiation of mixed carcinomas (adenoacanthomas) of the uterine cervix. Cancer 9: 941, 1956.

Korhonen MO: Adenocarcinoma of the Uterine Cervix. An evaluation of the available diagnostic methods. Acta Path Microbiol Scand Sect A Suppl 264: 1, 1978.

Leman MH Jr, Benson WL, Kurman RJ, Clark RC: Microinvasive carcinoma of the cervix. Obstet Gynecol 48: 571, 1976.

Litvak J: Latin American Cancer Research Information Project. Third International Symposium on Detection and Prevention of Cancer, New York, 1976.

Lohe KJ: Early squamous cell carcinoma of the uterine cervix: I. Definition and histology. Gynecol Oncol 6: 10, 1978.

O'Brien TG: The introduction of orithine decarboxylas as an early possible obligatory event in most skin carcinogenesis. Cancer Research 36: 7644, 1976.

Reagan JW, Ng ABP: The Cells of Uterine Adenocarcinoma, 2 nd ed. Baltimore: Williams & Wilkins, 1973.

Roche WD, Norris HJ: Microinvasive carcinoma of the cervix: The significance of lymphatic invasion and confluent patterns of stromal growth. Cancer 36: 180, 1975.

Sorvari TE:A histochemical Study of Epithelial Mucosubstances in Endometrial and Cervical Adenocarcinomas. Acta Path Microbiol Scand Suppl 207, 1969.

Table 1. Summary of some recent research on neoplasm, occurrence and mortality of carcinoma of the cervix.

Parameters	Concepts and investigations	Authors
NEOPLASM	Endometrial and tubal involvement by squamous carcinoma	Quizilbash et al. (1975)
	Vulvovaginal melanomas	Pantoja et al. (1976)
	Adenocarcinoma and pathological appraisal	Anderson et al. (1976)
	Uretric invasion by endometriosis	Way et al. (1976)
	Bony metastases from carcinoma. Occurrence diagnosis and treatment	Blythe et al. (1975)
	Cervical polyp, diagnostic and therapeutic approach with CO_2 hysteroscopy	David et al. (1978)
	Risk of cancer among an electrocoagulated population	Kauraniemi et al. (1978)
	Small cell cancer, pill seems safe for most women but those with dysplasia may have higher risk	van Nagell et al. (1978)
	Sociocultural factors associated with cancer in Nigeria	Emovon (1977)
	Microinvasive squamous carcinoma, definition, histologic analysis, late results of treatment	Seski et al. (1977)
	Microinvasive carcinoma	Fennell (1978)
	Blue nevus of cervix	Carinelli et al. (1978)
	Precancerous and cancerous lesions	Uyttenbroeck (1977)
	Cervical uterine and breast cancer with a favorable prognosis	Carsten (1977)
	Cervical adenocarcinoma and partial hydatidiform mole	Mazor et al. (1978)
	Cervical polyp, with CO_2 hysteroscopy	David et al. (1978)
	Risk among an electrocoagulated population	Kauraniemi et al. (1978)
	Verrucous carcinoma	Spratt et al. (1977)
	Small cell cancer	Van Nagell et al. (1977)
	Pill seems safe for most women but those with dysplasia may have higher risk	Van Nagell et al. (1978)
COMPLICATIONS	Secondary anaemia in malignancy haematologic changes after irradiation of cervical carcinoma	Einhorn et al. (1974)
	Pattern of incidence of primary tumours following cancer	Prior (1974)
	Urologic findings and complications	Marton et al. (1974)
	Response of hypertrophic pulmonary osteoarthropathy to radiotherapy	Steinfeld et al. (1974)
	Genital herpes in Black women with cervical carcinoma in Johannesburg	Freedman et al. (1974)
	Pelvic vascular bed isolation chemotherapy hemorrhage caused by advanced cancer	Hiroaka et al. (1977)
	Embolization of the hypogastric arteries	Smith et al. (1977)
CHEMICALLY INDUCED	Invasive squamous cell carcinoma in DES offspring	Lamb (1977)
	DES enigma	Baggish (1978)
	Squamous call neoplasia in female exposed to DES	Robboy et al. (1977)
	Transplacental carcinogenesis	Rice (1976)
	Effect of oral contraceptives	Moghissi (1977)
	Carcinoma and the pill	Collett et al. (1977)
	Squamous cel dysplasia and carcinoma *in situ* after prenatal exposure to DES	Robboy et al. (1978)
	Squamous cell carcinoma *in situ* after intrauterine DES exposure	Veridiano et al. (1978)
	Screening of DES exposed women	Edinger (1978)
	Effect of estradiol and prolactin incidence of 3-methylcholanthrene induced carcinomas in mice	Forsberg et al. (1976)
	Oral contraceptives carcinoma	Boyce et al. (1977)
	Age incidence and risk of diethylstilbestrol-related	Herbst et al. (1977)
	Examination of young women exposed to stilbestrol	Sandberg et al. (1977)
	Cancers and other abnormalities associated with exposure in utero to diethylstilbestrol	Adam et al. (1977)
	Questions and answers about DES	Adam et al. (1977)
	Cancers and other abnormalities associated with exposure in utero to diethylstilbestrol	Adam et al. (1977)
	Exposure in utero to diethylstilbestrol	Adam et al. (1977)
	Cancer risks from estrogen intake	Greenwald et al. (1977)
	Steroid contraceptive use and cervical dysplasia	Stern et al. (1977)
	Oral contraceptive steroid and IUD users and nonusers	Sandmire et al. (1976)
	Stilbestrol-adenosis-carcinoma syndrom, testosterone	Ulfelder (1976)

232

Table 1. Continued

Parameters	Concepts and investigations	Authors
	Diethylstilbestrol	Unfelder (1974)
	Ethinyloestradiol	Ulfelder (1974)
	Mestranol	Unfelder (1974)
	Oestrone	Unfelder (1974)
	Surface ultrastructural changes following 3,4 benzopyrene to mouse cervix	Williams et al. (1976)
	Exposure in utero to diethylstilbestrol and related synthetic hormones	Williams et al. (1976)
	Invasive squamous cell carcinoma	Lamb (1977)
	DES inigma	Baggish (1978)
	Squamous cell neoplasia controversy exposed to diethylstilbestrol	Robboy et al. (1977)
	Oral contraceptives, relations to mammary cancer benign breast lesions, andcervical cancer	Drill (1975)
	Cervical neoplasia after exposure to stilbestrol in utero	Jordon (1975)
OCCURRENCE	Continuing mass screening re-screening in Turku	Gronros et al. (1974)
	Cervical cytology declining morbidity and mortality	Cramer (1974)
	Incidence of endometrial cancer in the United States	Cramer et al. (1974)
	Geographic, endometrial cancer	Dunn (1974)
	Changing nature of endometrial cancer	Reagan (1974)
	Colposcopies Nicaraguan clinic	Guido et al. (1974)
	Cancer among Iowans	Bale (1975)
	Incident age distribution with clinical staging	Mould (1974)
	Increased incidence of adenocarcinoma	Davis et al. (1975)
	Gynecologic malignancies in immunosuppressed organ homograft recipients	Porreco et al. (1975)
	Retroperitoneal lymph-node metastases in untreated cancer, based on abdominopelvic exploration	Ucmakli et al. (1974)
	Incidence of cancer, South Africa	Te Groen et al. (1974)
	Incidence of cancer, Kingston, Jamaica	Persaud (1974)
	Changing epidemiology of premalignant lesions of the cervix	Fredricsson et l. (1977)
	Mass screening in Sweden	Kjellgren, (1977)
	Mass screening, incidence and mortality in Finland	Timonen et al. (1977)
	Carcinoma and dysplasia in Greenland	Nielsen et al. (1978)
	Cancer and duration of oral contraceptive use	Peritz et al. (1977)
	Pap testing and hysterectomy with high and low cervical cancer rates	Stern et al. (1977)
	Epidemiology of cancer of the cervix, vagina and vulva	Henson et al. (1977)
	Selective screening for cancerr Finnish mass screening system	Hakama et al. (1977)
	Adenocarcinoma, cervix in Jewish women	Menczer et al. (1978)
	Cytological monitoring of femal genital tract in women using Cu IUD	Luthra et al. (1977)
	Effect of Lippes loop and copper IUDs	Misra et al. (1977)
	Mass screening in Iceland and mortality carcinoma	Johannesson et al. (1978)
	Premalignant and malignant lesions	Bhaskaran et al. (1978)
	Carcinoma in Ibadan; coital characteristics	Adelusi (1977)
	Cervical cancer by marital status	Leck et al. (1978)
	Cancer morbidity in depressive persons	Niemi et al. (1978)
	Cervical neoplasia and the pill	Niemi et l. (1977)
	Cancer detection in working women	Raphael (1977)
	Cytological screening University Teaching Hospital	O'Dowd et al. (1977)
	Age patterns of Tswana omen, South Africa	Fragoyannis et al. (1977)
	Age patterns of Tswana women	Leiman (1978)
	Geographical pathology	Leiman (1977)
	Colpocytologic mass screening comparison by age groups	Canevini et al. (1977)
	Cytologic screening	Behmard et al. (1977)
	Cancer in women belonging to a cytologically screened population	Rylander (1976)
	British Columbia screening program	Boyes et al. (1977)
	Cervical cancer screening	Rochat (1976)
	Age at registration and age at death	West (1977)
	Microinvasive squamous carcinoma	Duncan et al. (1977)

234

Table 1. Continued

Parameters	Concepts and investigations	Authors
	Natural duration	Dolhay et al. (1976)
	Mortality in Canada relationship to screening for cancer of cervix	Miller et al. (1976)
	Survival in stage I and stage II	Welander et al. (1975)
	Mortality in relation to mass screening	Christopherson et al. (1977)
	Mortality can be prevented	Kessler (1976)
	Can deaths be reduced	Steiner (1976)
	Expectation of life in cancer survival with incomplete follow-up information	Hakama et al. (1977)
	Mortality from carcinoma	Miller (1978)
	Mortality from carcinoma	Yule (1978)
	Papanicolaou testing and hysterectomy prevalence in low-income communities, Los Angeles	Stern et al. (1977)
	Expectation of life in cancer survival with incomplete follow-up information	Hakama et al. (1977)
	Mortality from carcinoma	Miller (1978)
	Mortality from carcinoma	Yule (1978)
	Papanicolaou testing and hysterectomy prevalence in low-income communities in Los Angeles	Stern et al. (1977)

Table 2. Summary of some recent research on cytology ultrastructure, immunology, metabolism, enzymology and blood supply of carcinoma.

Parameters	Concepts and investigations	Authors
CYTOLOGY	Binoucleate cell; implications for automated cytopathology	Cambier et al. (1975)
	Electronic cell volume (Coulter volume) distribution of vaginal cervical cytology samples	Cassidy et al.
	Preparing cell suspensions from cervical smears with pepsine and ultrasonic treatment	Freni et al. (1975)
	Cytophohoria in cervical cytology	Muller et al. (1975)
	Endocervical smears to and cervical cancer detection	Shingleton et al. (1975)
	Evaluation of automatic nucleus finding routines thresholding of cervical cytology images	Taylor et al. (1975)
	Prenatal sex detection with endocervical smears: utilizing Y-bodyfluorescence	Rhine et al. (1975)
	Method for the collection and examination of the exfoliative cytology	Freund (1977)
	Cytological using copper intrauterine devices	Misra et al. (1977)
	False-negative smear; an instrumental error	Rubio (1977)
	Use of impulse cytophotometry in automated cervix cytology	Weiss et al. (1978)
	Cervical cytology screening	Sargeant et al. (1977)
	Cervical cytology clinic	Jenner (1978)
	Epithelial repair and regeneration, analysis of cells	Geirsson et al. (1977)
	Rapid-flow cytofluoremetry of exfoliated cells suspensions from mice	Silverman et al. (1977)
	Routine use of flow-through photometric prescreening in detection	Sprenger et al. (1977)
	A multi-spectral approach for scene analysis cytology smears	Aggarwal et al. (1977)
ULTRA-STRUCTURE	Scanning electron microscopy findings on the cervix uteri	Wagner et al. (1974)
	In situ and microinvasive adenocarcinoma	Williams et al. (1974)
	Surface ultrastructure of exfoliated cervical cells	Williams et al. (1974)
	Scanning electron microscopy of normal and abnormal exfoliated cervical squamous cells	Murphy et al. (1975)
	Koilocytosis in dysplastic and reactive cervical squamous epithelium	Okagaki et al. (1978)
	Morphometry heterochromatin distribution in cell nucleus in dysplasia carcinoma *in situ*	Bahnsen et al. (1977)
	Orthologic and pathologic surface structures of portio uteri	Hiersche et al. (1977)
	Ultrastructure of the epithelial borders in cervix	Pape et al. (1977)
	Statistical evaluation of frequency distribution quantitative morphology	Wagner et al. (1977)
	Flow-microfluorometric analysis of nuclei from various normal and malignant human epithelial tissues	Koss et al. (1977)
	Mucoepidermoid carcinoma	Dinges et al. (1977)
	Squamous cell carcinoma of Linac irradiation appearance of lysosome and radiosensitivity	Ihara et al. (1977)
ENZYMOLOGY	Glycolytic enzyme activity	Pederson (1975)
	Cytochemical acid phosphatase	Malvi et al. (1974)
	Enzymes of glucose metabolism	Marshall et al. (1978)
	Cytoenzymology on normal and pathological epithelium	Rimbolt (1977)
	Cytochemical of respiratory enzymes after irradiation	El-Fiky et al. (1977)
	Decreased amniotic fluid peroxidase in pregnant patients	DiMmitt (1976)
IMMUNOLOGY	Antibodies to herpesvirus hominis type 1 and 2 among women with neoplastic change	Peltonen (1975)
	Circulatory and cellular immune responses to squamous cell carcinma	Chiang et al. (1976)
	Carcinoembryonic antigen in intraepithelial neoplasia	van Nagell et al.
	Isoantigen loss in cervical neoplasia immunofluorescence and immunoperoxidase techniques	Bonfiglio et al. (1976)
	Antibodies to herpes simplex virus types 1 and 2; using indirect haemagglutination	Freymuth et al. (1975)
	Cell mediated response to herpes simplex virion and non-virion antigens with a depressed response to phytohemagglutinin	Sprecher et al. (1975)
	Cellular immunity to human basic myelin protein dysplasia and carcinoma *in situ*	Singer et al. (1975)

Table 2. Continued

Parameters	Concepts and investigations	Authors
	Radiation-induced immune changes	Yamagata et al. (1976)
	Herpesvirus type 2-related antigens and relevance to humoral and cell-mediated immunity	Aurelian et al. (1976)
	In vivo and *in vitro* measurements relationship of human squamous carcinomas to herpes simplex virus tumor-associated antigens	Hollinshead et al. (1976)
	Antibody to a virus-induced tumor-associated antigen (AG-4) in Japanese sera	Kawana et al. (1976)
	Herpes simplex virus-specific antigens in exfoliated cervical cells with and without cervical anaplasia	Pacsa et al. (1976)
	Antigens of carcinoma by immunofluorescence	Nelson (1974)
	Adenie arabinoside (ARA-A) blocked HSV-2 infected human skin fibroblasts for detection of serum mediated and cellular cytotoxicity	Paulileinikki et al. (1976)
	Depression of lymphocyte reactivity and influence of serum factors, phytohemagglutinin and mixed lymphocyte response	Balakrishman et al. (1975).
	Herpes simplex antibodies, antibodies to surface antigen of herpes simplex virus	Chirstenson et al. (1976)
	IgM antibody to tumor-associated antigen (AG-4) induced by herpes simplex virus type 2	Aurelian et al. (1976)
	Antibodies to herpes simplex virus in Jewish women	Menczer et al. (1975)
	Herpesvirus antibodies and antigens	Pacsa et al. (1975)
	Rosette-forming lymphocytes *in situ* carcinoma	Ashman et al. (1975)
	Clinical follow-up and cell-mediated cytotoxicity against Hela cells with invasive or preinvasive cancer	Saksela et al. (1976)
	Herpes type-2 virus antigens	Adelusi et al. (1976)
	Common antigens of herpes simplex virus 2 associated hamster tumors and human cancer	Ibrahim et al. (1976)
METABOLISM	Protein synthesis with ribosomes non-analogous aminoacyl tRNA	Dube et al. (1974)
	Prolactin-stimulating effect on 3H-thymidine incorporation in 3-methylcholanthrene-induced carcinomas in normal and estrogenized mice	Forsberg et al. (1974)
	In vitro effects sex hormones upon deoxyribonucleic acid synthesis in carcinoma	Hughes et al. (1975)
	Steroids and growth human cell line stemming from carcinoma	Wibe et al. (1976)
BLOOD	Carcinoembryonic antigen in cervical and vulvar cancer, serum levels and disease progress	DiSaia et al. (1976)
	Cell numbers and activities of lymphocyte subpopulations	Ueda et al. (1975)
	Isoantigen ABH in cervical intraepithelial neoplasia	Lill et al. (1976)
	Free serum amino acids with advanced carcinoma	Wilson et al. (1976)
	Plasma alpha-1 antitrypsin in early and late carcinoma	Latner et al. (1976)
	Secondary anemia in malignancy. Folic acid	Einhorn et al. (1971)
BLOOD	Angiogenesis of cervical neoplasia	Stafl et al. (1975)
SUPPLY	Oxygen supply of uterine cervix cancer and radiation response with reference to menstrual history	Siracka et al. (1974)
	Tissue circulation in cervix and prognosis of newborn infant	Colette et al. (1977)

Table 3. Summary of some recent research on etiology, microbiology, and immunology of carcinoma of the cervix.

Parameters	Concepts and investigations	Authors
ETIOLOGY	Promiscuity and pill: etiologic agents	Leppaluoto (1977)
	Simultaneous *in situ* carcinoma after immuno-suppressive therapy for transplantation	Leckie et al. (1977)
	Causes, new ideas	Singer et al. (1977)
	Herpes simplex virus and carcinoma	Thiry (1976)
	Association of herpes simplex virus	Simon (1976)
	Genital herpes	Roizman et al. (1976)
	Dye-light treatment of herpetic lesions	Gudson et al. (1974)
	Mycoplasma species in dysplasia clinic population	Lyons et al. (?)
	Herpes genitalis	Kaufman (1974)
	Causative role of herpesvirus type 2	Melnick et al. (1974)
	Preinvasive lesions to invasion	Green (1974)
	Carcinogenesis with herpes simplex virus type	Sentz et al. (1975)
	Herpes hom. (simplex) type 2 virus infection	Joncas (1974)
	Epidemiology and etiology including the detection of carcinogenic N-nitrosamines in the human vaginal vault	Harington (1975)
	Role of a high-risk male in, a correlation epidemiology and molecular biology	Singer et al. (1976)
	Herpesvirus and cancer	Oates (1976)
	Herpes simplex virus	Melnick et al. (1976)
	Model systems cancer	Munoz (1976)
	Immunology of herpes simplex virus infection	Nahmias et al. (1976)
	Herpes simplex virus type 2 in Cebus monkeys	Palmer et al. (1976)
	Serological and epidemiological of herpes simplex virus type 2	Rawls et al. (1976)
	Psychological factors etiology and treatment	Labrun (1976)
	Epidemiological survey	Deeley (1976)
	Surveillance for carcinogenesis in women using Cu IUD	Luthra et al. (1976)
	Cancer and early sexual intercourse	Peto (1976)
	Sexually transmitted cancers	Aurelian (1976)
	Herpes simplex virus 2	Ravich (1975)
	Pelvic exenterationa	Singh et al. (1976)
	Herpes simplex virus type	Rotkin (1976)
	Age at first coitus and choice of contraceptive related to neoplasia	Merritt et al. (1975)
	Cytological studies in women using copper intrauterine devices	Misra et al. (1977)
	Smoking and cancer; hypothesis	Schoenberg (1978)
	Smoking and cancer; hypothesis	Winkelstein (1977)
	Cancer a sexually transmitted disease cytologic screening in a prostitute population	Sebastian et al. (1978)
	Cervical infections and cervical carcinoma	Astedt et al. (1978)
	Dysplasias; epidemiological aspects age at first coitus and use of oral contraceptives	Meisels et al. (1977)
	Herpes simplex viruses to human malignancies	Rawls et al. (1977)
	Papillomaviruses squamous cell carcinomas	Hausen (1977)
	Statistical model natural history cervical neoplastic disease	Barron et al. (1978)
	Penile carcinoma combined with cervical biopsy	Reddy et al. (1977)
	Cytomegalovirus (CMV) cervical cancer; isolation of CMV from cell cultures derived from cervical biopsy	Melnick et al. (1978)
	Epidemiologic and endocrinologic aspects	Kodama et al. (1978)
	Sperm basic proteins in cervical carcinogenesis	Cameron et al. (1978)
	Sperm basic proteins in cervical carcinogenesis: socioeconomic class	Reid et al. (1978)
	Sperm basic proteins in cervical carcinogenesis	Sandler (1978)
	Epidemiological approaches herpesvirus cervical cancer	Melnick et al. (1978)
	Genital herpes-cervical cancer	Nahmias et al. (1978)
	Cytological and quantitative cytochemical post-radiation dysplasia	Olkowski et al. (1978)
MICROBIOLOGY	Biology and immunologic comparison HSV-2 isolate from cervical tumor cells	Aurelian et al. (1974)
	Herpesvirus hominis: from latency to carcinogenesis	Aurelian (1973)
	Antibodies to herpesvirus vype 2	Adelusi et al. (1975)

Table 3. Continued

Parameters	Concepts and investigations	Authors
	Herpesvirus antigens and cell-mediated immunity	Aurelian et al. (1975)
	Latent herpes cervicitis and mixed cervical carcinoma	Lauchlan (1978)
	Herpesvirus hominis type II to carcinoma, an animal model for induction of long-term latency of herpesvirus	Tobin et al. (1978)
IMMUNOLOGY	Premalignant and malignant uterine changes in immunosuppressed renal transplant recipients	Husslein et al. (1978)
	Measurement of of antibodies to herpesvirus types 1 and 2 in human sera by microradioimmunoassay	Jankowski et al. (1977)
	Sero-epidemiology of herpes type- 2 virus	Adelusi et al. (1977)
	Cellular immunity in squamous cell carcinoma	Levy et al. (1978)
	Stages of development of immunologic response in the reginal lymph nodes in invasive cancer	Koslowski et al. (1977)
	Exfoliative immunocytology	Efthymiou et al. (1977)
	Radioimmunoassay for tumor antigen of squamous cell carcinoma	Kato et al. (1977)
	Identifcation of beta-oncofetal antigen in neoplastic and normal tissues	Goldenberg et al. (1978)
	Rosette formation and inhibition in dysplasia and carcinoma *in situ*	Sawanobori et al. (1977)
	T and B lymphocyte subpopulations in pre-invasive and invasive carcinoma	Rand et al. (1977)
	Antibodies to herpesvirus type 1 and 1 among Japanese	Ozaki et al. (1978)
	Immunofluorescence characteristics of basement membrane in squamous carcinoma	Rubio et al. (1978)
	Complement-dependent cytotoxic antibodies	Christenson (1977)
	Herpes simplex virus type 2	Vardthananusara et al. (1978)
	Blocking plasma factors of migration inhibition factor	Favila et al. (1978)
	Antibodies to herpes simplex virus type 2 in husbands of patients with cervical carcinoma	Kunkel et al. (1978)
	Serum carcinoembryonic antigens	Ito et al. (1978)
	Carcinoembryonic antigen levels squamous cell carcinoma	Kjorstad et al. (1978)

Table 4. Summary of some recent research on diagnosis, analysis, classification and radiography of carcinoma of the cervix.

Parameters	Techniques and concepts	Authors
DIAGNOSIS	Endocervical smears & cancer detection	Shingleton et al. (1975)
	Screening	Milligan et al. (1975)
	Colposcopic evaluation of the abnormal, Papanicolaou test in pregnancy	DePetrillo et al. (1975)
	Adenoid cystic carcinoma presenting as a primary bronchial neoplasm	Ryden et al. (1974)
	Papancolaou smear	Shulman et al. (1974)
	Pap smear: take two	Shulman et al. (1975)
	Mathematical evaluation of flow-through cytophotometric data cervical cytology	Sprenger et al. (1974)
	Detection, diagnostic evaluation and treatment of dysplasis	Nelson et al. (1975)
	Control of cancer by cytologic screening	Dickinson (1975)
	Critical evaluation of cervical cytology	Aikat et al. (1974)
	Diagnosis and management of neoplasia	Kuptsow (1975)
	Cervical cytology in family planning	Shahanl (1974)
	Observer variation and quality control of cytodiagnosis	Evans et al. (1974)
	Quality control in cervical cytology	Husain et al. (1974)
	Evaluation of abnormal Papanicolaou smear	Roy et al. (1974)
	Mass cytological screening early detection	Devi et al. (1974)
	Office detection neoplasia	Buchsbaum et al. (1974)
	Malignant plasma cells in cervical smear	Figueroa et al. (1978)
	Screening, cervical disorders in previously screened women	Gad et al. (1977)
	Cytologic sampling techniques	Garite et al. (1978)
	Sample preparation for automated cervical cancer screening	Husain et al. (1978)
	Accuracy and consistency of the cytologic classification of squamous lesions	Kern et al. (1977)
	Solitary reticulum cell sarcoma with initial cytodiagnosis	Krumerman et al. (1978)
	Dimensionality reducing displays in cell image analysis	Sychra et al. (1977)
	Computer recognition of abnormal ectocervical cells countour and textural	Sychra et al. (1977)
	Study of automatic cytoscreening for uterine cancer. Data, improvement of CYBEST	Tanaka et al. (1977)
	Computer recognition of ectocervical cells classification accuracy and spatial resolution	Wied et al. (1977)
	Cytologic diagnosis of clear cell adenocarcinoma	Young et al. (1978)
	Diagnostic and therapeutic aspects	Ruponen (1977)
	Adenocarcinoma evaluation of available diagnostic methods	Korhonen (1977)
	Staging laparotomy and survival	Kademian et al. (1977)
	Vaginal pool smears	Loeb (1977)
	Conventional diagnostic tests for detection of recurrent carcinoma	Photopulos et a. (1977)
	Verrucous carcinoma diagnosis and management	Rorat et al. (1978)
	Clinical management of carcinoma *in situ* and microinvasive carcinoma	di Re et al. (1977)
	Pulse cytophotometric measurements on tumor cell suspensions and exfoliative material	Krug (1978)
	Image analysing for automated cytologic prescreening	Kunze et al. (1978)
	Colposcopic evaluation abnormal cervical smears	Benedet et al. (1977)
	Intraepithelial neoplasia teenager	Feldman et al. (1978)
	Evaluation and management	Nordqvist (1978)
	Colposcopy in management of cervical neoplasia	Herbeck et al. (1977)
	Colposcopy in the evaluation of abnormal vaginal vault smears	Benedet et al. (1977)
	Cervical cytology clinic	Jenner (1978)
	Qualitative DNCB skin test	Dutta et al. (1977)
	Diagnosis and management of pre and early cancers	Saraiya et al. (1978)
	Trends in cervical cytology	Heyerdahl-o'Dowd (1978)
	Office diagnosis and management of cervical dysplasia	Crapanzano (1978)
	Preparation of cervix and corpus carcinoma patients records for computer evaluation	Nemeth et al. (1978)
	Colposcopy in detection and management of patients with cervical intraepithelial neoplasia	Deppe et al. (1978)

Table 4. Continued

Parameters	Techniques and concepts	Authors
	Cytologic screening with nomgynecologic hospital admissions	DuToit et al. (1978)
	Colposcopy of cervical intraepithelial neoplasia	Kohan et al. (1977)
	Colposcopy and selective biopsy with abnormal cervical cytology	Knutzen et al. (1977)
	Management of noninvasive carcinoma	Frick (1978)
	Cytology, colposcopy, target biopsy and conization to the early diagnosis of precancerous and cancerous lesions	Cecchini et al. (1978)
	Numerical composition of cellular samples carcinoma *in situ*	Bibbo et al. (1975)
	Non-visual prescreening with flow-through cytophotometer	Freni (1975)
	Who is responsible for the false-negative smear?	Rubio et al. (1975)
	Induction of bleeding as clinical test for carcinoma	Kishi et al. (1975)
	Lymphography in carcinoma	Fuchs et al. (1975)
	Combining colposcopy and cytology prevention of cancer	Kanka et al. (1974)
	Scalene node biopsy in pretreatment staging	Perez-Mesa et al. (1976)
	Evaluation of Schiller test before conization	Rubio et al. (1976)
	Diagnostic and therapeutic efficacy of conization	van Nagell et al. (1976)
	Random sample size in flow-through photometric prescreening	Sprenger et al. (1976)
	Automation in cancer screening flow systems and other techniques	Husain et al. (1976)
	Colposcopic evaluation with abnormal cytology	Benedet et al. (1976)
	Diagnosis and management of microinvasive (stage IA)	Averette et al. (1976)
	In vivo and *in vitro* markers intraepithelial	Wilbanks (1976)
	Cone biopsy	Tobell (1976)
	Evaluation for automated cancer cell indentification	Imasato et al. (1975)
	Diagnosis of cervical neoplasia by nonspecialized colposcopist	Delgado et al. (1975)
	Cytology, colposcopy and directed biopsy limitations	Dolan et al. (1975)
	Personal screening method	Rounds et al. (1976)
	Scanning electron microscopy in cervical cytology	Allen et al. (1976)
	Cervical Pap smears diagnosis of cervical	Steinkamp et al. (1975)
	Cytology automation program of National Cancer Institute	Herman et al. (1976)
	Colposcopic evaluation lower genital tract	Swan (1976)
	Making of a colposcopist	Feldman et al. (1976)
	Coloscopy clinic	Krumhotz et al. (1976)
	Colposcopy in the detection and management	Odell (1976)
	Colposcopically directed biopsy and conization with histologic diagnosis	Savage (1975)
	Colposcopy screening in a family planning program	Toress (1976)
	Colposcopic evaluation	Trombetta (1976)
	Long-term follow-up of carcinoma *in situ*	Kolstad et al. (1976)
	Malignant melanoma	Puri et al. (1976)
	Papanicolaou smears	Sandmire et al. (1976)
	Colposcopic evaluation abnormal cytologic smears during pregnancy	Talebian et al. (1976)
	III in-bleomycin	Woolfenden et al. (1975)
	Early detection of cancer	Brown (1976)
	Scalene lymph node biopsy	Buchsbaum et at. (1976)
	Carcinoma *in situ* in pregnancy	Gilotra et al. (1976)
	Colposcopy directed biopsies and cold	Havadhanakul et al. (1976)
	Gastric cancer producing retrograde lymphaic drainage	Franco et al. (1977)
	Complementary cytology and colposcopy in detection program	Fritsches et al. (1977)
	Cytologic diagnosis of adenocarcinoma	Krumins et al. (1977)
	Cytophotometric premalignant and malignant cells cervix automated cytology	Nishiya et al. (1977)
	Flow-through photometric prescreening in detection	Sprenger et al. (1977)
	Cytology in the detection of malignant lymphoma	Whitaker (1976)
	Reinvestigation of crucial case where first diagnosis by mailing smear test disagrees with second diagnosis by cytology and/or biopsy	Noda et al. (1976)
	Negative smears in women developing invasive cancer	Rylander (1977)
	Evaluation of abnormal Pap smear	Homesley (1977)
	Procidentia uteri and its mythical protection against cancer	Pantoja et al. (1976)
	Cytological evidence long preclinical evolution	Boddington et al. (1976)

	Randomized comparative trail Ayre and the Armovical cervical spatulae	Bounds et al. (1976)
	Screening programs	Penner (1976)
	Screening programs: the SOGCs	Schmidt (1977)
	Immunodiagnostic potential of a virus-coded tumor-associated antigen (AG-4)	Aurelian et al. (1978)
	Discrepancy in clinical staging	Gad (1977)
	Histochemical diagnosis of precancerous states	Yakovleva et al. (1976)
	Colposcopy and the management of intraepithelial neoplasia	Kohan et al. (1977)
	Cytology and colposcopy	Pang et al. (1977)
	Fluorescent and Papanicolaou technique	Singh et al. (1976)
	Diagnostic aspects of herpes simples virus tumor-associated antigens	Notter et al. (1976)
	Cytology: routine screening in sexually active adolescent	Hein et al. (1977)
	Colposcopic evaluation intraepithelial neoplasia	Cruikshank et al. (1976)
	Genitourinary tuberculosis simulating carcinoma	Shobin et al. (1976)
	Colposcopy in the evaluation of abnormal Papanicolaou smears	Akerele (1977)
	Granuloma inguinale simulating advanced pelvic cancer	Jofre et al. (1976)
	Diagnosis and treatment of microinvasive carcinoma	Burghardt et al. (1977)
	Significance of age in the colposcopic evaluation with a typical Papanicolaou smear	Shingleton et al. (1977)
	Colposcopic evaluation of abnormal cervical cytology	Talebian et al. (1977)
	Colposcopy in management of neoplasia of cervix	Selim et al. (1977)
	Surgical therapy by cost-benefi analysis	Barnes et al. (1977)
	Mass screening in Ljubljana	Kovacic (1976)
	Metastatic carcinoma presenting as primary thyroid cancer	Martino et al. (1977)
ANALYSIS	Characterization and localization of carcinembryonic antigen in a squamous cell carcinoma	Goldberg et al. (1976)
	Virus genomes in cells by molecular hybridization	Hausen et al. (1975)
	Basic amino acids in cell nucleus	Herzog (1975)
	Content of Schick-positive cells of cervix	Petrova et al. (1976)
	Quantification of protein thiols	Bajardi et al. (1977)
	Quantitative determination of protein thiols	Bajardi et al. (1977)
	Glycosaminoglycan content during pregnancy and labor	on Maillot et al. (1977)
	Quanitification of protein thiols	Bajardi et al. (1977)
	Microspectrophotometric research of content ascorbic acid in carcinoma	Avtandilov et al. (1977)
	Fatty acid composition of lipids from subcellular fractions human malignant cervical and mouse fibrosarcoma	Banerjee et al. (1976)
	Lipid composition of subcellular fractions	Bhattacharyya et al. (1976)
	Cytochemical properties of cells as revealed by study of deoxyribonucle protein susceptibility to Feulgen hydrolysis	Zelenin et al. (1977)
	Quantification of protein thiols	Bajardi et al. (1977)
	Microspectrophotometric content ascorbic acid	Avtandilov et al. (1977)
RADIOGRAPHY	Projection difference index in lymphographic diagnosis of lymph node metastases	Kolbenstvedt (1975)
	Pretreatment lymphangiography	Leman et al. (1975)
	Arteriographic assessment and staging	Lang (1976)
	Lymphangiographic detection of scale node metastases from cervical carcinoma	Steinfeld et al. (1978)
	Intravenous pyelographic	Vengadasalam et al. (1978)
	Pelvic arteriography in assesing carcinoma	Stage et al. (1978)
	Prognostic lymphography in cervical cancer	Volterrani et al. (1978)
RADIONUCLIDE IMAGING	Psoas bed gallium uptake post irradiation abscess or metastasis	Smith et al. (1978)
	Thallium scintigraphy – radionuclide imaging of the uterus	Pertynski et al. (1977)
CLASSIFICATION	Stage I cancer and pelvic node metastasis replaced FIGO classifications on stage Ia	Boronow (1977)

242

REFERENCES

Adams E et al.: Vaginal and cervical cancers and other abnormalities associated with exposure in utero to diethylstilbestrol and related synthetic hormones. Cancer Res 37(4): 1249–51, 1977.

Adams E et al.: Questions and answers about DES exposure before birth. Information about cancers and other abnormalities. J Arkansas Med Soc 73(8): 313–5, 1977.

Adams E et al.: Vaginal and cervical cancers and other abnormalities associated with exposure in utero to diethylstilbestrol and related synthetic hormones. J Med Assoc State Ala 46(9): 39–41, 1977.

Adams E et al.: Vaginal and cervical cancers associated with exposure in utero to diethyl. J Med Soc 74(1): 68–70, 1977.

Adams E et al.: Vaginal and cervical cancers associated with exposure in utero to diethylstilbestrol. J Tenn Med Assoc 79(5): 340–1, 1977.

Adelusi B et al.: Antibodies to herpesvirus type 2 in carcinoma of the cervix uteri in Ibadan, Nigeria. Am J Obstet Gynecol 123(7): 758–61, 1975.

Adelusi B et al.: Herpes type 2 antigens in human cervical carcinoma. Obstet Gynecol 47(5): 545, 1976.

Adelusi B et al.: Sero-epidemiology of herpes type 2 virus and carcinoma of the cervix in Ibadan. Afr J Med Sci 95–102, 1977.

Adelusi B: Carcinoma of the cervix uteri in Ibadan; coital characteristics. Int J Gynaecol Obstet 5–11, 1977.

Adelusi B.: Haemoglobin genotype, ABO blood groups and carcinoma of the cervix. J Trop Med Hyg 152–4 1977.

Aggarwal RK, et al.: A multi-spectral approach for scene analysis of cervical cytology smears. J Histochem Cytochem 25 (7);668–80, 1977.

Aikat M et al.: Critical evaluation of cervical cytology. Indian J Med Res 62 (5): 655–61, 1974.

Akerele FA: The use of colposcopy in the evaluation of abnormal Papanicolaou smears in a large group practice. MD State Med J 36 (6): 55–7, 1977.

Allen JM et al.: The use of scanning electron microscopy in cervical cytology; results from the examination of 218 patients. In Johari O Becker RP (ed): Scanning electron microscopy, 1976.

Anderson MC et al.: Adenocarcinoma of the uterine cervix a clinical and pathological appraisal. Br J Obstet Gynaecol 83 (4): 320–5, 1976.

Ashman R et al.: Letter: Rosette-forming lymphocytes in cervical in situ carcinoma. Lancet 2 (7946): 1212, 1975.

Astedt B et al.: Cervical infections and cervical carcinoma (letter) Br Med J 2 (6131): 201–2, 1978.

Atkin NB et al.: Chromosome 1 in cervical carcinoma. Lancet 984, 1977.

Aurelian L et al.: Biologic and immunologic comparison of two HSV -2 variants; one an isolate from cervical tumor cells. Arch Gesamte Virusforsch 45 (1–2): 27–38, 1974.

Aurelian L et al.: Herpesvirus antigens and cell-mediated immunity in cervical cancer. In Crowell RD et al. (eds): Tumor virus infections and immunity. Baltimore: Univ Park Press, 1975.

Aurelian L et al.: IgM antibody to a tumor-associated antigen (AG-4) induced by herpes simplex virus type 2: its use in location of the antigen in infected cells. J Natl Cancer Inst 56 (3): 471–7, 1976.

Aurelian L et al.: Herpevirus type 2 related antigens and their relevance to humoral and cell – mediated immunity in patients with cervical cancer. Cancer Res 36 (2pt 2): 810–20, 1976.

Aurelian L et al.: Immunodiagnostic potential of a virus-coded tumor-associated antigen (AG-4) in cervical cancer. Cancer 39 (4 Suppl) 1834–49, 1978.

Aurelian L: Herpesvirus hominis; from latency to carcinogenesis? Johns Hopkins med J Suppl 2 0): 245–68, 1973.

Aurelian L: Sexually transmitted cancers. The case for genital herpes. J Am Vener Dis Assoc 2 (3): 10–20, 1976.

Averette HE et al.: Diagnosis of management of microinvasive (stage IA) carcinoma of the uterine cervix. Cancer 38 (1 suppl) 414–25, 1976.

Avtandilov GG et al.: The microspectrophotometric research of content ascorbic acid in carcinomas of the uterine cervix. Acta Histochem (Jena) 59 (2): 254–7, 1977.

Baggish MS, Editorial: The DES insigma, present precis. Conn Med 42 (6): 395–9, 1978.

Bahnsen J et al.: Morphometry studies of heterochromatin distribution in the cell nucleus in dysplasia and in carcinoma in situ (proceedings). Ach Gynaecol 524–5, 1977.

Bajardi F et al.: Quantification of protein thiols in normal and pathological cells of the epithelium of the protio uteri. Acta Cytol (Baltimore) 21 (4): 573–7, 1977.

Bajardi F et al.: Quantitative determination of protein thiols in normal dysplastic and atypical cervical cells (proceedings). Arch Gynaekol 224 (1–4): 525–6, 1977.

Balakrishman K et al.: Depression of lymphocyte reactivity and influence of serum factors from patients with cervical carcinoma on phytohemagglutinin and mixed lymphocyte response. 319–24 In Talwar GP (ed): Regulation of growth and differentiated function in eukaryote cells. New York: Raven Press, 1975.

Bale GS: Cervical cancer among Iowans. J Iowa Med Soc 65 (2): 53–56, 1975.

Banerjee M et al.: Fatty acid composition of lipids from subcellular fractions of human malignant cervical and mouse fibroasarcoma tissues. Indian J Cancer 13 (4): 355–60, 1976.

Barnes BA et al.: Evaluation of surgical therapy by cost-benefit analysis. Surgery 82 (1): 21–33, 1977.

Barron BA et al.: A statistical model of the natural history of cervical neoplastic disease; the duration of carcinoma in situ. Gynecol Oncl 6: 196–205, 1978.

Behmard S et al.: Cytologic screening for cervical cancer in southern Iran. Acta Cytol (Baltimore) 432–4, 1977.

Bender S: Carcinoma in-situ of cervix in sisters. Br Med J 1 (6008): 502, 1976.

Benedet JL et al.: Colposcopic evaluation of patients with abnormal cervical cytology. Br J Obstet Gynaecol 83 (3): 177–82, 1976.

Benedet JL et al.: The role of colposcopy in the evaluation of abnormal vaginal vault smears. Gynecol Oncol 5 (4): 338–45, 1977.

Benedet JL et al.: Colposcopic evaluation of pregnant patients with abnormal cervical smears. Br J Obstet Gynaecol 84 (7): 517–21, 1977.

Berget A et al.: Sensitivity of specificity of screening by cervico vaginal cytology. Dan Med Bull 26–9, 1977.

Berget A: Epidemiologic characteristics in patients with epithelial dysplasia, carcinoma in situ, and invasive carcinoma of the uterine cervix. The population screening for cervical carcinoma in Maribo Amt (county) 1967–1969. Dan Med Bull 252–9, 1975.

Bhaskaran C et al.: Premalignant and malignant lesions of cervix. Syamala Indian J Med Res 97–105, 1978.

Bhattacharyya M et al.: Studies in lipid composition of various subcellular fractions obtained from human normal and malignant cervix uteri. Indian J Cancer 51–6, 1976.

Bibbo M et al.: The numerical composition of cellular samples from the female reproductive Tract I. Carcinoma *in situ*. Acta Cytol (Baltimore) 19 (5): 438–47, 1975.

Bigelow JH et al.: The false-negative rate in screening for cervical cancer. In Proceedings of the IIASA Who Workshop on Screening for Cervical Cancer. Laxenburg, International Institute for Applied Systems Analysis, 1975.

Bigelow JH: Cervical screening research plan. Design of IIASAs proposed cervical screening study. pp 79–85. In proceedings of the Joint IIASA Who Workshop on screening for cervical cancer. Laxenburg, International Institute for Applied Systems Analysis, 1975.

Blythe JG et al.: Bony metastases from carcinoma of cervix. Occurrence diagnosis and treatment. 475–84, 1975.

Boddington MM et al.: Adenocarcinoma of the uterine cervix.; Cytological evidence of a long preclinical evolution. Br J Obstet Gynaecol 83 (11): 900–3, 1976.

Bonfiglio TA et al.: Isoantigen loss in cervical neoplasia. Demonstration by immunofluorescence and immunoperoxidase techniques. Arch Pathol Lab Med 100 (6): 307–14, 1976.

Boronow RC: Stage I cervix cancer and pelvic node metastasis: special reference to the implications of the new and the recently replaced FIGO classifications on Stage Ia. Am J Obstet Gynecol 127 (2): 135–7, 1977.

Bounds W et al.: A randomized comparative trial of the performance of the Ayre and the Armovical cervical spatulae. Br J Obstet Gynaecol 83 (12): 981–7, 1976.

Boyce JG wt al.: Oral contraceptives and cervical carcinoma. Am J Obstet Gynecol 128 (7): 761–6, 1977.

Boyes DA et al.: Recent results from the British Columbia screening program for cervical cancer. Am J Obstet Gynecol 692–3, 1977.

Brown DC: Early detection of cancer in women. Primary care 3 (2): 251–3, 1976.

Brown HL: Proceedings of the joint IIASA/WHO workshop on screening for cervical cancer. Sociological and organization issues. Factors affecting participation pp. 51–64. In proceedings of the Joine IIASA/WHO workshop on Screening for cervical cancer. Laxenburg, International Institute for applied Systems Analysis, 1975.

Buchsbaum HJ et al.: Office detection of cervical neoplasia. J Iowa Med Soc 64 (9): 387–90, 1974.

Buchsbaum HJ et al.: The role of scalene lymph node biopsy in advanced carcinoma of the cervix uteri. Surg Gynecol Obstet 143 (2): 246–8, 1976.

Burghardt E et al.: Diagnosis and treatment of microinvasive carcinoma of the cervix uteri. Obstet Gynecol 49 (6): 641–53, 1977.

Cambier JL et al.: The binocleate cell: implications for automated cytopathology. Acta Cyto (Baltimore) 19 (3): 281–5, 1975.

Cameron D et al.: Sperm basic proteins in cervical carcinogenesis. Lancet 366, 1978.

Canevini P et al.: Results of a colpocytologic mass screening and in-patient casework; comparison by age groups. Tumori 575–84, 1977.

Carinelli SG et al.: Blue nevus of the cervix. Tumor 64 (1): 95–8, 1978.

Carsten PM: Problems of granting annuities to patients with cervical uterine and breast cancer with a favorable prognosis (proceedings). Arch Gynaekol 224 (1–4), 1977.

Cassiy M et al.: Electronic cell volume (coulter volume) distribution of vaginal cervical cytology samples. Acta Cytol (Baltimore) 19 (2): 117–25, 1975.

Cecchini S et al.: Contribution of cytology, colposcopy, target biopsy and conization to the early diagnosis of precancerous and cancerous lesions of the cervix uteri. Tumori 64 (4): 389–99, 1978.

Chiang WT et al.: Circulatory and cellular immune responses to squamous cell carcinoma of the uterine cervix. Am J Obstet Gynecol 126 (1): 116–21, 9176.

Chivetta J et al.: Cervical cancer screening: presis and critique of a recent Canadian report. Med J Aust 1–8, 1977.

Christenson B et al.: Long-term follow-up studies on herpes simplex antibodies in the course of cervical cancer. II. Antibodies to surface antigen of Herpes simplex virus infected cells. Int J Cancer 17 (3): 318–25, 1976.

Christenson B: Complement-dependent cytotoxic antibodies in the course of cervical carcinoma. B Int J Cancer 694–701, 1977.

Christopherson WM et al.: Trends in mortality from uterine cancer in relation to mass screening. Acta Cytol (Baltimore) 21 (1): 5–9, 1977.

Christopherson WM et al.: Report from KMA cancer committee. J Ky Med Assoc, 1976.

Colette C et al.: Dynamic study of tissue circulation in the cervix uteri and the prognosis of the newborn infant. J Gynecol Obstet Biol Reprod (Paris 6 (4): 497–506, 1977.

Collett HJ et al.: Cervical carcinoma and the pill (letter). Lancet 1 (8061): 441–2, 1978.

From the National Cancer Inst. An update of the DES problem: Important information about vaginal and cervical cancers. Med Times 105 (11): 114 31d–34d passim, 1977.

Connon AF et al.: A comparitive investigation of cervical cytology in Central Australian full-blooded aboriginal women. Med J Aust, 1976.

Cramer DW et al.: Trends in the incidence of endometrial cancer in the United States. Gynecol Oncol 2 (2): 130–43, 1974.

Cramer DW: The role of cervical cytology in the declining morbidity and mortality of cervical cancer. Cancer 34 (6): 2018–27, 1974.

Crapanzano JT: Office diagnosis and management of cervical dysplasia (colposcopy and cryosurgery in 32 patients). J La State Med Soc 130 (5): 101–4, 1978.

Cruikshank DP et al.: Colposcopic evaluation of cervical intraepithelial neoplasia. J Reprod Med 17 (6): 327–30, 1976.

Czernobilsky B et al.: The prevalence of cervicitis, reserve cell hyperplasia squamous metaplasia, and cervical dysplasia in Jewish women. Obstet Gynecol 587–91, 1977.

David A et al.: The cervical polyp: a new diagnostic and therapeutic approach with CO_2 hysteroscopy. Am J Obstet Gynecol 130 (6): 662–4, 1978.

Davis JR et al.: Increased incidence of adenocarcinoma of uterine cervix. Obstet Gynecol 45 (1): 7983, 1975.

Deeley TJ: Cancer of the cervix uteri an epidemiological survey. Clin Radiol 27 (1): 43–51, 1976.

Factors associated with or predisposing on cervical cancer pp. 49–50. *In* Proceeding of Joint IIASA/WHO workshop on screening for cervical cancer. Laxenburg, International Inst for Applied Systems Analysis, 1975.

Delgado G et al.: Diagnosis of cervical neoplasia by the nonspecialized colposcopist. Gynecol Oncol 3 (2): 114–6, 1975.

DePetrillo AD et al: Colposcopic evaluation of the abnormal, Papanicolaou test in pregnancy. Am J Obstet Gynecol 121 (4): 441–5, 1975.

Deppe G et al.: Colposcopy in the detection and management of patients with cervical intraepithelial neoplasia. Mt Sinai J Med (NY) 45 (1): 75–80, 1978.

Devi NN et al.: The value of mass cytological screening programme in the early detection of cervical cancer. J Indian Med Assoc 63 (3): 92–5, 1974.

Dickinson LE: Control of cancer of uterine cervix by cytologic screening. Gynecol Oncol 3 (1): 1–9, 1975.

Dimmitt SK: Decreased amniotic fluid peroxidase activity in pregnant patients with cervical carcinoma. J Am Med Wom Assoc 31 (12): 51–6, 1976.

Dinges HP et al.: Mucoepidermoid carcinoma of the cervix uteri. Zentralbl Gynaecol 396–403, 1977.

di Re F et al.: Clinical management of cervical carcinoma *in situ* and microinvasive carcinoma. Arch Geschwulsforsch 47 (4): 346–54, 1977.

DiSaia PJ et al.: Carcinoembryonic antigen in cervical and vulvar cancer patients. Serum levels and disease progress. Obstet Gynecol 47 (1): 95–9, 1976.

Dolan TE et al.: Cytology, colposcopy, and directed biopsy: what are the limitations? Gynecol Oncol 3 (4): 314–24, 1975.

Dolhay B et al.: The natural duration of cervical carcinoma. Arch Gynaekol 220 (4): 289–92, 1976.

Drill VA: Oral contraceptives; relations to mammary cancer benign breast lesions, and cervical cancer. Annu Rev. Pharmacol 15: 367–85, 1975.

Dube DK et al.: Protein synthesis with ribosomes from normal and malignant cervix uteri and non-analogous aminoacyl–tRNA. Indian J Biochem Biophys 11 (2): 95–6, 1974.

Duncan ID et al.: Microinvasive squamous carcinoma of cervix in the Tayside region of Scotland. Br J Obstet Gynaecol 67–70, 1977.

Dunn JE Jr: Geographic considerations of endometrial cancer. Gynecol Oncol 2 (2–3): 114–21, 1974.

DuToit JP et al.: Cervical cytologic screening among females with non-gynecologic hospital admissions. Obstet Gynecol 51 (3): 342–6, 1978.

Dutta TK et al.: Qualitative DNCB skin test in cancer patients. Indian J Cancer 14 (4): 351–3, 1977.

Edinger DD Jr: Screening of DES-exposed women in Rhode Island 1974–1977. R.I. Med J 61 (3): 123–6, 1978.

Efthymiou CJ et al.: Exfoliative immunocytology of cervical carcinoma. Arch Pathol Lab Med 575–8, 1977.

Einhorn N et al.: Secondary anemia in malignancy. Folic acid in cervical carcinoma. Acta Radio (Suppl) (Stockh) 310 (0): 75–84, 1971.

Einhorn N et al.: Secondary anemia in malignancy. Prognostic significance of haematologic changes six years after irradiation of cervical carcinoma. Acta Radiol (Stockh) 13 (4): 281–7, 1974.

El-Fiky S et al.: Cytochemical studies of respiratory enzymes in carcinoma of the cervix uteri after irradiation by radium. Arch Geschwulsforsch 47 (2), 1977.

Emovon AC: Sociocultural factors associated with cervical cancer Bendel State, Nigeria. Int J Gynaecol Obstet 15 (3): 252–2, 1977.

Engineer AD et al.: Cytological studies in women using intrauterine contraception. Indian J Med Res 1255–60, 1976.

Ericsson JL et al.: The incidence of breast and cervix cancer in the Swedish population. pp 191–204. *In* Bostrom H et al., ed. Health control in detection of cancer. Stockholm, Almqvist & Witsell, 1976.

Evans DM et al.: Observer variation and quality control of cytodiagnosis. J Clin Pathol 17 (12): 945–50, 1974.

Everett VJ: Carcinoma of cervix in Dar es Salaam. East Afr Med J 711–20, 1975.

Favila L et al.: Blocking plasma factors of migration inhibition factor production in patients with cervical carcinoma. J Natl Cancer Inst, 1978.

Feldman MJ et al.: The making of a colposcopist. A safe and sensible approach. J Reprod Med 16 (2): 73–7, 1976.

Feldman MJ et al.: Intraepithelial neoplasia of the uterine cervix in the teenager. Cancer 41 (4): 1405–8, 1978.

Fennell R: Microinvasive carcinoma of the uterine cervix. Obstet Gynecol Surv 33 (6): 406–11, 1978.

Figueroa JM et al.: Malignant plasma cells in cervical smear. Acta Cytol (Baltimore) 22 (1): 43–5, 1978.

Forsberg JG et al.: Prolactin-stimulating effect on 3Hthymidine incorporation in 3-methylocholanthreene-induced cervical carcinomas in normal and estrogenized mice. J Natl Cancer Inst 53 (5): 1247–52, 1974.

Forsberg JG et al.: A synergistic effect of oestradiol and prolactin influencing the incidence of 3-methylochololanthrene induced cervical carcinomas in mice. Acta Pathol Microbial Scand 84 (5): 384–90, 1976.

Fragoyannis S et al.: Age patterns of Tswana woman S. Africa, with carcinoma of the cervix. S Afr Med J 493–4, 1977.

Franco MF et al.: Gastric cancer producing retrograde lymphatic drainage with positive cervical smear. Acta Cytol (Baltimore) 21 (3): 368–9, 1977.

Fredricsson B et al.: Is there a changing epidemiology of premalignant lesions of the cervix? Results of cytologic screening of pregnant women. Acta Obstet Gynecol Scan 435–9, 1977.

Freedman RS et al.: A Study of associated factors, including genital herpes in Black women with cervical carcinoma in Johannesburg. S Afr Med J 48 (41): 1747–52, 1974.

Freni SC et al.: Preparing cell suspensions from cervical smears with pepsine and ultrasonic treatment. Acta Cytol (Baltimore) 306–12, 1975.

Freni SC: Non-visual prescreening of cervical smears with a flow-through cytophotometer. Acta Cytol (Baltimore) 19 (5): 488–52, 1975.

Freund M: A method for the collection and examination of the exfoliative cytology of the human female reproductive tract from menstrual blood flow-case reports; cervical dysplasia. M Acta Cytol (Baltimore) 21 (4): 497–500, 1977.

Freymuth F et al.: Antibodies to herpes simplex virus types 1 and 2: a comparative study using indirect haemagglutination in carcinoma of the cervix and in other malignant conditions. Biomedicine (Express) 23 (7): 271–5, 1975.

Frick HC: Management of noninvasive carcinoma of the cervix. 2d. Surg Clin North Am 58 (1): 55–60, 1978.

Fritsches HG et al.: The importance of complementary cytology and colposcopy in a detection program. Acta Cytol (Baltimore) 21 (1): 10–3, 1977.

Fuch WA et al.: Lymphography in carcinoma of the uterine cervix. Acta Radio (Stockh) 16 (4): 353–61, 1975.

Gad C: Cervical carcinoma in Frederiksberg borough; the influence of population screening on mortality. Dan Med Bull 295–6, 1976.

Gad C: Cervical carcinoma in Frederiksberg borough: the influence of population screening on incidence and stage distribution of invasive cases. 86–95, 1976.

Gad C et al.: Population screening for cervical carcinoma in Frederiksberg borough; economic considerations. Dan Med Bull 60–5, 1977.

Gad C et al.: The limitations of screening effect. A review of cervical disorders in previously screened women. Acta Cytol (Baltimore) 21 (6): 719–22, 1977.

Gad C: Discrepancy in clinical staging of cervical carcinoma. Dan Med Bull 24 (1): 20–2, 1977.

Gardner JW et al.: Low incidence of cervical cancer in Utah. Gynecol Oncol 68–80, 1977.

Garite TJ et al.: An evaluation of cytologic sampling techniques. A comparative study. Acta Cytol (Baltimore) 22 (2): 83–5, 1978.

Geirsson G et al.: Epithelial repair and regeneration in the uterine cervix. An analysis of the cells. Acta Cytol (Baltimore) 21 (3): 371–8, 1977.

Gilotra PM et al.: Carcinoma in situ of the cervix uteri in pregnancy. Surg Gynecol Obstet 142 (3): 396–8, 1976.

Glass NJ: Economic aspects of screening for cervical cancer. pp. 65–74. In proceedings of the Joint IIASA/WHO workshop in screening for cervical cancer. Laxenburg, International Institute for Applied Systems Analysis, 1975.

Goldenberg DM et al.: Characterization and localization of carcinoembryonic antigen in a squamous cell carcinoma of the cervix. Gynecol Oncol 4 (2): 204–11, 1976.

Goldenberg DM et al.: Identification of beta-oncofetal antigen in cervical squamous cancer and its demonstration in neoplastic and normal tissues. Cancer Res 1246–9, 1978.

Green GH: The progression of preinvasive lesions of the cervix to invasion. NZ Med J 80 (525): 279–87, 1974.

Greenwald P et al.: Cancer risks from estrogen intake. NY State J Med 77 (7): 1069–74, 1977.

Gronroos M et al.: Experience of a continuing mass screening program. Screening and re-screening for cervical carcinoma in Turkey. Ann Chir Gynaecol Fenn 63 (6): 470–8, 1974.

Grunfeld K et al.: Evaluation of mortality data for cervical cancer with special reference to mass screening programs. Denmark Am J Epidemiol 101 (4): 165–75, 1975.

Gudson JP Jr et al.: Letter: The oncogenic potential of dyelight treatment of herpetic lesions. Am J Obstet Gynecol 120 (4): 569–70, 1974.

Guido C et al.: Analysis of 1000 Colposcopies performed in a Nicaraguan clinic. Comparison with results of 2000 Colposcopies performed in a Brazilian Hospital. Int Sur 59 (9): 475–7, 1974.

Hakama M et al.: Mass screening for cervical cancer in Finland 1963–71. Organization, extent, and epidemiological implication. Ann Clin Res 202–11, 1975.

Hakama M et al.: Cervical cancer screening programs. I. Epidemiology and natural history of carcinoma of the cervix. Can Med Assoc J 1003–12, 1976.

Hakama M et al.: Selective screening for cervical cancer. Experience of the Finnish mass screening system. Br J Prev Soc Med 238–44, 1977.

Hakama M et al.: Estimating the expectation of life in cancer survival studies with incomplete follow-up information. N Chronic Dis 585–97, 1977.

Harington JS: Epidemiology and aetiology of cancer of the uterine cervix including the detection of carcinogenic N-nitrosamines in the human vaginal vault. S Afr Med J, 1975.

Hausen H et al.: Recognition of virus genomes in cells by molecular hybridization. pp. 415–25 Zur. In Kolber AR ed. Tumor virus-host cell interaction. New York Plenum Press, 1975.

Hausen H: Human papillomaviruses and their possible role in squamous cell carcinomas. Zur Curr Top Microbiol Immunol 78: 1–30, 1977.

Havadhanakul P et al.: Comparison of colposcopy directed biopsies and cold knife conization in patients with abnormal cytology. Surg Gyncol Obstet 142 (3): 333–6, 1976.

Hein K et al.: Cervical cytology: The need for routine screening in the sexually active adolescent. J Pediatr 91 (1): 123–6, 1977.

Henson D et al.: An epidemiology study of cancer of the cervix, vagina and vulva based on the Third National Cancer Survey in the United States. Am J Obstet Gynecol 525–32, 1977.

Herbeck G et al.: Colposcopy in the management of early cervical neoplasia. Endoscopy 9 (4): 232–8, 1977.

Herbst AL et al.: Age-incidence and risk of diethylstilbestrol related clear cell adenocarcinoma of the vagina and cervix. Am J Obstet Gynecol 128 (1): 43–50, 1977.

Herman CJ et al.: Goals of the cytology automation program of the National Cancer Inst. J Histochem Cytochem 24 (1): 1–5, 1976.

Herzog RE: Proceedings: Quantitative determination of basic amino acids in the cell nucleus of cervix carcinoma and its early stages. Arch Gynekol 219 (1–4) 186–8, 1975.

Hesselius I et al.: Comparison between participants and non-participants at a gynaecological mass screening. Scan J Soc Med 129–38, 1975.

Heyerdahl-O'Dowd TD: Trends in cervical cytology. Ir Med J 71 (5): 147–51, 1978.

Hiersche HD et al.: Orthologic and pathologic surface structures of portio uteri (scanning electron microscopy study) Proceeding Arch Gynaekol 522–3, 1977.

Hiraoka O et al.: Pelvic vascular bed isolation chemotherapy in the management of hemorrhage caused by advanced cervical cancer. A report of four clinical cases. Gynecol Oncol 4 (1): 87–107, 1976.

Herpes simplex and cervical carcinoma. Med Lett Drugs Ther 19 (12:52), 1977.

Hollingshead AC et al.: In vivo and in vitro measurements of the relationship of human squamous carcinomas to herpes simplex virus tumor associated antigens. Cancer Res 36 (2pt2): 821–8, 1976.

Homesley HD; Evaluation of the abnormal Pap smear. Am Fam Physician 16 (3): 190–4, 1977.

Hughes TB et al.: In vitro effects of female sex hormones upon deoxyribonucleic acid synthesis in carcinoma of the cervix. Br J Obstet Gynaecol 82 (10): 846, 1975.

Husain OA et al.: Quality control in cervical cytology. J Clin Pathol 27 (12): 935–44, 1974.

Husain OA et al.: Automation in cervical cancer screening. Part 1: Fixed cell scanning system. Biomed Eng11 (5): 161–6, 1976.

Husain OA et al.: A sample preparation for automated cervical cancer screening. Acta Cytol (Baltimore) 22 (1): 15–21, 1978.

Husslein H et al.: Premalignant and malignant uterine changes in immunosuppressed renal transplant recipients. Acta Obstet Gynecol Scand 73–8, 1978.

Ibrahim An et al.: Common antigens of herpes simplex virus 2 associated hamster tumors and human cervical cancer. Proc Soc Exp Biol Med 152 (3): 343–7, 1976.

Ihara T et al.: Electron-microscopic changes in squamous cell carcinoma of the uterine cervix following Linac irradiation – special reference to appearance of lysosome and radiosensitivity. Acta Obstet Gynaecol, 1977.

Imasato Y et al.: Feature evaluation for automated cancer cell identification. Comput Biol Med 5 (3): 245–55, 1975.

Ito H et al.: Serum carcinoembryonic antigens in patients with carcinoma of the cervix. Obstet Gynecol 468–71, 1978.

James W: Letter: Cervical cancer and sexual behavior. Lancet 2 (7881): 657, 1974.

Maternal Health in Ohio: Maternal cases involving carcinoma of the cervix. Ohio State. Ohio State Med J 70 (12): 726–8, 1974.

Jankowski MA et al.: Measurement of antibodies to herpes virus types 1 and 2 in human sera by microradioimmunoassay. Acta Virol (Praha) 405–11, 1977.

Jenner GM: The extended role of a cervical cytology clinic.

246

Study of 1,000 cases from a hospital based well women clinic. Health Bull (Edinb) 36 (1): 19–24, 1978.

Jofre ME et al.: Granuloma inguinale simulating advanced pelvic cancer. Med J Aust 2 (23): 869, 872–3, 1976.

Johannesson G et al.: The effect of mass screening in Iceland on the incidence and mortality of cervical carcinoma. Int J Cancer 418–25, 1978.

Joncas JH: Carcinoma of the cervix and herpes hom. (simplex) type 2 virus infection. Rev Can Biol 33 (3): 223–8, 1974.

Jordon JA: Proc. Vaginal and cervical neoplasia after exposure to stilbestrol in utero. Br J Obstet Gynaecol 82 (7): 588, 1975.

Jurkovski NJ: Carcinoma of the uterine cervix. Design of a clinical epidemiological study. God Zb Med Fak Skophe 209–14, 1974.

Kademian MT et al.: Staging laparotomy and survival in carcinoma of the uterine cervix. Acta Radiol (Ther) (Stockh) 16 (4): 314–24, 1977.

Kanka J et al.: The advantages of combing colposcopy and cytology in the prevention of uterine cervix cancer. Acta Univ Carol (Praha) 20 (5–6): 279–84, 1974.

Kata H et al.: Radioimmunoassay for tumor antigen of human cervical squamous cell carcinoma. 1621–8, 1977.

Kaufman RH et al.: Herpes genitalis and its relationship to cervical cancer. CA 25 (5): 258–65, 1974.

Kauraniemi T et al.: Risk of cervical cancer among an electrocoagulated population. Am J Obstet Gynecol 131 (5): 533–8, 1978.

Kawana T et al.: Frequency of antibody of a virus-induced tumor associated antigen (AG-4) in Japanese sera from patients with cervical cancer and controls. Cancer Res 36 (6): 1910–4, 1976.

Kern WH et al.: The accuracy and consistency of the cytologic classification of squamous lesions of the uterine cervix. Acta Cytol (Baltimore) 21 (4): 519–23, 1977.

Kessler II: Mortality from cervical cancer: can it be prevented now? Compr Ther 2 (9): 38–47, 1976.

Kiricuta I et al.: Chromosomes in preinvasive lesions and invasive carcinomas of the cervix uteri. Morphol Embryol (Burcur) 261–6, 1977.

Kishi Y et al.: Induction of bleeding as simple clinical tests for cervical carcinoma. Acta Obstet Gynaecol Jpn 22 (1) 14, 1975.

Kjellgren O: Mass screening in Sweden for cancer of the uterine cervix. Results and epidemiologic effect. Acta Obstet Gynecol Scan 5–11, 1977.

Kjorstad DE et al.: Carcinoembryonic antigen levels in patients with squamous cell carcinoma of the cervix. Obstet Gynecol 536–40, 1978.

Knutzen VK et al.: Colposcopy and selective biopsy in patients with abnormal cervical cytology. Afr Med J 52 (12): 478–81, 1977.

Kodama M et al.: Relationship between epidemiologic and endocrinologic aspects of cervical cancer. J Natl Cancer Inst 67: 35–9, 1978.

Kohan S et al.: Colposcopy and the management of cervical intraepithelial neoplasia. Gynecol Oncol 5 (1): 27–39, 1977.

Kolbenstvedt A: Projection difference index in lymphographic diagnosis lymph node metastases. Acta Radiol 16 (2): 200–8, 1975.

Kolstad P et al.: Long-term follow-up of 1121 cases of carcinoma *in situ*. Obstet Gynecol 48 (2): 125–9, 1976.

Korhonen MO: Adenocarcinoma of the uterine cervix. An evaluation of the available diagnostic methods. Acta Pathol Microbiol Scand (Suppl) 68: 1–42, 1977.

Koss LG et al.: Flow-microfluorometric analysis of nuclei isolated from various normal and malignant human epithelial

tissues. A preliminary report. J Histochem Cytochem 565–72, 1977.

Kovacic J: Evaluation of mass screening for cervical cancer in Ljubljana region. Tumore 62 (3): 343–9, 1976.

Kozlowski H et al.: Stages of development of immunologic response in the regional lymph nodes in invasive cancer of the uterine cervix. Arch Geschwulstforsch 550–60, 1977.

Krug H: Pulse cytophotometric measurements of tumor cell suspensions and exfoliative material. Arch Geschwulstforsch 48 (2): 145–9, 1978.

Krumerman MS et al.: Solitary reticulum cell sarcoma of the uterine cervix with initial cytodiagnosis. Acta Cytol (Baltimore) 22 (1) 46–50, 1978.

Krumholtz BA et al.: Coloscopy clinic: an evaluation of 500 new patients. J Reprod Med 16 (1): 31–4, 1976.

Krumins I et al.: The cytologic diagnosis of adenocarcinoma in situ of the cervix uteri. Acta Cytol (Baltimore) 21 (2): 320–19, 1977.

Kunkel M et al.: Antibodies to herpes simplex virus type 2 in husbands of patients with cervical carcinoma. Lancet 585–6, 1978.

Kunze KD et al.: An image analysing method for automated cytologic prescreening of cervix carcinoma and its prestages; demonstration and preliminary results. Arch Geschwulstforsch 48 (2): 131–9, 1978.

Kuptsow PC: Changing trends in the diagnosis and management of cervical neoplasia. J Am Ostoepath Assoc 74 (7): 621–30, 1975.

Labrum AH: Psychological factors in the etiology and treatment of cancer of the cervix. Obstet Gynecol 19 (2): 419–30, 1976.

Lamb EJ: Invasive squamous cell carcinoma of the cervix in DES a diethylstilbestrol-exposed offspring. Am J Obstet Gynecol 129 (8): 924–5, 1977.

Lang EK: Arteriographic assessment and staging of carcinoma of the cervix. Panminerva Med 18 (304): 114–6, 1976.

Laskey PW et al.: Uterine cervical carcinoma in Connecticut, 1935–1973 evidence for two classes of invasive disease. J Natl Cancer Inst 1037–43, 1976.

Latner Al et al.: Plasma alpha-1 antitrypsin levels in early and late carcinoma of the cervix. Oncology 33 (1) 12–4, 1976.

Lauchlan SC: Latent herpes cervicitis and mixed cervical carcinoma. Am J Obstet Gynecol 109–10, 1978.

Lawrence RA: Screening for cervical cancer (letter A1) Br Med J 754, 1976.

Leadly PJ et al.: Cervical cancer deaths in Maine. A retrospective case study. J Main Med Assoc 66 (2): 55–64, 1975.

Leck I et al.: Incidence of cervical cancer by marital status. J Epidemiol Community Health 108–10, 1978.

Leckie GB et al.: Simultaneous *in situ* carcinoma of the cervix, vulva and perineum after immunosuppressive therapy for transplantation. Br J Obstet Gyn 143–8, 1977.

Leiman G: Cervical cancer screening in a Johannesburg family planning centre. 1975.

Leiman G: Age patterns of Tswana women with carcinoma of the cervix. L Afr Med J 310, 1978.

Leiman G: Geographical pathology of cancer of the uterine cervix. Persaud V Trop Geogr Med 335–45, 1977.

Leman MH Jr et al.: Pretreatment lymphangiography in carcinoma of the uterine cervix. Gynecol Oncol ((4): 354–60, 1975.

Leppaluoto PA: Promiscuity and pill: etiologic agents in the genesis of cervical malignancy. Acta Cytol (Baltimore) 21 (2): 182, 1977.

Levy S et al.: Cellular immunity in squamous cell carcinoma of the uterine cervix. Am J Obstet Gynecol 160–4, 1978.

Lill PH et al.: Isoantigen ABH in cervical intraepithelial neoplasia. Am J Clin Pathol 66 (5): 767–74, 1976.

Loeb RA: Vaginal pool smears. (Letter). Am Fam Physician 16 (6) 13, 1977.

Luthra UK et al.: Surveillance for carcinogenesis in women using Cu-IUD for contraception. Indian J Med Res 63 (12): 1787–93, 1976.

Luthra UK: Epidemiology of cervical cancer in India. pp. 161–6 In Hirayama T, ed. Cancer in Asia, Baltimore, Univ Park Press, 1976 W3GA 163 no 18.

Luthra UK et al.: Cytological monitoring of female genital tract in women using Cu IUD. Indian J Med Res 216–22, 1977.

Lyons JF et al.: Mycoplasma species in a dysplasia clinic population. Am J Obstet Gynecol 120 (4): 554–6

Malvi SG et al.: A cytochemical study of acid-phosphatase in carcinoma of the cervix uteri. Indian J Cancer 11 (1): 81–7, 1974.

Marshall MJ et al.: Enzymes of glucose metabolism in carcinoma of the cervix and endometrium of the human uterus. Br J Cancer 37 (6): 990–1001, 1978.

Martino E et al.: Metastatic cervical carcinoma presenting as primary thyroid cancer. Case Reprot Tumori 63 (1): 25–30, 1977.

Marton I et al.: Urologic findings and complications in 759 cases of uterine cervix cancer. Neoplasma 21 (5): 583–9, 1974.

Mazor B et al.: Cervical adeno-carcinoma and partial hydatidiform mole. Acta Obstet Gynecol Scand 75 (3): 273–6, 1978.

Meisels A et al.: Dysplasias of uterine cervix: epidemiological aspects: Role of age at first coitus and use of oral contraceptives. Cancer 40 (6): 3076–81, 1977.

Melnick JL et al.: The causative role of herpesvirus type 2 in cervical cancer. Cancer 34 (4) suppl: 1375–85, 1974.

Melnick JL et al.: Studies on herpes simplex virus and cancer. Cancer Res 36 (2pt2) 845–56, 1976.

Melnick JE et al.: Epidemiological approaches to determining whether herpesvirus is the etiological agent of cervical cancer. Prog Exp Tumor Res 49–69, 1978.

Melnick JL et al.: Association of cytomegalovirus (CMV) infection with cervical cancer: isolation of CMV from cell cultures derived from cervical biopsy. Intervirology 10: 115–9, 1978.

Menczer J et al.: Antibodies to Herpes simplex virus in Jewish women with cervical cancer and in healthy Jewish women of Israel. J Natl Cancer Inst 55 (1) 13–6, 1975.

Menczer J et al.: Adenocarcinoma of the uterine cervix in Jewish Women a distinct epidemiological entity. Cancer 2464–7, 1978.

Merritt CG et al.: Age at first coitus and choice of contraceptive method: preliminary report on a study of factors related to cervical neoplasia. Soc Biol 22 (3): 255–60, 1975.

Miller AB: Mortality from carcinoma of the cervix. Lancet 469–70, 1978.

Milligan C et al.: Screening for cervical cancer. Am J Nurs 75 (8): 1343–4, 1975.

Misra JS et al.: Cytological evaluation of long term effect of Lippes loop and copper IUDs. Indian J Med Res 942–5, 1977.

Misra JS et al.: Cytological studied in women using copper intrauterine devices. Acta Cytol (Baltimore) 21 (4): 514–8, 1977.

Moghissi KS: Effect of oral contraceptives and endometrial and cervical cancer. J Toxicol Environ Health 3 (1–2): 243–65, 1977.

Mould RF: The pattern of incident age distribution with clinical staging for cancer of the cervix in England and Wales from 1945 to 1969. J Obstet Gynecol Br Commonw 81 (8): 644–9.

Muller Koboid-Wolterbeck AC et al.: Letter Cytophohoria in cervical cytology. Acta Cytol (Baltimore) 19 (2): 89–91, 1975.

Munoz N: Model systems for cervical cancer. Cancer Res 36 (2pt2) 892–3, 1976.

Murphy JF et al.: Scanning electron microscopy of normal and abnormal exfoliated cervical squamous cells. Br J Obstet Gyne 44–51, 1975.

Nahmias AJ et al.: Immunology of herpes simplex virus infection: relevance to herpes simplex virus vaccines and cervical cancer. Cancer Res 36: 836–44, 1976.

Nahmias AJ et al.: The genital herpes-cervical cancer hypothesis 10 years later. Prog Exp Tumor Res 11739, 1978.

Naik KG: Cervical carcinoma in Zambia. Int Surg 110: 1, 1977.

Neighbor RM et al.: Incidence of cervical cancer in perimenopausal and postmenopausal woman detected by Papanicolaou smears. Am J Obstet Gynecol 348–51, 1976.

Nelson DS: Antigens of carcinoma of the cervix uteri. A study by means of immunofluorescence. Clin Exp Immunol 16: 53–62, 1974.

Nelson JH Jr et al.: Detection, diagnostic evaluation and treatment of dysplasis and early carcinoma of the cervix. CA 25: 134–51, 1975.

Nemeth G et al.: Preparation of cervix and corpus carcinoma patients records for computer evaluation. Methods Int Med 17: 113–5, 1978.

Nielsen NH et al.: Carcinoma of the uterine cervix and dysplasia in Greenland. Acta Pathol Microbiol Scand 36–44, 1978.

Niemi T et al.: Cervical neoplasia and the pill (letter). Lancet 825–6, 1977.

Niemi T et al.: Cancer morbidity in depressive persons. J Psychosom Res 117–20, 1978.

Nishiya I et al.: Cytophotometric study of premalignant and malignant cells of the cervix in an approach towards automated cytology. Acta Cytol 21: 271–5, 1977.

NOda S et al.: Reinvestigation of crucial cases where first diagnosis by mailing smear test disagrees with second diagnosis by cytology and/or biopsy. Acta Obstet Gynaecol. Jpn 23: 173–8, 1976.

Noller KL et al.: Clear-cell adenocarcinoma of the vagina and cervix: survival data. Am J Obstet Gynecol 124: 385–8, 1976.

Notter MF et al.: Comparative diagnostic aspects of herpes simplex virus tumor-associated antigens. J Natl Cancer Inst 57: 483–8, 1976.

Nordqvist SR: Evaluation and management of cervical cancer. Compr Ther 4: 19–23, 1978.

Oates JK: Herpesvirus and cervical cancer (Letter) Br Med J 1: 900, 1976.

Odell LD: The use of the colposcope in the detection and management of patients with early cervical neoplasia. J Reprod Med 16: 235–41, 1976.

O'Dowd MJ et al.: An evaluation of cervical cytological screening in the University Teaching Hospital. Med Z Zambia 117–21, 1977.

Okagaki T et al.: Koilocytosis in dysplastic and reactive cervical squamous epithelium. An ultrastructural study. Acta Cytol 95–8, 1978.

Olkowski ZL et al.: Cytological and quantitative cytochemical studied of post-radiation dysplasia. Strahlentherapie 53–9, 1978.

Onuigbo WI: Carcinoma of the uterine cervix in Nigerian Igbos. Gynecol Oncol 255–8, 1976.

Ory HW et al.: Cervical neoplasia in residents of low-income housing project: an epidemiologic study. Am J Obstet Gynecol 275–7, 1975.

248

Ozaki Y et al.: Antibodies to herpes virus type 1 and 2 among Japanese cervical cancer patients. Gan. 119–22, 1978.

Pacsa AS et al.: Herpes virus antibodies and antigens in patients with cervical anaplasia and in controls. J Natl Cancer Inst 55: 775–81, 1975.

Pacsa AS et al.: Herpes simplex virus-specific antigens in exfoliated cervical cells from women with and without cervical anaplasia. Cancer Res 36: 2130–2, 1976.

Palmer AE et al.: A preliminary report on investigation of oncogenic potential of herpes simplex virus type 2 in Cebus monkeys. Cancer Res 26: 807–9, 1976.

Pang JC et al.: Cytology and colposcopy in the diagnosis of cervical neoplasia. Gynecol Oncol 5: 134–41, 1977.

Pantoja E et al.: Some clinical features of vulvovaginal melanomas with case reports. Bol Assoc Med PR 68: 13–6, 1976.

Pantoja E et al.: Procidentia uteri and its mythical protection against cervical cancer. Historical review. Bol Assoc Med PR 68: 252–6, 1976.

Pape C et al.: Ultrastructure of the epithelial borders in the cervix uteri area (Proceedings) Arch Gynaekol 526–7, 1977.

Paulileinikki ES et al.: Adenine arabinoside (ARA-A) blocked HSV-2 infected human skin fibroblasts as targets for the detection of serum mediated and cellular cytotoxicity in patients with cervical carcinoma. Clin Exp Immunol 25: 264–9, 1976.

Pederson SN: The glycolytic enzyme activity of the human cervix uteri. Cancer 35: 469–74, 1975.

Peltonen R: Antibodies to herpesvirus hominis types 1 and 2 among women with neoplastic change of uterine cervix. Acta Obstet Gynecol Scan 54: 369–72, 1975.

Penner DW: Cervical cancer screening programs (letter). Can Med Assoc J 115: 725–9, 1976.

Perez-Mesa C et al.: Scalene node biopsy in the pretreatment staging of carcinoma of the cervix uteri. Am J Obstet Gynecol 1: 93–5, 1976.

Peritz E et al.: The incidence of cervical cancer and duration of oral contraceptive use. Am J Epidemiol 462–9, 1977.

Persaud V: Incidence of cancer of the uterine cervix in Kingston, Jamaica, 1958–1970. West Indian Med J 23: 8–14, 1974.

Persaud V: Epidemiology of cancer of the uterine cervix in Jamaica. West Indian Med J 171–8, 1975.

Pertynski T et al.: 201 Thallium Scintigraphy – a new method for radionuclide imaging of the uterus. Nuklearmedizin 16: 245–7, 1977.

Peto R: Cervical cancer and early sexual intercourse (letter). Int J Epidemiol 5: 97, 1976.

Petrova AS et al.: Content of Schick-positive substances in the cells of cervix tumors. Lab Delo 3: 144–6, 1976.

Photopulos GJ et al.: Evaluation of conventional diagnostic tests for detection of recurrent carcinoma of the cervix. Am J Obstet Gynecol 129: 535–5, 1977.

Porreco R et al.: Gynecologic malignancies in immunosuppressed organ homograft recipients. Obstet Gynecol 45: 359–64.

Prior P: The pattern of incidence of primary tumors following cancer of the uterine cervix (Proceedings). Br J Cancer 30: 173, 1974.

Puri S et al.: Malignant melanoma of the cervix uteri. Obstet Gynecol 47: 459–62, 1976.

Quizilbash AH: In situ and microinvasive adenocarcinoma of the uterine cervix. A clinical, cytologic and histologic study of 14 cases. Am J Clin Pathol 64: 155–70, 1975.

Quizilbash AH et al.: Endometrial and tubal involvement by squamous carcinoma of the cervix. Am J Clin Pathol 64: 688–71, 1975.

Rand RJ et al.: T-and B-lymphocyte subpopulations in preinvasive and invasive carcinoma of the cervix. Clin Exp Immunol 421: 8, 1977.

Raphael M: Cancer detection in working women: a report on 7450 subjects. Med J Aust 557: 60, 1977.

Rawls WE et al.: Serological and epidemiological considerations of the role of herpes simplex virus type 2 in cervical cancer. Cancer Res 36, 829: 35, 1976.

Rawls WE et al.: Relation of herpes simplex viruses to human malignancies. Curr Top Microbiol Immunol 77: 7–95, 1977.

Reagan JW: The changing nature of endometrial cancer. Gynecol Oncol 2: 144–51, 1974.

Reddy CR et al.: A study of 80 patients with penile carcinoma combined with cervical biopsy study of their wives. Int Surg 549–53, 1977.

Reid BL et al.: Sperm basic proteins in cervical carcinogenesis: Correlation with socioeconomic class. Lancet 60: 2, 1978.

Rhine SA et al.: Prenatal sex detection with endocervical smears: successful results utilizing Y-bodyfluorescence. Am J Obstet Gynecol 122: 155–60, 1975.

Rice JM: Transplacental carcinogenesis. In Gynecology and Obstetrics. Castelazo-Ayala L et al. eds (Amsterdam: Excerpta Medica, 1976 pp. 115–24.

Robboy SJ et al.: Squamous cell neoplasia controversy in the female exposed to diethylstilbestrol. Hum Pathol 8: 483–5, 1977.

Robboy SJ et al.: Squamous cell dysplasia and carcinoma in situ of the cervix and vagina after prenatal exposure to diethylstilbestrol. Obstet Gynecol 51: 528–35, 1978.

Rochat RW: The prevalence of cervical cancer screening in the United States in 1970s. Am J Obstet Gynecol 478: 83, 1976.

Roizman B et al.: Does genital herpes cause cancer. A midway assessment. In Sexually Transmitted Diseases. RD Catterall and CS Nichols, eds. (London: Academic Press, 1976).

Rorat E et al.: Verrucous carcinoma of the cervix: a problem in diagnosis and management. Am J Obstet Gynecol 130: 851–3, 1978.

Rotkin ID: Another view of Herpes Simplex Virus type 2. (Letter). JAMA 235: 2188–9, 1976.

Rounds DE et al.: Prospects for a personal screening method for cervical carcinoma. Gynecol Oncol 4: 125–32, 1976.

Roy M et al.: New concepts in the evaluation of the abnormal Papanicolaou smear. J Fam Pract 1: 10–3, 1974.

Rubio CA et al.: Who is responsible for the false-negative smear? (Letter). Acta Cytol 19: 319, 1975.

Rubio CA et al.: A critical evaluation of the Schiller test in patients before conization. Am J Obstet Gynecol 1: 96–6, 1976.

Rubio CA: The false negative smear; an instrumental error? Acta Cytol 21: 500–1, 1977.

Rubio CA et al.: The immunofluorescence characteristics of the basement membrane in squamous carcinoma of the uterine cervix. Histopathology 67: 73, 1978.

Ruponen S: Diagnostic and therapeutic aspects of cervical carcinoma. Based on the material of 991 cases. Acta Obstet Gyneco Scan 68: 42, 1977.

Ryden SE et al.: Adenoid cystic carcinoma of the cervix. Presenting as a primary bronchial neoplasm. Am J Obstet Gynecol 120: 846–7, 1974.

Rylander E: Cervical cancer in women belonging to a cytologically screened population. Acta Obstet Gynecol Scand 361–6, 1976.

Rylander E: Negative smears in women developing invasive cervical cancer. Acta Obstet Gynecol Scand 56: 115–8, 1977.

Saksela E et al.: Clinical follow-up and the cell-mediated

cytotoxicity against HeLa cells in patients with invasive or preinvasive cervical cancer. Med Biol 54 (3): 217–22, 1976.

Sandberg EC et al.: Examination of young women exposed to stilbestrol in utero. Am J Obstet Gynecol 128 (4): 364–70, 1977.

Sandler B: Sperm basic proteins in cervical carcinogenesis. Lancet 208–9, 1978.

Sandmire HF et al.: Carcinoma of the cervix in oral contraceptive steroid and IUD users and nonusers. Am J Gynecol 125 (3): 339–45, 1976.

Sandmire HF et al.: Experience with 40,000 Papanicolaou smears. Obstet Gynecol 48 (1): 56–60, 1976.

Saraiya U et al.: Experience with diagnosis and management of pre and early cancers of the cervix. Int Surg 63 (2): 107–7, 1978.

Sargeant EJ et al.: Cervical cytology screening: experience of a general hospital. Can Med Assoc J 117 (9): 1026–7, 1977.

Savage EW: Correlation of colposcopically directed biopsy and conization with histologic diagnosis of cervical lesions. J Reprod Med 15 (6): 211–3, 1975.

Sawanobori S et al.: Rosette formation inhibition in cervical dysplasia and carcinoma *in situ*. Cancer Res 4332–5, 1977.

Schmidt OA: Cervical cancer screening programs: The SOGCs view (letter). Can Med Assoc J 116 (9): 971–2, 1977.

Schoenberg BS: Smoking and cancer of the uterine cervix; hypothesis (letter). Am J Epidemiol 107 (4): 353–4, 1978.

Sebastian JA et al.: Cancer of the cervix a sexually transmitted disease. Cytologic screening in a prostitute population. Am J Obstet Gynecol, 1978.

Selim MA et al.: Indications for the experience with colposcopy in the management of neoplasia of cervix. Surg Gynecol Obstet 145 (4): 529–32, 1977.

Sentz WB et al.: Cervical carcinogenesis with herpes simplex virus type 2. Obstet Gyn 46 (2): 117–21, 1975.

Seski JC et al.: Microinvasive squamous carcinoma of the cervix. Definition, histologic analysis, late results of treatment. Obstet Gynecol 50 (4): 410–4, 1977.

Shahanl SM: Role of cervical cytology in family planning. J Biosoc Sce 6 (3): 383–5, 1974.

Shingleton HM et al.: The contribution of endocervical smears to cervical cancer detection. Acta Cytol (Baltimore) 19 (3): 261–4, 1975.

Shingleton HM et al.: The significance of age in the colposcopic evaluation of women with atypical Papanicolaou smears. Obstet Gynecol 49 (1): 61–4, 1977.

Shobin D et al.: Genitourinary tuberculosis simulating cervical carcinoma. J Reprod Med 17 (5): 305–8, 1976.

Shulman JJ et al.: The Papanicolaou smear: an insensitivie casefinding procedure. Am J Obstet Gynecol 120 (4): 446–51, 1974.

Shulman JJ et al.: The Pap smear: take two. Am J Obstet Gynecol 121 (8): 1024–8, 1975.

Silverman AD et al.: Rapid-flow cytofluoremetry of exfoliated cervicovaginal cell suspensions from mice. Acta Cytol (Baltimore) 21 (1) 63–7, 1977.

Silverstone H: Squamous papilloma of the cervix uteri. A two year prospective cytological study. Med J Aust, 1975.

Simon J—W: The association of Herpes simplex virus and cervical a review. Gynecol Oncol 1976.

Singh K et al.: An unusual complication of pelvic exenrationa. J Urol 116 (1): 114–5, 1976.

Singh M et al.: Comparative study of fluorescent and Papanicolaous techniques for detection of carcinoma of cervix uteri. Indian J Med Res 64 (12): 1783–7, 1976.

Singer A et al.: Cellular immunity to human basic myelin protein in women with dysplasia and carcinoma *in situ* of the cervix. Br J Obstet Gynaecol 82 (10): 820–5, 1975.

Singer A et al.: A hypothesis; The role of a high-risk male in the etiology of cervical carcinoma; a correlation of epidemiology and molecular biology. Am J Obstet Gynecol 126 (1): 110–5, 1976.

Singer A et al.: Causes of cervical carcinoma; New Ideas. Compr Ther 2 (9): 29–37, 1977.

Siracka E et al.: Oxygen supply of uterine cervix cancer and radiation response with special reference to menstrual history. Neoplasma 21 (4): 433–9, 1974.

Smith DC et al.: Embolization of the hypogastric arteries in the control of massive vaginal hemorrhage. Obstet Gynecol 49 (3): 317–22, 1977.

Smith RW et al.: Psoas bed gallium uptake in a patient with carcinoma of the cervix post irradiation-abscess or metastasis. Clin Nucl Med 3 (6): 230, 1978.

Singer A et al.: A hypothesis; The role of a high-risk male in the etiology of cervical carcinoma; a correlation of epidemiology and molecular biology. Am J Obstet Gunecol 126 (1): 110–5, 1976.

Singer A et al.: Causes of cervical carcinoma; New Ideas. Compr Ther 2 (9): 29–37, 1977.

Siracka E et al.: Oxygen supply of uterine cervix cancer and radiation responses with special reference to menstrual history. Neoplasma 21 (4): 433–9, 1974.

Smith DC et al.: Embolization of the hypogastric arteries in the control of massive vaginal hemorrhage. Obstet Gynecol 49 (3): 317–22, 1977.

Smith RW et al.: Psoas bed gallium uptake in a patient with carcinoma of the cervix post irradiation-abscess or Metastasis. Clin Nucl Med 3 (6): 230, 1978.

Snyder RN et al.: Dysplasia and carcinoma *in situ* of the uterine cervix prevalence in very young women (under age 22). A one year study in a health plan population. Am J Obstet Gynecol 751–6, 1976.

Spratt DW et al.: Verrucous carcinoma of the cervix. Am J Obstet Gynecol 129 (6): 699–700, 1977.

Spreacher-Goldberger S et al: Letter: Cell mediated response to herpes simplex virion and non-virion antigens in patients with cervical carcinoma with a depressed response to phytogemagglutinin. Biomedicine (express) 23 (9): 399–401, 1975.

Sprenger E et al.: The mathematical evaluation of flow-through cytophotometric data in processing cervical cytology. Beitr Pathol 153 (3): 289–96, 1974.

Sprenger E et al.: The significance of random sample size in flow-through photometric prescreening in cervical cytology. Beitr Pathol 157 (2): 142–6, 1976.

Sprenger E et al.: Routine use of flow-through photometric prescreening in the detection of cervical carcinoma. Acta Cytol (Baltimore) 21 (3): 435–40, 1977.

Stafl A et al.: Angiogenesis of cervical neoplasia. Am J Obstet Gynecol 121 (6): 845–52, 1975.

Stage AH et al.: The use of pelvic arteriography in assessing carcinoma of the cervix. Obstet Gynecol 52 (2): 151–4, 1978.

Steiner C: Can deaths from cancer of the cervix be reduced in Georgia? J Med Assoc Ga 65 (10): 391–4, 1976.

Steinfeld AD et al.: The response of hypertrophic pulmonary osteoarthropathy to radiotherapy. Radiology 113 (3): 709–11, 1974.

Steinfeld AD et al.: Lymphangiographic detection of scalene node metastases from cervical carcinoma. AJR 130 (2): 371–2, 1978.

Steinkamp RC et al.: Comparison of cervical pap smears with subsequent diagnosis of cervical carcinoma an analysis of

250

Arkansas health department pap smears for 1970 and 1971. J Arkansan Med Soc 72 (4): 168–71, 1975.

Steinkamp RC: Mortality rates from carcinoma of the uterine cervix in Arkansas. J Arkansas Med Soc 71 (10): 312–3, 1975.

Stern E et al.: Pap testing and hysterectomy prevalence; a survey of communities with high and low cervical cancer rates. Am J Epidemiol 296–305, 1977.

Stern E et al.: Papanicolaou testing and hysterectomy prevalence in low-income communities; a survey in Los Angelos county. Natl Cancer Inst Monogr 113–9, 1977.

Stern E et al.: Steroid contraceptive use and cervical dysplasia: increased risk of progression. Science 196 (4297): 1460–2, 1977.

Sumithran E: Rarity of cancer of the cervix in Malaysian Orang Asli despite the presence of known risk factors. Cancer 1570–2, 1977.

Swan RW: Colposcopic evaluation of the female lower genital tract. J Mill State Med Assoc 17 (7): 181–3, 1976.

Sychra JJ et al.: Dimensionality reducing displays in cell image analysis. Acta Cytol (Baltimore) 21 (6): 747–52, 1977.

Sychra JJ et al.: Computer recognition of abnormal extocervical cells. Comparison of the efficacy of contour and textural features. Acta Cytol (Baltimore) 21 (6): 765–9, 1977.

Talebian F et al.: Colposcopic evaluation patients with abnormal cytologic smears during pregnancy. Obstet Gynecol 47 (6): 693–6, 1976.

Talebian F et al.: Colposcopic evaluation of patient with abnormal cervical cytology. Obstet Gynecol 49 (6): 670–4, 1977.

Tanaka N et al.:Fundamental study of automatic cytoscreening for uterine cancer. V. Data Analysis for Improvement of CYBEST. Acta Cytol (Baltimore) 21 (4): 536–8, 1977.

Tarlowski L et al.: Comparison of late mortality in women 'cured' of endometrial and cervical cancer. Ann Med Sect Pol Acad Sci 20 (1): 5–14, 1975.

Taylor J et al.: Development and evaluation of automatic mucleus finding routines: thresholding of cervical cytology images. Acta Cytol (Baltimore) 19 (3): 289–98, 1975.

TeGroen LH et al.: A preliminary investigation into the incidence of cancer of the cervix. S Afr Med J 48 (57): 2341–5, 1974.

Thiry L: Herpes simplex virus and carcinoma of the cervix. Eur J Cancer 851–8, 1976.

Timonen S et al.: Cervical Cancer. Mass screening, incidence and mortality in Finland. Acta Obstet Gynecol Scand 13–9, 1977.

Tobell HM: Cone biopsy of the cervix. Clin Obstet Gynecol 19 (1) 1–15, 1976.

Tobin SM et al.: Relation of herpesvirus hominis type II to carcinoma of the cervix. An animal model for the induction of longterm latency of herpesvirus hominis type II. Obstet Gynecol 707–12, 1978.

Torres JE: Colposcopy screening for cervical cancer in a family planning program. J Reprod Med 16 (5): 246–8, 1976.

Trimbolt de Estevez O: Cytoenzymology on normal and pathological epithelium of human cervix. Cell Mol Biol 22 (3–4): 323–u, 1977.

Trombetta GC: Colposcopic evaluation of cervical neoplasis in pregnancy. J Reprod Med 16 (5): 243–5, 1976.

Ucmakli A et al.: Retroperitoneal lymph-node metastases in untreated cancer of the uterine cervix. An analysis based on abdominopelvic exploration. Radiology 113 (1): 173–5, 1974.

Ueda D et al.: Changes in cell numbers and activities of lymphocyte subpopulations in the progress of uterine cervical cancer. Osaka City Med J 21 (2): 97–109, 1975.

Ulfelder H: The stilbestrol-adenosiscarcinoma syndrome. Cancer 38 (1 Suppl) 426–31, 1976. Testosterone. pp 209–17.

In Evaluation of carcinogenic risk of chemicals in man. Stockholm, Karolinski Ins, 1974. Diethylstilbetrol (Stilboestrol) 55–76.

In Evaluation of the carcinogenic risk of chemicals to man Stockholm Karolinski Inst, 1974. Ethinyloestradiol 77–85.

In Evaluation of the carcinogenic risk of chemicals to man. Stockholm, Karolinski Inst, 1974. Oestrone, 123–32.

In Evaluation of the carcinogenic risk of chemicals to man. Stockholm Karolinski Ins, 1974.

Uyttenbroeck F: Precancerous and cancerous lesions of the cervix uteris. Chirurgie 1–3–(8) 669–78, 1977.

Van Nagel JR Jr et al.: Carcinoembryonic antigen in intraepithelial neoplasia of the uterine cervix. Am J Obstet Gynecol 126 (1) 205–9

Van Nagell JR Jr et al.: Diagnostic and therapeutic efficacy of cervical conization. Am J Obstet Gynecol 124 (2): 134–9, 1976.

Van Nagell JR Jr et al.: Small cell cancer of the uterine cervix. Cancer 40 (5): 2243–9, 1977.

Van Nagell JR Jr et al.: Cervical cancer: pill seems safe for most women but those with dysplasia may have higher risk. Fam Plann Perspec 19 (3): 165–6, 1978.

Vardthananusara C et al.: Herpes simplex virus type 2 and carcinoma of cervix uteri. J Med Assoc Thai 14–9, 1978.

Vengadasalam D et al.: Intravenous pyelographic studies in carcinoma of cervix. J Med Assoc Tahi 61 Suppl 1: 271, 1978.

Veridiano NP et al.: Squamous cell carcinoma in situ of the vagina and cervix after intrauterine DES exposure. Obstet Gynecol 52 (1 Suppl) 30S–33S, 1978.

Volterrani F et al.: Prognostic value of lymphography in cervical cancer. Tumori 64 (3): 295–304, 1978.

Von Maillot K et al.: Glycosaminogylcan content of the cervix uteri during pregnancy and labor (proceedings). Arch Gynaekol 224 (1–4) 220–1, 1977.

Wagner R et al.: Proceedings: Scanning electron microscopy findings on the cervix uteri. Verhdtsch Ges Pathol, 1974.

Wagner H et al.: Statistical evaluation of frequency distribution in quantitative morphology. Verh Anat Ges 77–81, 1977.

Way S et al.: Uretic invasion by endometriosis. Br J Urol 48 (1): 38, 1976.

Way S: Letter: Carcinoma-in situ of cervix in sisters. Br Med J 1 (6013): 834, 1976.

Weiss H et al.: Some methodical remarks on the use of impulse cytophotometry in automated cervix cytology. Arch Geschwulstforsch 48 (3): 205–11, 1978.

Welander CE et al.: Factors affecting survival in stage I and stage II carcinoma of the cervix. Obstet Gynecol 46 (4): 439–43, 1975.

West RR: Cervical Cancer; Age at registration and age at death. Br J Cancer 236–41, 1977.

Whitaker D: The role of cytology in the detection of malignant lymphoma of the uterine cervix. Acta Cytol (Baltimore) 20 (6): 510–3, 1976.

Wibe E et al.: Steroids and growth of a human cell line stemming from a carcinoma of the uterine cervix. Mol Cell Endocrinol 5 (5): 359–64, 1976.

Wied GL et al.: Computer recognition of ectocervical cells. Classification accuracy and spatial resolution. Acta Cytol (Baltimore) 21 (6): 753–64, 1977.

Wilbanks GD: In vivo and in vitro markers of human cervical intraepithelial neoplasia. Cancer Res 36 (7PT2): 2485–94, 1976.

Williams AE et al.: Proceedings: The surface ultrastructure of exfoliated cervical cells. Br J Cancer, 1974.

Williams AE et al.: Surface ultrastructural changes following the application of 3,4 benzopyrene to the mouse cervix. Johari O, Becker RP ed. Scanning electron microscopy, 1976.

Williams AE et al.: Exposure in utero to diethylstilbestrol and related synthetic hormones. Association with vaginal and cervical cancers and other abnormalities. JAMA 236–(10) 1107, 1976.

Wilson EA et al.: Free serum amino acids in patients with advanced cervical carcinoma. Gynecol Oncol 4 (3): 311–3, 1976.

Winkelstein W Jr: Smoking and cancer of the uterine cervix. Hypothesis. Am J Epidemiol 106 (4): 257–9, 1977.

Wollfenden JM et al.: Evaluation of carcinoma of the cervix using III inbleomycin. Obstet Gynecol 46 (3): 347–52, 1975.

Yakovleva IA et al.: Histochemical methods in the diagnosis of pre-cancerous states and early formes of cancer of the uterine cervix. Folia Histochem Cytochem (Krakow) 14 (4): 243–7, 1976.

Yamagata S et al.: Radiation-induced immune changes in patients with cancer of the cervix. Br J ObstetGynaecol 83 (5): 400–8, 1976.

Young QA et al.: The cytologic diagnosis of clear cell adenocarcinoma of the cervix uteri. Acta Cytol (Baltimore) 22 (1) 3–6, 1978.

Yule R: Mortality from carcinoma of the cervix. Lancet 1031–2, 1978.

Zelenin AV et al.: Peculiarities of cytochemical properties of cancer cells as revealed by study of deoxyribonucleaoprotein susceptibility to Fueulgen Hydrolysis. J Histochem Cytochm 25 (7): 580–4, 1977.

SUBJECT INDEX

256

258